Mixed Economies
of Welfare

A comparative perspective

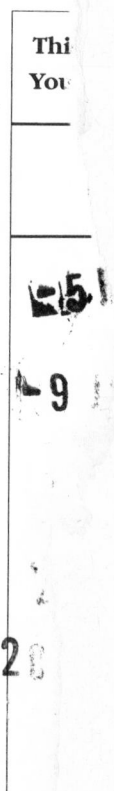

Mixed Economies of Welfare

A comparative perspective

Norman Johnson
University of Portsmouth

PRENTICE HALL EUROPE

London   New York   Toronto   Sydney   Tokyo
Singapore   Madrid   Mexico City   Munich   Paris

First published 1999 by
Prentice Hall Europe
Campus 400, Maylands Avenue
Hemel Hempstead
Hertfordshire, HP2 7EZ
A division of
Simon & Schuster International Group

Typeset in 10/12pt Times by
Hands Fotoset, Ratby, Leicester

Printed and bound in Great Britain by
T. J. International Ltd.

Library of Congress Cataloging-in-Publication Data

A catalog record for this book is available
from the publisher

British Library Cataloguing in Publication Data

A catalogue record for this book is available from
the British Library

ISBN 0–13–354002–2

---

1 2 3 4 5   03 02 01 00 99

For Ruth, David, Karen,
Neil and Christopher

CONTENTS

PREFACE

It is more than ten years since the publication of *The Welfare State in Transition* (Johnson, 1987). Too much has happened in those ten years for this to be a second edition of that book. The general format is the same, but although small parts of the original book have found their way into this one, the book has been almost entirely re-written; it is essentially a new book and this is the reason for the different title.[1] The general introductory chapter on the welfare state has been dropped, because several good books on the history and development of the welfare state have appeared in the 1990s (Alcock, 1996; Deakin, 1994; Glennerster, 1995; Hill, 1993; Lowe, 1993; Sullivan, 1996; Timmins, 1995).

There have been changes in world politics which have profoundly affected both welfare state 'geography' and the provision, finance and regulation of welfare in established welfare states. The most dramatic of these changes are those in Central and Eastern Europe and the former Soviet Union with the replacement of totalitarian, centrally-planned regimes and the development of mixed economies of welfare. In 1987, changes of this order could not really have been predicted. Still less predictable was the unification of Germany. The rapid economic development in South-East Asia has produced more newly emerging welfare states, although further development may have been curtailed in the wake of the serious financial crisis affecting this part of the world in 1997/98. All these developments have taken place within the context of increasing globalisation and the greater competition between more open economies. One aspect of the globalisation process is the greater influence of multinational companies and international financial institutions. The nation state's capacity to act autonomously has diminished, but by no means disappeared. On a less than global scale, the European nations have taken several steps towards greater integration within the European Union, and shortly after the publication of this book the European Monetary Union will be in existence.

The coverage of the book has been widened to take account of these changes, but there are still some areas which receive less than their fair share of attention. The most obvious of these are the developing nations. Although the research and literature in these parts of the world has been growing in recent years, there is still a relative shortage of information. There is rather more on international and indigenous development agencies and this is reflected in Chapter 4.

Welfare states survived a further period of recession in the early 1990s, and when economic conditions improved, governments in Western Europe were obliged to control and reduce deficits in preparation for entry into the European Monetary Union. There has been a great deal of talk about the need for retrenchment, and some has been achieved, in the sense at least that the rate of growth of social expenditure has slowed down. Efforts to contain public expenditure in the long term are linked with a concern about demographic changes, especially the continued growth in the number and proportion of elderly people in the advanced industrial nations, and the costs associated with this growth. The continued popular support for the welfare state has, however, restricted the degree of retrenchment that political leaders believed they could attempt without running unacceptable political risks. There have been cuts, however, and the result has been growing inequality and widening social divisions in many parts of the world.

Scholarship in social policy has advanced on several fronts. One welcome change has been the greater acceptance of the need to study the inter-relationships between different policy areas: the most fruitful outcomes have resulted from studies incorporating aspects of both social and economic policy. Some specific areas have been the subject of particularly intense research attention: among the areas relevant for this book are gender studies, families and carers, the voluntary sector, markets and quasi-markets and developments in local and central government.

Many of these studies had a comparative focus, and the

considerable expansion of comparative work in social policy over the last twenty years represents one of the most significant developments in the subject. This expansion has been particularly noticeable in the countries of the European Union: among the major benefits for scholars is the supply of information on social affairs from the European Commission including both its routine publications and those flowing from its special initiatives on such issues as poverty and social exclusion, family policies, equal opportunities, regional policy, the voluntary sector and training.

In attempting to examine mixed economies of welfare from a comparative perspective, this book follows the trend towards cross-national studies. The book aims to explain the changes that have occurred in welfare states since the early 1970s and to consider some of the policy dilemmas that have arisen. To this end, each of the chapters begins with an introduction to set the scene, followed by an examination of the theoretical and conceptual perspectives relating to the sector under discussion. The main body of the chapter analyses the major changes in the sector and there is an issue-based conclusion which also highlights the policy dilemmas identified in the course of the chapter. The influence of ideology and values is given prominence throughout.

Although each of the sectors has its own chapter, the important point to bear in mind is the relationships between the sectors. In a sense, the significance of one sector is fully understood only when its relationships with other sectors are understood: only then, can its place in the production and delivery of welfare be assessed. An important consideration is the degree to which changes in one sector lead to changes in the others. For example, the strong development of commercial provision (Chapter 3) has an impact on voluntary organisations which may be competitors for custom and contracts. Government policies and government retrenchment clearly affect all of the other sectors: retrenchment leaves room for commercial and voluntary providers and places greater caring responsibility on families, and government policies may specifically encourage such developments. One of the themes of this book is the extent to which changes in mixed economies of welfare are the result of government policies and retrenchment of public services. Another strand identified in the book is the increasing influence on social policy of international financial institutions, especially the World Bank and the International Monetary Fund.

However, changes in the welfare mix are not simply the result of the initiatives of governments and international institutions: a top-down approach has to be considerably modified by taking into account change stemming from social movements and from those lower down in the political system. Chapter 4, dealing with the voluntary sector, identifies the important role played by voluntary organisations in advocacy. For example, mental health groups, or groups made up of or representing older people, disabled or chronically sick people, homeless people, carers or children and young people, put pressure on decision-makers to implement policies favouring the particular group, or to abandon policies thought to be damaging to the interests of the group. Equally, advocacy groups may promote specific causes, such as penal reform or environmental protection. The same chapter also discusses self-help, user and citizen involvement and empowerment.

Bottom-up change is most clearly seen in Central and Eastern Europe where popular pressure resulted in the overthrow of un-popular regimes. Less dramatically, social movements can also be influential: feminism and consumerism are good examples of move-ments which have become increasingly effective over the last twenty years. The particular significance of the women's movement is recog-nised in different parts of the book, but principally in Chapter 5.

Chapter 5 also demonstrates that there are long-term changes over which governments and international financial institutions have little influence. We have already had cause to mention the growing numbers and proportion of older people in the populations of all advanced industrial nations, but other trends are important. Changing patterns of marriage and partnership represent one such trend. Fewer and later marriages, smaller families and the greater frequency of divorce all have implications for informal care. So too, does the increased participation of women in the labour market.

Nationally and internationally, the debate about mixed economies of welfare is far from over, and the importance of the debate has not diminished, connected as it is to a worldwide reappraisal of the role of the state. The book contains six chapters. An introductory chapter sets the scene: it analyses some of the problems besetting welfare states and the views of some of its critics; it examines the continuing support for the welfare state; it explains what is meant by 'mixed economies of welfare' and considers their underlying ideology and values. Chapters 2–5 are devoted to the different sectors

contributing to mixed economies: the state, commercial under-
takings and the market, the voluntary sector and the informal sector.
The final chapter attempts to draw the material together.

Notes

1. Chapter 3 uses some material originally published in Johnson, N. (ed.)
   (1995) *Private Markets in Health and Welfare,* Oxford: Berg, but the new
   material outweighs the re-used elements.

ACKNOWLEDGEMENTS

I wish to thank colleagues at the University of Portsmouth and elsewhere for their support and encouragement. I am grateful for the help and patience of successive editors at Prentice Hall, beginning with Clare Grist, and most recently, Penelope Woolf. Three readers made helpful comments, and I hope that they feel that I have taken their views fully into account. I have been fortunate enough to spend time with many colleagues from other countries, learning a great deal in the process. There are too many to mention individually. As always, my greatest debt is to my wife, Ruth, who has contributed to this book in so many ways: without her help, the book might never have been completed.

CHAPTER 1

INTRODUCTION

There has never been a time when welfare states were free from criticism. The conservative right criticised them for interfering with markets and damaging both the economy and individual self-reliance and self-respect. There was much talk in conservative circles of welfare dependency. The welfare state was seen as the enemy of freedom – Hayek's road to serfdom epitomising this view. Marxist critics argued that there was a contradiction between capitalism and welfare. The welfare state worked primarily in the long-term interests of capital, although concessions to working class pressure might be necessary to legitimate capital accumulation. Fabian friends of the welfare state frequently highlighted its shortcomings, pointing to the persistence of poverty and inequality and to large areas of unmet need. Yet for all this criticism there was little talk of crisis or retrenchment in the 1950s and 1960s; still less was there any talk of the dismantling of the welfare state. The criticisms of the New Right and of the Marxists were not taken very seriously, and the Social Democratic and Fabian criticisms were used as arguments for improving and extending welfare provision.

This comfortable, not to say complacent, view of the welfare state began to be eroded in the early and mid-1970s to such an extent that in 1984 an influential book by Mishra, *The Welfare State in Crisis*, opened with the following sentence: 'In varying degrees and forms, the welfare state throughout the industrialised west is in disarray'. More than twenty years after the onset of the problems which allegedly gave rise to the welfare state's predicament, there is continuing talk of crisis. Esping-Andersen (1996, p. 1), for example,

1

writes: 'It cannot be for lack of prosperity that *welfare states are in crisis*' (emphasis added). Whether the word 'crisis' is appropriately applied to chronic rather than acute problems is open to question. It could be, of course, that talk of crisis occurs only when there is a recession. Thus, the early 1980s and the early 1990s might be characterised as periods of crisis, with the intervening period, between 1985 and 1990 and the period after 1995 seen as periods of growth and greater economic confidence. In this interpretation there are recurring crises interspersed with periods of stability. The early part of this chapter will analyse the factors that are said to have precipitated the alleged crisis in the 1970s, considering whether there are any new elements present in the 1990s. The emphasis is on *problems* rather than *crisis*, because the evidence for a crisis is equivocal. Crisis would show itself in at least two major ways: a retreat on the part of governments from the welfare state with partial dismantling of basic programmes and a diminution in popular support for welfare services. The later part of the chapter will examine the meaning and significance of the term 'mixed economies of welfare'.

It is possible to identify four major groups of problems facing welfare states in the 1980s: economic problems, problems of government and fiscal problems combining to create legitimation problems. It should be stressed that much of the discussion of these problems takes the form of criticisms of state welfare. The discussion is not so much about practicalities as about ideology. In what follows, the views of both the New Right and Marxists are given some prominence, because in their different ways these two ideological groups have been among the sternest critics of the welfare state.

Economic problems

The first sign of impending trouble for the welfare state was the oil crisis of 1973, which sparked off or intensified a world recession. In the period between the mid-1970s and the middle of the following decade most advanced industrialised countries experienced lower rates of economic growth, higher levels of unemployment and lower rates of investment. This presents a stark contrast to the low rates of unemployment, the relatively high rates of capital formation and the substantial economic growth which characterised the 1950s and 1960s.

In the 1950s and 1960s governments in most countries generally believed that social provision benefited the economy, by providing an educated and healthy workforce and maintaining people as *consumers* when they were unemployed, sick or retired. This view began to be questioned with the onset of recession and as Keynesian economic theories were abandoned in favour of monetarism. High social expenditure was identified as contributing significantly to economic decline by diverting resources from the 'productive' to the 'non-productive' sectors of the economy; by reducing incentives to work and invest; and by creating large numbers of welfare dependents. In other words, the welfare state was less the *victim* of economic problems than their *cause.*

The debate gave rise to some very odd bedfellows with a surprising degree of agreement between policy analysts from the right and left of the political spectrum. For example, O'Connor (1984), an American Marxist, supported the view that in the long term the welfare state would reduce opportunities for capital accumulation: he wrote of an 'accumulation crisis' in the United States stemming from the 'dominant national ideology' of individualism. Individualism legitimates the struggle for more: higher wages and the production of consumption or wage goods as opposed to capital goods. A similar process occurs in social policy. There is a demand for more benefits and services of higher quality. These processes necessarily reduce surplus value for appropriation by capital. Consequently, in the developed countries, 'average profit rates and the profit share of national income . . . declined and average unemployment and/or inflation rates increased' (p. 1).

The economic problems came to the fore again in the recession of the early 1990s. The question being asked was whether welfare states could continue to finance systems of social protection at present levels. The OECD (1994) issued the following warning:

> The risks remain, as do the programmes that have evolved in response to them. But the economic context has changed. All countries now are confronted by increasing demands on their social policy expenditures while, at the same time, they face growing resource constraints and, often, budget deficits. And the current recession has underscored the serious financial pressures affecting systems of social protection.
>
> (p. 7)

The worst of the recession in Western Europe had passed by 1995, but economic concerns remained paramount as countries tried to reduce budget deficits in order to meet the criteria for membership of the European Monetary Union in 1999.

Of particular concern in all industrialised countries is the increasing proportion of older people in their populations and the possible economic consequences of what the European Commission (1995, p. 13) has called 'the impending demographic time-bomb'. The ratio of older people to those of working age will go on increasing until well into the next century. This has implications for retirement pensions and for expenditure on health and social services, but as we shall see in Chapter 5, informal care will also be affected.

The final economic consideration is the impact of globalisation on welfare states at different stages of development.[1] One facet of globalisation is the increasing influence of international financial institutions on the policy choices of individual countries. This is most obvious in Central and Eastern Europe, Latin America and more recently in South-East Asia, but it is not restricted to these areas. Globalisation also implies less protected, more open economies, and Esping-Andersen (1996) argues that more economic openness

> entails tougher competition and greater vulnerability to international trade, finance and capital movements. Governments' freedom to conduct fiscal and monetary policy 'at will' is therefore more constrained: profligate deficit spending to maintain employment or pursue redistributive ambitions will be punished . . .
>
> (p. 256)

The mature welfare states of Western Europe find themselves in competition with Japan and South Korea, and in Japan, at least, wage costs are higher than in the 'tiger economies' of Thailand and Indonesia. In order to compete with low-wage economies, the countries of Europe and North America have adopted a variety of strategies in relation to unskilled labour. Esping-Andersen (1996) identifies three different approaches with 'Europe opting for an exit strategy, subsidizing workers to leave the labour market; North America and Britain favouring a wage deregulation strategy, thus bringing down relative wage costs; and Scandinavia stressing a retraining strategy and welfare state jobs, the latter mainly a source of women's employment' (p. 258). It would be a mistake to apply this categorisation too inflexibly. It is mainly a matter of emphasis, and most governments adopt a mixture of approaches. All of them have retraining schemes, for example: the Labour Government which came to power in 1997 in the UK is placing increased emphasis on training and retraining. The European Commission (1996, p. 15) says that 'all states continue to be active with the various employment promotion schemes which they developed or extended during the recession years'.

Problems of government

Since the early 1970s political science has been much exercised by the problems of government growth leading to overload. For the New Right the growth of government is an unmitigated disaster. In particular, the intervention of governments in the economy and in the provision of welfare services has been a failure. In each capitalist country a long list of deficiencies of the welfare state is compiled as evidence of this failure. The massive expenditure of resources and effort has brought little benefit and caused a great deal of harm: governments become overloaded to the point of inefficiency and ineffectiveness.

Brittan (1977) and King (1975) were the overload theorists most frequently cited by the neo-liberals in the 1970s and 1980s. Brittan (1977) claims that the problem of overload stems from the operation of the 'political market'. The businessman or businesswoman attempts to maximise profit, the politician attempts to maximise votes and the bureaucrat attempts to maximise the size of his/her bureau.

Demand-side pressures for government growth have two sources. First, powerful pressure groups and the electorate generally urge governments to increase and improve provision. Second, competitive party politics encourages political parties to make ever more extravagant promises in an attempt to win electoral support. Keynesian economic policies and Beveridge-style welfare policies were responsible in the post-war years for the growth of government. Keynes made deficit budgeting and increased government borrowing and spending respectable. The initial success of these policies exacerbated the problem of overload in the long term because it increased the prestige of government and encouraged people to believe that there need be no limit to its munificence.

Supply-side pressures leading to big government also have two sources. First, there is what might be termed 'administrative accretion': once programmes are initiated they gain a momentum of their own. New programmes do not always replace those already in existence, so that the functions of the government agency concerned grow year by year. Second, bureaucrats have a vested interest in expanding their departments and resisting any reduction in its resources and responsibilities. Professional providers of services, too, have an interest in extending services. Public bureaucracies work in the interests of the providers rather than consumers. These arguments were reinforced by the work of the adherents of the public choice school of economics (Downs, 1957, 1967; Buchanan and Tullock, 1962; Niskanen, 1971, 1978) who sought to apply economic theory to the behaviour of governments. More particularly, they argued that the methods employed in the analysis of markets could be applied to the public sector. The behaviour of bureaucrats was just as self-interested as the behaviour of individuals in the market. The difference was that bureaucrats were not subject to the discipline of the market and the necessity of making a profit.

The consequences of government overload, according to King (1975), include a serious decline in government effectiveness and an increase in the number of policy failures. This raises the possibility that 'mass dissatisfaction with the consequences of our present political arrangements could grow to the point where the arrangements themselves were seriously called in question' (p. 287). A further problem is that as the governmental system becomes larger and more complex, the difficulties of co-ordination and control increase. Among other things, this means greater freedom from political control for administrative and professional staff. It is curious that Offe, a Marxist, analyses the aetiology of the 'ungovern-ability crisis' in terms similar to those used by the overload theorists, particularly King: he blames the growing pressure of expectations and the diminished steering capacity of the state. The ungovern-ability crisis according to Offe stems from a contradiction between the functions of the state in facilitating the accumulation of capital and its functions in relation to legitimation. Class conflict is at the base of this contradiction.

The New Right use overload theories and the extremely one-sided evidence of policy failures to argue for rolling back the state and returning to *laissez-faire* policies; a return to the marketplace and

more reliance on families and voluntary effort. Government intervention is said to be the negation of freedom, a close parallel being
drawn between economic freedom in the market and freedom in
general. State-provided social services, attempts by the state to
reduce inequality and to maintain high levels of employment are all
rejected as being unattainable except at too high a cost in terms of
freedom. What the New Right is advocating, therefore, is a welfare
state based on residual principles with government restricted to the
protection of individuals from coercion, the administration of justice
and mediation in disputes, the provision of basic amenities and
compensation for external or neighbourhood effects and, finally, the
protection of those members of society who cannot be regarded as
'responsible individuals'.

Space has been devoted to theorists active in the 1970s, because
they provided a foundation for more recent contributions which have
developed and modified the earlier work. The New Right in Britain
have continued the critique of big government (Green, 1996; Marsland, 1996). Other writers without new right connections, and indeed
directly opposed to new right ideas, have been critical of the central
state. Communitarianism (see Chapter 5) certainly anticipates a
reduced role for government.

Le Grand (1991), certainly no friend of the New Right, has
attempted to construct a theory of government failure comparable to
the theory of market failure by freely adapting the work of Wolf
(1988). The theory is mainly concerned with efficiency in three
spheres of government activity: provision, subsidy and regulation.
Government provision of goods and services may be inefficient
because very often government providers are monopolies free from
competition both actual and potential. The absence of competition
reduces the pressure to keep cost to a minimum. Where government
providers are not monopolies and are forced to compete, the level of
efficiency will depend upon the kinds of organisation with which
they are competing. If their competitors are profit-maximising
organisations, then government providers will be forced to reduce
costs to a minimum. If competitors are other government agencies or
non-profit organisations, the effect on costs will be less, although
inter-departmental competition in government may have its own
benefits in terms of service quality.

Government subsidies may result in over-provision. As Le Grand
argues: 'if the commodity is provided at any price below cost, there

will be excess demand for the commodity: that is, there will be a demand for the commodity that is in excess of the demand that it would be socially efficient to provide' (p. 12). The government then has to choose between satisfying the inflated demand or rationing by means of imposing restrictive eligibility criteria (e.g. means tests) or relying on waiting lists.

Government, at least in theory, can regulate for quantity, quality, price and market structure. This implies, however, that the regulators have perfect knowledge, or at least that there is no information deficit with the providers or sellers having more information than the regulators. Those responsible for providing a service are more likely to be knowledgeable about the economics of providing it, and it might be in their interests to conceal or even falsify information relating to costs, for example. Furthermore, there are high costs attached to regulation. For example, monitoring and evaluation are difficult to implement and costly. A balance has to be struck between a need for flexibility, innovation and entrepreneurial motivation and the need for regulation. Le Grand is careful to emphasise that 'a study of government failure does not imply that governments always fail; still less that markets always succeed. . . . Governments sometimes succeed: a fact that should not be lost to view in the current glare of the market's bright lights' (p. 19).

Recent changes to the structure of government in many countries may go some way to meeting the criticisms, and there is less discussion in the late 1990s about the problems of big government. Indeed, the main problem may now be fragmentation of government. There is further discussion of these issues in Chapter 2, and here only the main elements of the changes will be identified. The first element is sometimes referred to, rather inelegantly, as deconcentration. This is the breaking up of central government departments by hiving off some of their functions into semi-autonomous executive agencies. The second element is the importation into the public sector of some of the values and practices of the private sector. This implies a greater emphasis on: (i) consumerism with citizens redefined as customers; (ii) markets and quasi-markets and competition; (iii) contracts; (iv) performance indicators with more attention being given to outputs rather than process; (v) reduced or attenuated political accountability. Osborne and Gaebler (1992) characterise the changes taking place in American governance as the transformation of the public sector by a new entrepreneurial spirit. The third

element is decentralisation with a greater emphasis on re
and local administration.

These changes do not go as far as the New Right w
wished. The New Right have never been interested in reforming the
public sector – they want to see its curtailment and partial replacement. The scale of government activity is closely related to the state's
financial and administrative capacity (Pierson, 1994). Something has
been said in this section about administrative capacity, and we now
turn to fiscal capacity.

Fiscal problems

The New Right relate the fiscal problems of welfare states to the
notion of government overload – governments are overstretching
their resources by attempting too much. Marxists agree with this, but
argue that the fiscal crisis is one manifestation of the contradictions
in capitalism and, more specifically, the contradiction in state
intervention in a capitalist system. The fiscal problems for both the
Right and Left are the financial aspect of the problems of government identified in the last section. As the welfare state develops,
people's expectations rise and pressure groups are established to
protect and promote particular interests and causes. Electoral
competition between parties leads to promises of more and better
services and benefits which become increasingly difficult to fulfil.
The fiscal problem is to try to achieve a balance between expenditure
arising from attempts to satisfy citizens' demands for public goods
and services and their willingness to pay for them in the form of taxes.
Governments increase taxes in order to pay for services, and
eventually there is resistance to any further increases. Governments
are therefore faced with a dilemma: they are popular if they provide
services and they are unpopular if they increase taxes. In the United
States, citizens' dissatisfaction with rising taxes led to what have been
referred to as tax rebellions. The best known of these took place in
California in 1978 when Proposition 13 was passed imposing tax
limitations, and since then many other states have followed suit.

Reference has already been made to O'Connor's identification of
an accumulation crisis. Some years earlier (1973) he also identified a
fiscal crisis. O'Connor's analysis starts from the idea that the state in

capitalist society has two major functions – capital accumulation and legitimisation – which may be in conflict. The state assists capital accumulation in two ways: through public expenditure on the economic infrastructure (e.g. transport, water supplies, sewage) and by meeting the costs of reproducing labour power through, for example, the provision of education, housing and health services. The state bears these two forms of costs, but the resulting profits are privately appropriated. It is this which creates a fiscal gap. The fiscal problem is exacerbated by continued pressure upon governments to spend more: 'Every economic and social class and group wants government to spend more and more money on more and more things. But no one wants to pay new taxes or higher rates on old taxes. Indeed, nearly everyone wants lower taxes' (p. 1). These words are prophetic, given the tax revolts that began five years after the publication of O'Connor's work on the fiscal crisis.

The perceived popularity among electorates of lower taxes, has led to the prominence of fiscal issues in election campaigns in many countries. This has been very plain in the most recent elections in the UK and the United States. For example, taxation was a major issue in the 1997 General Election in the UK, with both parties claiming that a vote for their opponents was a vote for higher taxes. Only the Liberal Democrats promised a very small increase in income tax. The political danger of going back on election promises not to increase tax has caused problems for the government in dealing with inflationary pressure: between May and August 1997 interest rates were raised on four occasions.

Now that it is no longer considered acceptable to follow the Keynesian practice of budgeting for a deficit when economic conditions seem to call for it, there is a general concern about deficits. If deficits are to be avoided and public borrowing to be restricted, then a lowering of taxes leaves governments with the sole option of reducing expenditure. Since social expenditure is the largest single item in any budget, lower taxation means reduced benefits and services. The gap can be bridged temporarily by the sale of public utilities as has happened in the UK, Italy and France. In the European Union (EU), one of the conditions for entry to the European Monetary Union is a deficit in 1997 of no more than 3 per cent of Gross Domestic Product (GDP). France, Germany, Italy and Spain were forced to cut expenditure in 1997, although the simplest measure would have been to increase taxation. This is a very clear indication of the political imperative of not increasing taxes. The situation in Germany is interesting in that Chancellor Kohl is dependent on the support of the Free Democratic Party which has given a firm undertaking to resist tax increases.

When President Clinton took office in 1992 the American deficit stood at $290 billion, a record high. In spite of substantial tax cuts the deficit by 1996 had been reduced to $107 billion – a cut of 63 per cent. There was an increase in 1997 to $125 billion, but by 2002 this deficit will have been converted to a $17 billion surplus. Between 1997 and 2002 taxes will be cut by a total of $98 billion, and expenditure will be cut by $388 billion.

It is not unreasonable to talk of fiscal problems, if not a fiscal crisis. Even in the United States, tax cuts have been made possible only by huge reductions in expenditure. The real problem is the lack of political will to raise taxes. Pierson (1994) notes that the visibility of a tax makes a difference to the amounts of tax that can be safely extracted:

> There is, however, significant evidence that the structure of taxation has an impact on how much money governments can raise, and hence on how much is available for social programs. . . . The less visible the tax system (e.g., high reliance on indirect and payroll taxes than on income taxes) the more revenue a government can generate without provoking a taxpayer backlash.
>
> (p. 37–8)

To some extent the same point could be made about cuts in expenditure.

Legitimation problems

The economic, governmental and fiscal problems of the welfare state that we have so far identified give rise to legitimation problems. If, because of economic, administrative and fiscal problems, the welfare state cannot deliver what it promises, or what people expect of it, then it may begin to lose mass support; there may be a loss of legitimacy. There is a crucially important distinction to be drawn, however, between the existence of problems and a crisis. Problems will only lead to crisis if they cannot be contained or resolved and result in a loss of stability threatening the political and economic institutions of a society.

Habermas (1976; 1984) is one writer who has attempted to integrate the different forms of crisis tendencies said to be affecting advanced capitalist society. His analysis is Marxist with a distinctive, individual flavour; his theoretical framework is that of systems theory. There are three systems: the economic, the politico-administrative and the socio-cultural. Each system has its attendant crisis tendencies. The economic system is subject to output crises if it does not produce the necessary quantity of goods and if profits decline. The political system has both input (loyalties) and output (decisions) crisis tendencies. The crisis arising from output problems is termed a rationality crisis: the administrative system fails to provide the decisions required to steer the economic system. There is a contradiction between the need in advanced capitalist societies for administrative economic planning on the one hand and private ownership of the means of production on the other. Turning to political inputs, Habermas stated that 'the political system requires an input of mass loyalty that is as diffuse as possible' (1976, p. 46). If this loyalty is not secured, then a legitimation crisis occurs; Habermas refers to this as a 'legitimation deficit' which implies that 'it is not possible by administrative means to maintain or establish effective normative structures to the required extent' (1976, p. 47).

In advanced capitalism the state becomes more active; it intervenes more in the economy in the interests of capital, providing global planning and the necessary economic infrastructure and bearing the costs of both 'unproductive' commodities and social service provision. To some extent, therefore, the market becomes politicised, and the increased involvement of the state increases disproportionately the need for legitimation. Habermas says, however, that up to this stage in his argument he has succeeded only in identifying legitimation problems, and these do not in themselves constitute a crisis. Legitimation difficulties will be sharpened into a legitimation crisis only if there are failures in the socio-cultural system which result in a motivation crisis:

> A legitimation crisis can be predicted only if expectations that cannot be fulfilled with the available quantity of value or, generally, with rewards conforming to the system, are systematically produced. A legitimation crisis must be based on a motivation crisis – that is, a discrepancy between the need for motives declared by the state, the

educational and the occupational systems on the one hand, and the motivation supplied by the socio-cultural system on the other.

(1976, pp. 74–5)

The most important motivations provided by the socio-cultural system are, according to Habermas, 'the syndromes of civil and familial-vocational privatism'. Civil privatism implies a very weak form of democracy from which genuine participation is excluded because it would expose the contradictions of the system, especially that between socialised forms of production and private appropriation of profits. Familial-vocational privatism, which complements civil privatism, 'consists in a family orientation with developed interests in consumption and leisure on the one hand, and in a career orientation suitable to status competition on the other' (1976, p. 75). Civil and familial-vocational privatism rest on pre-bourgeois traditions and core components of bourgeois ideology, which are being eroded by changes in the social structure. It is this erosion which could precipitate a crisis. It should be stressed, however, that Habermas does not argue that there is a crisis. He asserts that there are certainly legitimation problems, but that a crisis would occur only if these problems could not be solved or successfully contained.

Reduced public support?

Undeniable confirmation of a crisis in the welfare state would be evidence of a large-scale withdrawal of public support. But the weight of evidence points in the opposite direction. Taylor-Gooby (1991) is unequivocal:

> First, the welfare state is extremely popular. A large number of surveys indicate a strong enthusiasm for the key institutions of state welfare and their willingness to pay increased sums in taxes to support them. . . . There is growing evidence that support for state welfare increased among all social and political groupings and became more unified as the 1980s progressed.
>
> (p. 111)

The evidence indicated virtually no difference between social classes in the proportions supporting higher taxes and spending.

Thanks to the annually published *British Social Attitudes* reports complete series of figures are available from 1983. The survey in 1995 (Brook *et al.*, 1996) confirmed earlier findings of general support for extra spending, but with different levels of support for different services and benefits. Health, education, pensions and benefits for disabled people are easily the most popular candidates for extra resources with police, in fifth place, some distance behind. Benefits for single parents were not at all popular and un-employment benefits were also low on people's lists of priorities for extra expenditure. As in earlier surveys, people in 1995 expressed a general willingness to pay extra taxes in return for improvements in services. An innovation in the 1995 survey was to test whether people's general willingness to pay extra taxes persisted when the specific consequences for the individuals concerned were made apparent. The results showed a fall in the popularity of tax and expenditure increases, but with health and education holding up well. Brook *et al.* say:

> It remains the case that, even when the personal tax consequences of spending choices *are* clearly spelled out, some two in every three people still say they would be willing to pay more in tax to support improvements in the NHS, a majority (albeit a smaller one) would be prepared to pay more taxes to improve education, and a substantial minority (40 per cent) would pay more in taxes to improve policing.
> (p. 192)

Unfortunately, pensions and disability benefits were not included in this part of the survey, although one suspects that they, too, might have fared well.

The relationship between support for increased public expenditure and support for private provision for those who can afford it is interesting. Taylor-Gooby (1985; 1991) has emphasised that support for the private market does not necessarily mean antipathy towards the state: people can simultaneously support both market and state provision, which appears to indicate support for a mixed economy of welfare with both public and private sectors playing a part. Brook *et al.* (1996) went one step further by questioning people who actually used private health and education about their support for higher public expenditure and higher taxes. It has to be remembered that those using private services are richer and more likely to vote Conservative. Even so, 54 per cent of those using private health care supported increased expenditure on the NHS, and the proportion of those using private education who supported increased public expenditure on education actually exceeded the proportion favouring increased public expenditure among parents whose children attended a state school. Brook *et al.* suggest that this may be because parents who send their children to private schools 'have opted only reluctantly for the private sector, feeling they have been faced with little choice' (1996, p. 200).

The discussion so far has been concentrated mainly on Britain. Esping-Andersen, on a broader front, however, talks about 'the vast popular majorities in favour of the welfare state that opinion polls and election results regularly identify' (1996, p. 267). This appears to indicate that the positive attitudes demonstrated in Britain are replicated to varying degrees in other countries. The European Commission (1995), for example, says that 'attachment to the existing system of social support remains deeply entrenched in popular opinion' (p. 7). One would anticipate lower support for increased public expenditure in the United States and Australia, and rather more in the Scandinavian countries.

The most recent comparative work on attitudes to government and health and welfare provision is in *International Social Attitudes* (ISA) (Jowell *et al.,* 1993). A paper by Taylor-Gooby in ISA summarises some of the evidence on what citizens want from the state. One of the questions asked people to say whether they thought the government was *definitely* responsible for providing: health care, a decent pension, decent housing and decent unemployment benefits. The widest support was given to health care and pensions. The proportions considering that the government had a definite responsibility to provide health care varied from 40 per cent in the United States to 88 per cent in Italy. Apart from West Germany (57 per cent) all the other European nations[2] in the survey did not fall below 75 per cent. It was a broadly similar picture in relation to pensions with 40 per cent of Americans thinking it a definite government responsibility, 54 per cent of West Germans taking this view and none of the other European nations falling below 77 per cent. Decent housing was thought to be a government responsibility by only 21 per cent of Americans and 24 per cent of West Germans whereas the other European nations varied between 35 per cent and 56 per cent. There was a slight change in relation to unemployment benefits: although the United States came bottom of the list with 14 per cent, Hungary was next lowest with 21 per cent; the other European nations (including West Germany) varied between 32 and 52 per cent. A second question, including a slightly different group of nations,[3] asked respondents to say whether there should be more or less government spending on a range of nine items. People were asked to calibrate their answers on a five-point scale from much less to much more. Surprisingly, a postscript was added to the 'much more' category which warned respondents: 'Remember that if you say "much more", it might require a tax increase' (Taylor-Gooby, 1993, p. 90). In view of the wording of the question, it is surprising that so many people selected the 'much more' option . Unfortunately only those selecting much more government expenditure are reported upon: it would have been helpful to have had a complete breakdown of the answers. In the case of health care Australia (16 per cent) came bottom of the list followed by the United States (20 per cent) and Norway (25 per cent). The remaining five nations varied between 36 and 59 per cent. In the case of pensions, Australia was again at the bottom (12 per cent) followed again by the United States (13 per cent) and West Germany and Norway (both with 16 per cent). The respondents from Northern Ireland were the most willing for much more to be spent on pensions (43 per cent). Taylor-Gooby sums up the results:

> Reassuringly, calls for extra spending follow the pattern set by opinions on where state responsibility should lie. So again we see substantially more support for increased spending generally in Hungary and Italy, followed by Northern Ireland and Britain, though in this case little support for extra spending in Norway, except on the environment. Americans and Australians . . . are the least keen on increased state spending, although there is considerable commitment to more investment in education in the USA (probably associated with the widespread commitment to an ideology of opportunity there), and to law and order in Australia.
>
> (1993, p. 91)

These figures need to be treated with some caution: we really do need to know how many people supported *some* extra expenditure.

The evidence relating to the United States is contradictory. On the one hand, the ISA figures seem to support the traditional view of the United States as a welfare state laggard, with Americans showing much less trust of government, and particularly central government, than is found in Western Europe. The characterisation of the United States as a 'reluctant welfare state' has a long history. Wilensky and Lebeaux (1965) were among the first to analyse the American attitude to the welfare state in their well-known work distinguishing between residual and institutional models of welfare. Almost thirty years later, and after the extensions of state involvement in welfare in the 1960s, Salamon (1992) says: 'reflecting a deep-seated tradition of individualism and an ingrained hostility to centralized institutions, Americans have resisted the worldwide movement toward exclusively governmental approaches to social welfare provision' (p. xv). On the other hand, there is equally strong evidence for a quite different view, and there are indications of a disjunction between the views of the general public and those of the government. Navarro (1994), for example, says that government action is more acceptable to the American public than is sometimes supposed:

> In summary, for many years, poll after poll showed that the majority of Americans did not want cuts in social and welfare programs or in programs for the elderly, the poor, and the needy. Nor did they want a weakening of the health protection of the worker, the consumer, and the environment. Also, and contrary to widely held belief, the majority of Americans favored more, not less, government intervention in supporting people's lives and welfare. For example, in the health sector, most Americans were willing to pay even higher taxes if those taxes were spent on health services.
>
> (p. 13)

Pierson (1994) indicates increasing support for social programmes during the whole of the 1980s following a decline in the late 1970s. He says that 'the well-publicized cutbacks in AFDC and other programs during 1981 produced an immediate reaction. Within months, poll results indicated a liberal turn in public opinion – a trend that was to continue throughout the 1980s' (p. 149).

This presents a dilemma for those wishing to understand US social policy. Why is it that clearly stated public preferences are not translated into practical reforms? Why is it that the Republican Party, vehemently opposed to government extension, was able to gain such a clear victory in the Congressional elections in 1994? Why did Clinton believe that a promise 'to end welfare as we know it' was a likely vote-winner in the Presidential elections of 1996? I have no convincing answers to these questions. One *possible* explanation for the discrepancy is that welfare issues are not those that influence the way people choose to vote: perhaps they are more influenced by promises of economic prosperity or lower taxes or by law and order issues. The fate of Clinton's health reforms may also provide a clue. There seems to be little doubt that more radical reforms than Clinton's proposals, with a single payer along the lines of the Canadian system, commanded majority support (see Navarro 1994, p. 195). However, ranged against even the modest Clinton health plan were some of the most powerful interest groups in America – big industrial firms and the insurance giants. It is these institutions that determine health policy in the United States.

The true test of a legitimation crisis in the welfare state is the degree to which public support for its principles has been withdrawn. The weight of the evidence so far considered in this chapter points to one conclusion: that public support for the welfare state has not diminished. It is true that recipients of means-tested benefits and some stigmatised groups, such as lone mothers, do not attract much public sympathy but this has always been the case. If the object of governments' rhetoric has been to undermine public confidence in the welfare state, then it has been singularly unsuccessful.

General popular support for the welfare state should not, however, lead to the complacent conclusion that all is well. Nor is it necessary, on the other hand, to accept the New Right's rejection of the *principles* of the welfare state and their call for root and branch change. It is quite reasonable simultaneously to support the welfare state in principle, but to be critical of particular aspects of its operation.

Walker (1993), in a paper dealing with the personal social services for older people in the UK, identifies growing dissatisfaction with *certain aspects* of the provision:

> While the postwar period up to the end of the 1970s may have been characterized by policy consensus among politicians the users of the social services were increasingly dissenting. Disillusionment with certain aspects of the social services set in gradually and during the 1980s, has become more and more outspoken. The residualization policy has articulated some of the criticisms of the social services and has, thereby, gained some legitimacy from them.
>
> (1993, p. 74)

These comments, while relating to particular services in the UK, can be applied to other services and other countries. Indeed, the paper by

Walker appears in a study of nine countries with similar concerns, although in none of the others has residualisation been so prominent a feature of government policy (Evers and Svetlik, 1993).

Walker discusses four sets of grassroots criticisms: bureaucratic structure; feminist concerns; lack of adequate support for carers; failure to recognise the specific needs of ethnic minority groups. All of these issues get an airing in subsequent chapters of this book, and all that is called for here is brief reference to each of them.

One criticism, then, is that the welfare state is over-bureaucratic, over-centralised, over-authoritarian and too dominated by professionals. The system is said to be unresponsive to people's varied and changing needs, and clients have little or no control over the services: they are passive recipients rather than active participants. Two questions suggest themselves: (i) are these unavoidable features of the welfare state? (ii) are other configurations of services likely to be free from these faults? There is nothing inevitable about a centralised system. Many services in most countries are regionally or locally administered, and during the last two decades decentralisation has been a consistent theme in Western Europe, the United States and Canada. In Central and East European countries, formerly among the most highly centralised nations, decentralisation is proceeding slowly because local administrative structures have to be established. Empowerment is now the fashionable term for participation and it is just as imprecise. It would be a mistake to under-estimate the difficulty of empowering the users of statutory services, and there is always the danger of rhetoric exceeding achievement, but there is no reason to suppose that, given the political commitment, progress cannot be made.

The claim that other configurations of services, making greater use of voluntary and commercial agencies, would be less bureaucratic and more responsive to user needs still requires to be substantiated. The big service-providing voluntary organisations, for example, are scarcely less bureaucratic than their statutory counterparts, and they may be no more inclined or able to give user-involvement a high priority. Similarly, large commercial enterprises may be more remote than local government agencies.

Feminist analysis in the last twenty years has provided many new insights into the workings of the welfare state. Wilding (1992) identifies its significance:

Feminist analysis raises a wide range of questions about policies, starting from a concern for the position of women. Those questions are important for commitment to equal opportunities. Those questions are also important for a broader evaluation of the 'welfare state'. They supply Social Policy with a new armoury of critical questions and a new agenda.

(p. 112)

In the next chapter, feminist views of the state are considered. In summary, feminists claim that most of the standard treatments of the state are flawed, because they fail to recognise the extent to which the state is gendered. Feminist writers are critical of some of the assumptions about the role of women built into the welfare state. For example, Beveridge assumed women would be dependent upon their husbands' earnings and that their chief roles would be as wives and mothers in the home. In a very real way, women's rejection of this role has highlighted the relationship between work and home life. There is a mass of literature on the dependence of the welfare state on the caring work of women. Feminist analysis is critical of the gender inequalities in the welfare state and notions of inequality have been widened considerably. For example, Glendinning and Millar (1992) and Millar (1996) have demonstrated the preponderance of women among those living in poverty and women's greater dependence on state benefits. Pahl (1989) has shown that studies of inequality are deficient in not taking into account the control and distribution of money in marriage, and more generally in households. A range of studies indicate the distortion produced by talking about equal opportunities in terms of the labour market without taking into account inequalities in the domestic economy. In spite of the sometimes devastating feminist critique of the welfare state, most feminists working in the field of social policy are not opposed to the principle of sate welfare: they argue for reform and changed attitudes, not retrenchment.

Financial and other support for carers is examined in Chapter 5 where evidence of the gender bias in caring is discussed. It is not simply that women take most of the responsibility for child care, but they are also involved in caring for frail elderly and disabled relatives. Belatedly, welfare states are beginning to recognise the importance of carers in social and health care, but as Chapter 5 demonstrates, support varies considerably from country to country. Carers, who have long been critical of their treatment in welfare states, have in a number of countries begun to form mutual support groups.

Ethnic minorities exist in all countries, and in all countries they experience discrimination in a wide variety of contexts: income distribution, work and training, housing, social security. The groups include: Turkish and other 'guest workers' in Germany; North Africans in France; Koreans in Japan; Gypsies in Central and Eastern Europe; Afro-Caribbeans, Chinese, Indians and Pakistanis in the United Kingdom; African Americans and Hispanics in the United States; Aboriginals and South-East Asians in Australia and Maoris in New Zealand. Each of these groups has specific needs which they justifiably claim are not being met, or even considered, in the welfare states of which they are a part.

The welfare state, then, is certainly not without its critics, including those who question its principles and those who question its practice. There is also criticism of its outcomes and achievements. Critics point to shortages of supply in relation to demand, the persistence of poverty and inequality, poor housing, and inadequate responses to the individual needs of older and disabled people and deprived children. It is, of course, relatively easy to identify failings since shortage in relation to demand is universal, but it is possible to argue that the welfare state is to a large extent a victim of its own success. It is the success of state services which has raised people's expectations of them and created the gap between demand and supply.

The critics provided governments with a ready-made target to blame for economic problems. Governments anxious to reduce public expenditure, or at least reduce its rate of growth, could use the arguments of critics of state welfare to justify their actions. The European Commission (1994; 1995; 1996), the OECD (1994), the World Bank (1994) and the International Monetary Fund all highlight the need for public expenditure restraint. Hill (1996), in a comparative analysis of social policy, says the 'debates about social policy cut-backs, or at least restraint upon the growth of social policy, have become fairly universal' (p. 293). His analysis leads him to suggest that 'there has been a shift, even amongst welfare state supporters, from a commitment to the advancement of statism to a mixed "economy of welfare"' (p. 294). We can no longer delay a discussion of the meaning and implications of this term.

Mixed economies of welfare

In order to avoid confusion, it should be emphasised that the term 'mixed economies of welfare' is one of two terms in general use to describe the same phenomenon: the alternative is 'welfare pluralism'. The term 'welfare pluralism' first came into general use in Britain following the Wolfenden Report (1978) on the future of voluntary organisations. The term used in this book, mixed economies of welfare, is of slightly more recent origin, but the meaning of the two terms is identical and they can therefore be used interchangeably.

We first need a broad, uncomplicated definition which will serve as a basis for further expansion and elucidation. One definition that meets the criteria is that proposed by Knapp *et al.* (1994):

> A mixed economy has two principal dimensions: alternative modes of provision and sources of funding. Together they define the broad arrangements for the delivery and purchase of services, ranging from a centrally planned welfare state, with everything provided and funded by the state, to a market 'free-for-all' with users or their relatives buying services from a variety of profit-seeking suppliers.
>
> (p. 124)

It should be noted that the definition allows for a range of possibilities between two extreme positions: one where the state is entirely dominant and the other where the market is in the ascendancy. A second feature of the definition, closely connected to the first, is that two sectors – the voluntary sector and the informal sector – are omitted. A third significant aspect of the definition is that it links provision and financing: the two are very closely connected in that decisions about the mode of provision necessarily imply particular forms of funding. It could also happen that decisions about funding are the driving force with modes of provision responding to changes in funding.

In a mixed economy of welfare, there are four sectors involved in the production and delivery of welfare: the state sector; the commercial sector; the voluntary (non-profit or third) sector; the informal sector (family, friends and neighbours). It must be stressed that there is nothing new in this. Welfare states have always been mixed and the same four sectors have always been present. The crucial consideration is not the existence of these four sectors, but the *balance* between them which varies along the following dimensions:

● Between one country and another: compare, for example, the Scandinavian countries which have large state sectors and relatively small private sectors with the United States where the state sector is more limited and the private sector more extensive.
● Between one time and another: for example, there was a significant expansion of the state sector in Western Europe after the Second World War and a relative decline in more recent years. The history of the commercial sector is to some extent the reverse of this.
● Between one service and another: compare, for example, the dominance of the state sector in education in most countries with the dominance of the commercial sector in housing.
● Between one component of a service and another: compare, for example, hospitals (voluntary or non-profit sector dominance) and nursing homes (commercial sector dominance) in health care in the United States.

The above variations, however, are based on *provision* of services, and two further aspects of the production, delivery and consumption of welfare need to be incorporated into the analysis: *finance* (or funding) and *regulation*. Table 1.1 gives a very broad indication of the relationships among all three elements in four different approaches. It should be stressed that the different approaches are not intended to constitute descriptions of particular welfare states: they are models or ideal types, used for purposes of analysis rather than description. In the state-oriented approach the government is responsible for provision, finance and regulation – the former communist societies of Central and Eastern Europe came closest to this approach. In traditional mixed economies the government is joined as a provider by the voluntary sector and this brings in an element of private funding, although voluntary agencies often rely heavily on government finance. Anheier and Seibel (1998), from whose work this table is taken,[4] say that this approach is typical of countries 'where the principle of subsidiarity governs the relationship between both sectors, as it does in The Netherlands and Germany'. A feature of the relationships in traditional mixed economies is the corporatist division of labour between the government and the voluntary sector. In contemporary mixed economies, commercial suppliers join the government and the voluntary sector. Anheier and Seibel say that this model differs from the traditional form in two respects: the relationships are competitive rather than corporative and roles are not specifically assigned. Given the advance of market provision in many countries, more welfare states will exhibit some of the characteristics of this model. Australia, Japan, New Zealand, the United States, the United Kingdom, some of the countries of South America and some in South-East Asia are already all or part of the way along this route. In the market-oriented approach, the government is not involved in welfare, even in a regulatory role. Even the most committed of the New Right do not contemplate such a totally unregulated free-for-all.

Anheier and Seibel apply the categories in Table 1.1 to countries in Central and Eastern Europe. They say that:

> Few Central Eastern European countries would regard either the government or the market-oriented approach as the only feasible option both in practical as well as political terms, although the free market ideology and the promise of socialist stability are attractive to different segments of their populations.
>
> (1998, p. 186)

They hypothesise that the former East Germany will follow the traditional mixed economy approach, that Poland will have a centralised system uneasily fluctuating between a traditional mixed economy of welfare and a state-oriented approach. Hungary will adopt an approach fairly close to the contemporary mixed economy model. Although Anheier and Seibel do not cover the Czech Republic and Slovenia, I would speculate that they, too, will follow the contemporary mixed economy route.

Table 1.1   Approaches to service delivery

Approach	Provision	Finance	Regulation
State-oriented	Government	Government	Government
Traditional mixed economy	Government Vol. agencies	Government Private sources	Government Self-regulated assocs
Contemporary mixed economy	Government Vol. agencies Commercial suppliers	Government Private sources Fees and charges	Government Self-regulated assocs Markets
Market-oriented	Commercial suppliers	Fees and charges	Markets

Source: Modified form of Anheier and Seibel (1998)

Although Table 1.1 is useful, it has at least one serious weakness: while it identifies the participants in provision, finance and regulation, it says nothing about the balance between them (including the power balance) or the extent of their participation. For example, we learn that in contemporary mixed economies finance comes from three sources, but each of these are closely related: thus the role of government finance is likely to be of paramount importance. A large part of the funding of the voluntary sector in many countries is from government. The same may be true of commercial enterprises when they enter into contracts with public sector agencies. The government is also likely to retain a dominant role in regulation. Indeed, the entry into the market of a greater diversity of suppliers for client groups some of which will include vulnerable people, may necessitate an increase in the government's role in regulation.

The maintenance of a split between provision, on the one hand, and finance and regulation, on the other, is a common theme in analyses of mixed economies of welfare. The general aim is to reduce the state's role as a direct provider of services, but to retain its role in finance and regulation. In this way, state agencies become enablers rather than providers. Osborne and Gaebler (1992) talk of catalytic government, and borrowing a phrase from Savas (1987), they say that the government should be concerned with steering the boat not with rowing it. Public agencies remain responsible for ensuring that services are provided, but they purchase services from the independent sector, the term now used to denote the combined resources of the commercial and voluntary sectors. Increasingly, services are provided on the basis of contracts which may or may not result from a process of competitive tendering. Contracting for social and health care, which is intended to induce efficiency through competition, and simultaneously extend choice and empower consumers, is furthest advanced in the United States and the UK, but is being developed in many other countries throughout the world. The issues surrounding contracting are addressed more fully in Chapters 2, 3 and 4.

The term 'mixed economies of welfare' may be viewed as neutral, since it does not imply any particular mix, but its use is far from neutral. The movement towards mixed economies is part of a world-wide reappraisal of the role of the state. In the process, the ethos of public service and the structure of the state are also undergoing change. It is difficult to imagine a more important issue for public policy. It is not being claimed that mixed economies of welfare, on their own, could bring about such major structural changes, but they are an important component in a broad sweep of changes. Part of the reason for the popularity of mixed economies of welfare with conservative governments is that they can be used to legitimate policies of 'rolling back the state'. This had particular appeal to Reagan and his successors in America (including Democrat Clinton) and Mrs Thatcher and her successors in the UK, but President Chirac in France and Chancellor Kohl in Germany have both expressed support for similar policies. It is ironic that among the most vigorous attempts to reduce the role of the state were those made by a Labour Government in New Zealand.

An essential feature of 'rolling back the state' are the attempts that have been made by all governments to reduce (or more realistically, to contain) public expenditure. There was certainly a hope that mixed economies of care would help to reduce public expenditure, but unless services were to be discontinued, the resources to provide them had to be found and sometimes costs were simply transferred from the state to individuals, families and the voluntary sector. As will be seen in Chapter 5, community care means care by families, and if public services are cut then extra costs have to be borne by relatives. If a voluntary agency has traditionally provided a vital service and the public funding agency, because of financial stringency, cuts or fails to increase the contract price, the voluntary agency has two options: either to reduce provision or to maintain service levels and subsidise the public authority.

It is primarily in attitudes towards the state that the ideological element in mixed economies of welfare comes most clearly into focus. Different approaches to the analysis of the state are considered in Chapter 2, but it may be worth indicating briefly at this point how different ideological perspectives on the state are likely to be reflected in views of mixed economies of welfare. Since most ideological groups do not specifically refer directly to mixed economies, an element of speculation is involved. A good treatment of welfare state ideology is to be found in George and Wilding (1994) who identify six ideological positions: the middle way, democratic socialism, Marxism, the New Right, feminism and greenism. The brief outline which follows uses George and Wilding's categories.

The middle way, represented in Britain by Keynes and Beveridge and traditional one-nation Conservatives, has strong affinities with pluralism and is the most firmly committed to mixed economies of welfare. Its adherents acknowledge the importance of markets, but recognise that they need to be managed and regulated. George and Wilding say that 'this group has few doubts that the state must play a major role in welfare but there is a critical approach to the nature and extent of that role' (pp. 46–7). The group give enthusiastic support to the welfare role of the voluntary and informal sectors.

The social democratic approach is represented by Tawney, Titmuss, Townsend, Crosland and the Fabians in Britain and by Social Democratic parties in Europe and elsewhere. The democratic socialists are less suspicious of the state than are the adherents of the middle way, and the state would retain a dominant position in mixed economies of welfare. This group now accepts the role of markets, but would accord them a less significant role in welfare than middle-way supporters, and insist on their modification and regulation. There is support for universal services, which contrasts with the selective approach of the middle way. The voluntary sector would play an essentially supplementary and complementary role.

At its more radical end, democratic socialism shades into Marxism. Traditional Marxists would see mixed economies of welfare as evidence of the capitalist state's ability to change forms while retaining substance: it does not alter power relationships and the capitalist system, with its inherent contradictions, is maintained. Mixed economies of welfare are likely to be interpreted as little more than attempts to reduce welfare expenditure. The voluntary sector is becoming more market-oriented and simultaneously drawn into government. Marxism, at its most moderate end is virtually indistinguishable from democratic socialism. Indeed, Eurocommunism, in so far as it is Marxist at all, may be less radical in some respects than democratic socialism. The idea that revolution is the only sure way of ensuring the triumph of socialism has been abandoned in favour of the democratic parliamentary route. Markets, although treated with considerable scepticism, are reluctantly accepted.

The New Right has already been given substantial space earlier in this chapter, and there will be more in other chapters. Members of the New Right welcome any reduction in the role of the state and just about any extension of markets. They therefore find mixed economies of welfare preferable to state-dominated systems, but they are to be regarded as a very small step in the right direction; indeed, it could even be counter-productive from their point of view if policy-makers believe that the welfare mix has undergone sufficient change. The continuation, or even expansion, of the state's role as regulator and in finance is deprecated. Markets and families with some help from voluntary organisations (especially self-help groups) should be the main means of satisfying needs. The kind of welfare arrangements favoured by the New Right would replace state domination with market domination.

Feminism takes several different forms (Dale and Foster, 1986; Williams, 1989; George and Wilding, 1994). A division is usually made between liberal, socialist and radical feminism. Liberal feminists are mainly concerned with equal opportunities and rights. Socialist feminists see women's disadvantages stemming from their position within an exploitative capitalist system which favours men. Radical feminists are concerned with the oppression of women by men in a male-dominated political, social and economic system. Radical and socialist feminists are in agreement that the state works in the interests of men, but they disagree about whether the state can *ever* work in the interests of women. One of the main contributions of feminism has been to identify and analyse caring roles within families which are predominantly, although not exclusively, carried out by women. There has been pressure to have work in the domestic economy given equal recognition with paid work in the labour market, and for more to be done to enable women to participate fully and equally in the labour market. Many women see the mixed economy of welfare as detrimental to their interests in so far as it means more reliance on the unpaid work of carers. More is said on this issue in Chapter 5.

Greenism has little to say directly about mixed economies of welfare, but it has plenty to say about the welfare state which, it claims, takes too little account of environmental issues. They advocate decentralisation to small local units and participatory structures and processes. The Greens have been particularly influential in Germany and they are making some headway in other countries. Many environmental projects involve collaboration between the state, the market and the voluntary sector – mixed economies in action.

This discussion of ideology emphasises again that the balance between sectors is the crucial element in mixed economies of welfare, and the different ideological groups disagree about exactly where the balance should be struck. We have already seen how the question of balance is complicated by a division between provision, finance and regulation. Decentralisation and deconcentration further complicate matters. When relationships are studied in detail in specific instances (see Evers and Svetlik, 1993; 6 and Vidal, 1994) what is revealed is an enormously complex array of different arrangements. Like most social phenomena, mixed economies of welfare do not fall into neat patterns.

There is no formula to work out the 'right' balance: what is right in one situation or in one country will not be right in other situations and countries. This book is an attempt to analyse the strengths and weaknesses of each of the sectors and to examine how the sectors inter-relate. An international approach is taken to demonstrate the different ways in which the mixed economy of welfare is interpreted. A separate chapter is devoted to each of the sectors, beginning with the state. This will be followed by chapters on the commercial sector, the voluntary sector and the informal sector.

Notes

1. A very good discussion of globalisation is to be found in Esping-Andersen (1996), Chapter 9.
2. The countries in this part of the survey comprised: Britain, West Germany, East Germany, Hungary, Italy, Ireland, Norway, N. Ireland and USA.
3. The countries comprised: Australia, Britain, West Germany, Hungary, Italy, N. Ireland, Norway and USA.
4. This is a modified version of Anheier and Seibel's tabulation. It should be noted that they use the terms traditional and contemporary pluralism.

CHAPTER 2

THE STATE AND
SOCIAL WELFARE

Introduction: defining terms

Before looking in more detail at the role of the state in social welfare some consideration must be given to what is meant by the state. The state is an abstraction in that there is no single entity that can be said to constitute the state, and this makes an analysis of its involvement in welfare something of a problem. It is, however, possible to identify the institutions of the state. The focus in this approach is on *governmental* institutions – those concerned with promulgating laws, rules and regulations and ensuring that these are enforced. There is scope for disagreement about precisely which institutions should be included, and the scope for such disagreement may be widened by the increased fragmentation of government. It is also possible to identify the *functions* of the state, although disagreement about functions is much more fundamental than disagreement about the choice of institutions. Marxists, for example, maintain that the function of the state in the long run is to serve the interests of the dominant class – the owners of capital – and to support the capitalist system. This contrasts with early pluralist views that the function of the state is to act as a neutral arbiter between competing interests, and with the view of the New Right that the function of the state is to provide the legal framework for free competition and the development of individualism and self-reliance.

Dunleavy and O'Leary (1987, p. 2) say that the state has five main characteristics:

- it is a 'recognizably separate . . . set of institutions, so differentiated from the rest of its society as to create identifiable public and private spheres';
- within its territory, the state is the supreme power;
- the state's sovereignty extends to everyone living within its territory;
- 'the modern state's personnel are mostly recruited and trained for management in a bureaucratic manner';
- it has the power to levy taxes.

Schwarzmantel (1994) identifies a similar set of characteristics:

> The state . . . can be described as a set of institutions constituting a specialised apparatus of domination. Not only is the modern state in this sense distinct from the society over which it rules, but it is also a centralised apparatus of power, which rules over a territorially demarcated area and which possesses a monopoly of rule making.
>
> (p. 8)

One of the interesting similarities between these two definitions is that they both see the necessity of differentiating between state and society. Two observations may be made about the 'identifiable public and private spheres'. The first is that their relative size will vary from country to country. Second, the distinction between public and private is by no means clear-cut, even in liberal democracies, and in totalitarian states civil society and the state are not clearly differentiated. Furthermore, as will be seen shortly, there are some theoretical approaches which deny the existence of a clear dividing line between state and society.

Before turning to the theoretical approaches, it might be worth recalling what was said in the preceding chapter about the impact of increasing globalisation on the autonomy of the nation state. Globalisation is said to diminish the capacity of nation states to decide policies without reference to global economic pressures. Furthermore, policies may be thwarted by developments beyond the control of individual nation states. Esping-Andersen (1996, pp. 256–7) suggests that the freedom of governments to design discrete social policies has been eroded, because 'it is increasingly world finance which defines what is possible and desirable'. While there is some justification for these fears, it is possible to exaggerate the nation state's loss of autonomy. The state is still the most significant al institution. As Hutton (1997, p. 30–1) asserts, 'the balance of power between the nation state and the world market is very complex', and there are no other participants with the same power as the state.

Theories of the state

There are numerous theories of the state. Dunleavy and O'Leary (1987) for example, identify five different approaches: pluralism, the New Right, elite theory, Marxism and neo-pluralism. Schwarzmantel (1994) adds feminist views of the state and also includes communist and fascist states as rivals to the liberal democratic state. In the space available there is no possibility of attempting anything more ambitious than a brief sketch of some of these different theories of the state. Five schools of thought on the state will be discussed: pluralist, elitist, the New Right, Marxist and feminist.

Pluralist views

The principal components of pluralist politics are elections, representative democracy, political parties and pressure groups. The state, if it is mentioned at all, consists of the formal institutions of government. References tend to be to 'the political system' rather than to 'the state'.

Schwartzmantel (1994) sums up the main characteristics of pluralism:

> In its broadest terms, pluralism is a view of the political structure of liberal-democracy which emphasises the diffusion of power in such systems. . . . Pluralism suggests a solution to the problem of how to achieve popular power and at the same time limit the power of the state. This solution lies through participation in a network of groups and associations, which form multiple and competing centres of power.
>
> (p. 48)

As the quotation indicates, pluralism is both normative, purporting to demonstrate how the political system *should* be organised, and explanatory, claiming to describe accurately how the political system actually works.

The theoretical base of pluralism is the group theory of politics stemming largely from the work of Bentley in the early part of the twentieth century who made the bold claim that 'there are no political phenomena except group phenomena' (1908, p. 222). Bentley was attempting to provide an alternative to the formal, institutional, rather static approach to politics and to move away from atomistic individualism. The theory is concerned with the group rather than the individual, and it is more concerned with processes than with institutions. An often-quoted passage sums up Bentley's approach:

> When the groups are adequately stated, everything is stated. When I say everything I mean everything. The complete description will mean the complete science, in the study of social phenomena, as in any other field.
>
> (1908, pp. 208–9)

Bentley's theories have been refined and modified by Truman (1951), Dahl (1956; 1982) and Lindblom (1977) but the classic statements of pluralism still rest on the central notion of competing groups. Power is widely distributed among a plurality of interest groups, each of which seeks to mobilise political support. Power is defined in terms of decision-making by asking which groups or individuals participated in the decision-making process and whose view prevailed? What concessions did the different groups have to make in order to extract an acceptable outcome? In this way, the policy-making process consists of bargaining among groups, and particular policy decisions are based on compromise and accommodation. Such a process means that policy changes are incremental.

In this view of politics the government is a mediator, an impartial umpire or broker concerned with the 'authoritative allocation of values' (Easton, 1953). The whole system rests on an underlying consensus on what are seen as central values – democracy, the rule of law and respect for private property, for example. When pluralists speak of democracy, they are referring to representative democracy with elections as a means of making choices between competing political parties. Such a system allows for only periodic participation by the mass of the citizenry and the choice is restricted to 'bundles of policies'. The representative system is a relatively blunt instrument for expressing specific preferences – a task more effectively accomplished by interest groups. Thus, territorial and functional

representation are both required for the achievement and maintenance of a democratic society.

Pluralists view the state, especially the centralised state, with some
suspicion. Too much power in the hands of government, or one arm
of government, is inimical to democracy, and means of dispersing
power must be sought. The interest group system is the surest way of
achieving power dispersal, but it is not sufficient on its own. Pluralists
therefore favour federal political systems over unitary ones and
argue for as much decentralisation as possible. A further safeguard is
a separation of powers, so that no single arm of government can
completely dominate the others. They accept that this will lead to
fragmentation, although they prefer the term diversity. But, like
some post-modernists, they hold that diversity is something to be
celebrated, not condemned.

The pluralist approach has been the subject of much criticism –
especially the theory's treatment of power. Bachrach and Baratz
(1962), for example, criticised the concentration on decision-
making, arguing that non-decisions were as important as decisions.
The power to keep items off the political agenda was crucial. Lukes
(1974), while acknowledging the contribution of Bachrach and
Baratz, claimed that their formulation of power is deficient in
two respects: it fails to take account of the structural element in
power, and it does not recognise that power may be exercised
when there is no conflict. It is a significant exercise of power to
prevent conflict arising in the first place. This is done by manipu-
lating people into believing that the power-holders are acting in
everyone's best interests. People acquiesce in actions which are not
in their real interests but only in their interests as defined by the
power-holders.

Wide dispersal of power is essential to the pluralist case, but both
elite and Marxist theorists claim that power is concentrated in very
few hands. Feminist theories of the state maintain that power is
largely in the hands of men. Pluralists do not deny that power is
unevenly distributed, and they recognise that there is a danger of
some groups becoming too dominant while other sections of society,
being unorganised, are excluded from the policy-making process.
The system is said, however, to have two built-in safeguards. The first
is overlapping membership or multiplicity of interests. For example,
motorists are also pedestrians; on a bigger scale, industrialists are
also sons and daughters and possibly mothers and fathers, and as

individuals they may belong to environmental, sporting or welfare groups. The second protection is that the development of powerful groups gives rise to the emergence of groups in opposition, and those currently unorganised constitute potential groups who may be activated if their interests appear to be threatened by the activities of an existing group. These restraints have not prevented business interests becoming and remaining the dominant influence in policy-making.

In response to the criticisms, and in order to take account of contemporary developments, pluralists have modified their theories. Dunleavy and O'Leary (1987) group these modifications together under the title of neo-pluralism. To deal with the criticism of the dominant position of business in the interest group system, the idea of a dual polity has been developed. The dual polity thesis argues that the state is indeed partly controlled by the democratic processes of electoral competition, interest group pressure and representative assemblies. The other side of the duality is the direct influence of business on government policy. However, the influence of business, the argument continues, is restricted largely to the economic field. This pre-supposes that clear distinctions can be made between economic and other policies. With regard to social policy, this is a contestable view to say the least. Furthermore, the dual polity thesis ignores the penetration of for-profit businesses in health and welfare provision.

Another major modification of pluralist theory is the reduced emphasis on the institutions of representative government and the development of an alternative model of the professionalised state. Dunleavy and O'Leary (1987) summarise the model in the following passage:

> The 'professionalized state model' argues that Western democracies remain pluralist in their mode of operation because of the development of internalized controls among more expert and professionalized state officials, the fragmentation of government to create interactive policy-making systems, and the growth of issue-specific forms of public participation.
>
> (p. 300)

Expert and professionalised state officials may form the basis of a new power elite, and it is to elitist theories of the state that we now turn.

Elitist views

Elitist views have a long history, going back to Plato's *Republic* in which government would be the responsibility of specially selected and trained guardians. The origins of modern elitism can be found in the writings of Mosca (1896), Michels (1911) and Pareto (1916). The theories claimed to apply to all societies at all times. They also claimed to disprove the claims of both democratic and Marxist theory. Democratic theory did not accord with reality and the Marxist dream of a classless, egalitarian society was an impossibility. The basis of their theory is stated in this well-known quotation from Mosca:

> In all societies – from societies that are very meagrely developed and have barely attained the dawnings of civilisation, down to the most advanced societies – two classes of people appear – a class that rules and a class that is ruled. The first class, always the less numerous, performs all political functions, monopolises power and enjoys the advantages that power brings, whereas the second, the more numerous class, is directed and controlled by the first. . . .
>
> (trans. 1939, p. 50)

Although the theories of Mosca, Michels and Pareto vary, all three would accept that the few invariably govern the many: there are those who lead and those who are content to follow. Popular sovereignty, democracy, can never be achieved. Michels is specifically concerned with the organisation of political parties which, he claims, are subject, like any other organisation, to the 'iron law of oligarchy'. The party leaders are self-perpetuating groups of decision-makers. Mosca and Pareto divide their elites into two sections. Mosca's division is into upper and lower strata, with a small upper stratum responsible for major policy decisions and the remainder responsible for more mundane work. Pareto's division is into a governing elite and a non-governing elite. The governing elite are those who make the major political decisions, and the non-governing elite are those who occupy leading positions in society, but have no role in decision-making.

Elites gain and retain power through a mixture of manipulation, deception and coercion. They bolster their positions by appearing to work in the interests of the masses. Lukes' (1974) third dimension of power is of some relevance here. Mosca emphasises their cohesion and superior organisation as important factors in the retention of power by elites. Pareto lays greater emphasis on psychological factors. A stable elite would contain the right balance between what he called 'lions' (those willing to use force) and 'foxes' (those relying on cunning and manipulation). Mosca, Michels and Pareto thought of the mass as gullible, apathetic and uninterested in politics.

Elites may be open (liberal) or closed (autocratic). Open elites recruit new talent from below, either from second level elites or from the masses. Closed elites, denying themselves the chance of renewal, will ultimately atrophy and decay, and are likely to be overthrown to be replaced by a new elite. Revolution merely replaces one elite with another in what Pareto called 'the circulation of elites'.

In contemporary societies, elites may be more diverse. Mills (1956) said of the American political system that power was concentrated in the hands of inter-related elites who use it for their own ends. Mills identified big business, the military and the political coterie surrounding the president as forming the main components of an elite which took all the big decisions. The interlinking of these groups was so close that it was possible to talk of a single power elite, although concentration on the apparatus of democratic politics served to cloak this. The composition of elites will vary from country to country, but might include: political leaders, top administrators, business, the labour movement, religious leaders and those controlling the media.

It is clear that classical pluralism and classical elitism are diametrically opposed, but there are ways in which the two can be partially reconciled. For an example of one such attempt at reconciliation we can turn to the work of Schumpeter (1944) who agreed with Michels that parties might very well be oligarchies, but claimed this did not make democracy impossible. Political parties represent rival elites who have to compete for electoral support.

Corporatism also offers opportunities for combining elements of pluralism with elements of elitism. Corporatism emphasises the importance of key or peak associations in negotiation with the state. In advanced industrial capitalism the competitive pressure groups posited by pluralism are partially replaced (the degree depending on the country concerned) by corporate groups which 'are defined by their location in the social and economic division of labour: their identity is given by the *function* that their members perform in society and the economy' (Cawson, 1982, p. 38). The main characteristics of corporatism are identified by Cawson:

one of the most important features of corporate representation is that the organisations are involved in negotiation with the state not simply to press their demands, but to act as agents through which state policy is implemented. . . . In a corporatist model of policy-making, representation (of demands) and implementation (of policies) are fused with a mutually dependent bargaining relation-ship in which favourable policy outcome are traded for co-operation and expertise.

(1982, pp. 38–9)

Corporatist arrangements are most frequently found in the economic field in which tripartite discussions take place between both sides of industry (in Britain the Trades Union Congress and the Confederation of British Industry) and the government. Such discussions do not have to be tripartite, however. For example, the Joint Commission in Austria has four participant organisations. In Denmark, Finland, Germany, Norway, Sweden and Japan peak welfare associations are involved in discussions of social policy. The restriction of discussion and negotiation to peak groups gives the corporatist system a strongly elitist flavour. In social policy, for example, health and welfare professionals and producer groups are involved in the bargaining process, but consumers are largely excluded.

New Right views

Classical liberal theory sees freedom or liberty as the supreme moral value: there can be no trade-offs against other values such as equality. Indeed, as Friedman and Friedman (1980) argue, the pursuit of equality is to be avoided:

A society that puts equality – in the sense of equality of outcome – ahead of freedom will end up with neither equality nor freedom. The use of force to achieve equality will destroy freedom, and force, introduced for good purposes, will end up in the hands of people who use it to promote their own interests.

(p. 181)

At the risk of over-simplification, freedom is seen as the absence of external restraint, and particularly freedom from state intervention. The New Right see the state as the potential enemy of a free society.

This view comes out most strongly in the work of Hayek from 1944 to the 1980s. His best known and most polemical work is *The Road to Serfdom* (1944) in which he argued that social democracy, socialism and the welfare state all led to greater state intervention and this posed a serious threat to liberty and a free society. Hayek, like other liberals, strongly supports capitalism and the operation of free markets both of which are essential to liberal democracy. On no account is the state to interfere in the economic sphere. Thus, classical liberal theory supports the notion of a nightwatchman or minimal state limited to the enforcement of contracts and the protection of its citizens from theft, fraud or violence.

But the New Right is an amalgam of not entirely consistent strands. Gamble (1988) in an analysis of Thatcherism in the UK, says that the twin aims of the Conservative governments in the 1980s were the development of a free economy and a strong state. We therefore have a New-Right inspired government embarking on a programme of greatly increased government intervention in many areas and deregulation in others. The strong interventionist state was required to restore the authority of the state and ensure the compliance of other agencies and interests. King (1987) in an analysis similar to that of Gamble, argues that New Right theories consist of two conflicting elements: a liberal element which emphasises freedom from state control, individualism and free markets and a conservative element which emphasises authority and order and the use of government to achieve these. In the United States, a third element would need to be added – the religious right. Stoesz and Midgley (1991), in relation to the United States, claim that 'despite rhetorical antipathy toward government, the radical right has demonstrated increasing sophistication in using the state to advance its objectives' (p. 39).

The theoretical base of the New Right has been strengthened, particularly in the United States, as a result of its adoption since the early 1970s by public choice theorists. Not all public choice theorists are New Right enthusiasts, but many of them are (e.g. Buchanan, Niskanen, Tullock). Public choice theorists are economists who attempt to adapt traditional economic analysis and apply it to the 'political market'. If entrepreneurs seek to maximise profit, then politicians seek to maximise their vote and bureaucrats seek to maximise their budgets. This can be used as an argument for small government.

Among the most interesting and influential arguments for a minimal state in recent years have been those propounded by Nozick in *Anarchy, State and Utopia* (1984). As the title indicates, the book is divided into three parts, but the main argument is contained in the first two parts, and we will concentrate on them.

In the first part Nozick rejects anarchy. Anarchists hold that the state is immoral because it uses coercion to enforce rights and violates the absolute rights of life, liberty and property. The state, the main source of injustice, should be replaced by decentralised, non-hierarchical, communal institutions and assemblies. Nozick argues that a minimal state is possible without infringing anyone's rights. The minimal state would develop out of a state of nature. In such a state most would behave according to moral principles, but nevertheless disputes and abuses would occur. In these circumstances 'people would begin to set up private protection associations. Eventually one of these would become the dominant protection agency, which would acquire a monopoly of force within a geographical area and be responsible for protecting everyone's rights within its territory'. At this stage a minimal state will have emerged without anyone having taken a specific decision to form it. Nozick borrows Adam Smith's notion of 'the invisible hand' to explain these developments.

In the second part of the book Nozick argues that a minimal state is all that is justified. Any state which attempts to be more than minimal necessarily violates individual rights. To argue this point Nozick develops a novel theory of justice based on entitlement. People are entitled to what they have so long as its acquisition did not involve the infringement of anyone else's rights. Any attempt by the state to interfere with entitlement would be illegitimate. Redistributive welfare state policies are to be deprecated because they damage entitlement rights. There is no moral justification for taking from A (who is wealthy) to give to B (who is poor). Furthermore, people are under no obligation to help those less fortunate than themselves. Nozick sums up his views as follows:

> Our main conclusions about the state are that a minimal state, limited to the narrow functions of protection against force, theft, fraud, enforcement of contracts, and so on, is justified; that any more extensive state will violate persons' rights not to do certain things and is unjustified. . . . Two noteworthy implications are that the state may not use its coercive apparatus for the purpose of getting some citizens

to aid others, or in order to prohibit activities to people for t
good.

(1984, p. ix)

This is an alarming philosophy with considerable appeal to the New Right. It is a philosophical indictment of the welfare state, providing the ammunition for those who wish to roll back the state.

Marxist views

Marxism has been particularly rich in theories of the state. There are innumerable variations, but the common core is that state power in capitalist society is based on class; that political power and class power are closely linked, and that the state principally serves the interests of the dominant class and facilitates capital accumulation. It is important to recognise the class-based nature of the state, because in the classless, communist society the state as an instrument of class domination would become redundant and would wither away. In *The Communist Manifesto* Marx and Engels (1977, p. 44) stated that the executive of the modern State is but a committee for managing the common affairs of the whole bourgeoisie'. *The Manifesto* is a polemical work, and such a stark, uncompromising view of the role of the state is not to be found in Marx's other works. A more typical view (shared by Marx himself and most present-day Marxists) is that the state has a dual role of serving the long-term interests of capital, but also, to a degree, serving the interests of the community as a whole. This apparent paradox is one of the contradictions of the capitalist state.

It is important to consider the means by which the capitalist class retains its dominance. The basic reason is its control over the means of production and the economic power that this bestows. Miliband (1969) makes the connection between economic and political power:

> The most important political fact about advanced capitalist societies . . . is the continued existence in them of private and ever more concentrated economic power. As a result of that power the men . . . in whose hands it lies enjoy a massive preponderance in society, in the political system and in the determination of the state's policies and actions.
>
> (p. 265)

Miliband contends that the power of the capitalist class is secured by its members' occupation of key positions. Those who occupy the top positions in industry, the media, the universities and the state, are drawn from the same dominant class. Furthermore, the state is dependent upon the capitalist class for its resources.

Poulantzas (1973) questioned Miliband's approach of establishing who occupies elite positions, claiming that this was irrelevant. Poulantzas argued that it was the structure of capitalist society and the balance of power among classes within it which determined the class bias of the state. One of the features of the capitalist state was that the different classes were not unified but split into fractions, strata and sub-categories. The economically dominant class was made up of fractions with different and sometimes opposing interests. The state needed to be 'relatively autonomous' from the specific interests of particular fractions if it were to be in a position to protect the long-term interests of the capitalist class. In the short term, the state may introduce changes in the face of opposition from sections of the capitalist class. The idea of the relative autonomy of the state runs through Marxist literature, but Dunleavy and O'Leary (1987, p. 258) identify two different interpretations: autonomy from the capitalist class or autonomy from the capitalist mode of production.

Offe (1984) departs from both Miliband and Poulantzas in postulating a quite different relationship between the state and the capitalist class. The state is not allied with specific classes: 'While it does not defend the specific interests of a single class, the state nevertheless seeks to implement and guarantee the collective interests of all members of a class society *dominated by capital'* (p. 120). The state itself is excluded from accumulation, but it depends upon the accumulation process for the revenues it needs to further its political ends. It is therefore in the state's *own interest* to create the conditions most conducive to capital accumulation. It must conceal its dependence on capital accumulation, and seek to legitimate its activities through the democratic process of elections and the provision of welfare services.

The structuralist Marxist, Althusser (1972), says that economic power is translated into political power by a combination of repression, coercion and the control of ideology, and emphasises the relationship between what he calls the repressive and ideological apparatuses of the state. The repressive apparatus consists of the police and the armed forces; the ideological apparatus includes the mass media, educational institutions, religious organisations, trade unions and the family. For Althusser, the appearances of democracy were a sham designed to deceive the masses into believing that they were participating in the political system. Gramsci (1971) writing in prison between 1929 and 1935 emphasised the ideological hegemony of the bourgeoisie, which made concessions to the working class without disturbing the power structure.

Many more theorists than are mentioned in this summary have contributed to Marxist theories of the state. Furthermore, those writers who have been identified have been treated too briefly to do them justice. Readers interested in pursuing their ideas in greater depth are advised to go to the original texts.

Feminist views

It is difficult to write about the feminist view of the state, since there are several different kinds of feminism, each with slightly different concerns and with different agendas.[1] One thing upon which all groups would be in agreement, however, is that the other theories of the state that we have so far considered are flawed because they fail to recognise the extent to which the state is gendered. Pluralists ignore the fact that the influential positions in interest groups are occupied by men; elitist theories take little account of the pre-dominance of men in elites; although contemporary Marxists are prepared to recognise the importance of gender relations in social analysis, Marxism has traditionally emphasised class divisions, some-times to the exclusion of other sources of social cleavage. Feminists maintain that despite the rhetoric of democracy and equality of opportunity, state power is largely in the hands of men. Radical feminists talk of the patriarchal state which simultaneously rests upon and bolsters systems of patriarchy in the wider society and in the economy. The state plays a crucial role in reproducing patri-archal power. This analysis of the distribution of power goes well beyond the demands of liberal feminists for equal opportunities and equal social, legal and political rights, and it widens the discussion among socialist feminists about the relationships between class and gender inequalities. However, Lewis (1992) argues that states are not all equally patriarchal. She identifies three models illustrated by Britain and Ireland as highly male-dominated, Sweden where male domination is much less apparent, with France falling somewhere between the two. Lewis quotes Hernes (1987) and Kolberg (1991) as examples of those among Scandinavian feminists who insist on the possibility of a woman-friendly state: Kolberg 'has dismissed any idea that the Scandinavian welfare state might be patriarchal, insisting that it has increased women's independence, empowerment and emancipation' (p. 170).

Some socialist feminists (e.g. Ehrenreich and English, 1979; Barrett, 1981) reject the notion of patriarchy as being unhelpful as a means of describing gender inequalities in capitalism. The term, they contend, should be restricted to pre-capitalist societies. The more usual position, however, is a combination of both approaches, with socialist feminists, including Marxists, arguing that although patriarchy provides useful explanations and insights, it has to be seen in association with class relations in capitalist society. Dale and Foster (1986) explain this dual approach: '. . . capitalism and patriarchy *together* shape women's position. Patriarchy is not seen as more important than capitalism, and men are not the main enemy' (p. 56).

In the 1970s socialist feminists concentrated their attention on the degree to which particular family and gender relations benefited the capitalist system and those who controlled it. Unpaid domestic labour assisted employers, by bearing some of the costs of producing an effective labour force – women were encouraged to remain in the home to provide the male labour force with food, clothing and a haven for relaxation and rest: they would also provide care during periods of sickness. Another function which aided capitalism was the *reproduction* of the labour force: the bearing and raising of children. At first glance, it might appear that the greater participation of women in the labour market has weakened this argument somewhat, but the preponderance of *part-time* work among women, at least outside Scandinavia, has to be taken into consideration. Part-time work may be seen as allowing women to continue their roles as home-makers and carers. There is ample evidence demonstrating that the greater proportion of women in the labour force has had little impact upon the division of domestic and caring work in the home. The relationship between paid work and unpaid work is still a major concern of feminists as is the state's role in encouraging or discouraging greater equity in both areas by intervening in the labour market or less directly through various welfare measures, especially

social security. Some of the debates surrounding these issu
considered in Chapter 5.

The growth of state intervention

State involvement in welfare goes back several centuries, but the
welfare state as we understand it today can be traced back to the late
nineteenth century. Kuhnle (1981, p. 126) states that 'Most writers
trace the initiation of the welfare state, or at least the beginning of
the present stage of development, to Bismarck's large-scale social
insurance schemes of the last quarter of the nineteenth century'.
Different countries developed services at different rates, at different
times and with different priorities.

Nevertheless, by 1900 Germany already had sickness insurance,
industrial accident insurance and old age pensions. By 1911 every
country in Western Europe had some form of workers' compensation scheme. In 1913 Sweden was the first country to introduce a
pensions insurance scheme covering the entire population, but by
that time Australia, Austria, Belgium, Denmark, France, Germany,
Italy, The Netherlands, Norway, Switzerland and Britain all had
some form of sickness insurance which financed both cash benefits
and some health care services. Membership of the schemes was
compulsory for certain categories of workers in Austria, Germany,
The Netherlands, Norway and Britain; elsewhere membership was
voluntary but with some subsidisation from the state. Unemployment insurance, introduced in Britain in 1911, came later elsewhere;
for example, not until 1927 in Germany, not until 1935 in the United
States, and not until 1944 in Canada.

It would take far too long to chronicle the gradual and fitful
development of the welfare state from the nineteenth century to the
present time, and I will now turn to the post-war period when all
capitalist countries accepted the principle of the welfare state,
although to different extents and with varying degrees of enthusiasm.
The foundations for the welfare state laid during the sixty years
before the outbreak of the Second World War were now consolidated as the range of state provision expanded. The late 1940s saw
the beginning of a period of social reform which continued unabated
until the end of the 1960s. This period may be considered the heyday

of the welfare state. In the immediate postwar period every capitalist country co-ordinated and extended its social security system, and benefits were increased. In West European countries coverage became increasingly comprehensive and universal. In the United States social security expanded more gradually than it did in Europe, and it was not until the 1960s that provision became a little less selective, and in 1965 Medicaid (for poorer people) and Medicare (for older people) were introduced. Almost everywhere expenditure on health and education rose absolutely and as a proportion of GDP. Housing programmes were launched in most countries, and governments began to take a more active role, through subsidies, loans and allowances.

The war itself had a direct and indirect impact on the extension of the welfare state in the 1940s. The privations of war were not evenly distributed among the population. Nevertheless, in a total war all suffer some discomfort, and there was a greater sense of solidarity so that class barriers, even if only temporarily, were reduced. Those enduring privations believed that their present sacrifices must be compensated for by a higher standard of living, full employment and the provision of more and better social services when the war was over. At a more mundane level, war accustomed people to greater central government intervention and higher rates of taxation, both of which were required for post-war developments in social provision.

There is another side to this picture. All countries had experienced severe unemployment in the world depression beginning in 1929. One of the lessons to be drawn from the economic problems of the 1930s was that mass, long-term unemployment and the chaos resulting from runaway inflation lead to the growth of political extremism. Fascism was seen as a direct consequence of economic dislocation; and full-employment policies, improved social security provisions and better housing, education and health services were seen as one possible way of avoiding the re-emergence of fascist regimes. If resurgence of fascism was seen as one danger, the spread of communism was seen as another, especially in the United States. American foreign policy was directed towards the achievement of stability in Europe. Democratic welfare states would help to ensure stability and provide an effective barrier against the spread of communism.

Governments may have been concerned with what they perceived as the dangers of fascism and communism, but ordinary people were concerned with re-establishing their lives with greater security and prosperity than they had enjoyed before the war. Many remembered the hardship and degradation of inter-war unemployment and the inadequate, sometimes harsh, responses of governments to it. They now wanted assurance that there would be no return to such conditions, and they voted for political parties whose promises of full employment and improved social security seemed to be the most genuine.

Social reform after the Second World War was made possible by the very high rates of economic growth experienced by all advanced industrial societies, although not all countries were equally success-ful. In a paper examining the post-war development of public expen-diture in Western Europe and North America, Kohl (1981) writes:

> The rapid economic growth of the recovery period after World War II enabled Western democracies to increase public spending in almost all fields because of greater fiscal resources. . . . Most authors, whether conservative or radical, agree that social expenditures have been the outstanding component in the secular rise of public expenditures, accounting for the large share of general growth during the past decades.
>
> (pp. 307–8)

At the same time as public expenditure was growing, Keynesian economics seemed to offer governments the opportunity to manage aggregate demand and thus control levels of unemployment and inflation. There were thus four major influences at work in the period after 1945:

1. The direct and indirect impact of the war and the desire for stability in Western Europe as a defence against both commun-ism and fascism.
2. Memories of inter-war unemployment and the unwillingness of electorates, at least in Western Europe, to return governments not committed to full-employment policies and social reform.
3. Unprecedented and sustained economic growth.
4. The acceptance of Keynesian economic theories.

At the time when Western Europe, Australia, Canada, New Zealand and the United States were establishing welfare states, the countries of Central and Eastern Europe turned to communism forming a block largely dominated (with the exception of Yugoslavia) by the Soviet Union. China also became communist. All these countries became one-party, totalitarian states with the Communist Party controlling the state apparatus. The pattern being established in the West did not commend itself to the new leaders in Central and Eastern Europe. Separate welfare institutions were unnecessary, since socialism would solve any problems that arose. The welfare of the people would be achieved by guaranteed work and heavily subsidised food, clothing, housing and transport. Following the downfall of the communist regimes in 1989/90, most governments embraced neo-liberal economics and set about constructing welfare systems. The charms of neo-liberalism may now be wearing a little thin, at least with the electorates, and in some countries former Communist leaders have re-established themselves in government. This is not, however, an attempt to return to the pre-1990 position, and economic and social restructuring are still on the agenda. The former East Germany (GDR) is something of an exception to this pattern: since German re-unification the welfare systems of West Germany (FDR) have been extended to the whole country.

The services established in the 1940s in the non-communist countries were further developed, with some brief setbacks, throughout the 1950s and 1960s, gradually consuming a larger share of government spending and of GDP. Summing up the development of the welfare state in 1983, Heidenheimer, Heclo and Adams (1983) state:

> The data are far from perfect, but the overall trends in Europe and the United States are clear and consistent for the last hundred years: a rising share of total economic resources has been absorbed by taxation and devoted to public spending. Of all public spending, a growing share (except in years of war) has gone to social programs . . . national variations within these trends are important, but the overall movements stand out as long-term themes for every developed nation.
>
> (p. 10)

When this statement was made, there was already much talk of the crisis of the welfare state and the rate of increase in public social expenditure as a percentage of GDP had already been checked. A fuller analysis of changes in public expenditure is to be found on pages 50–71, but in very broad terms, social expenditure as a proportion of GDP continued to rise substantially until about 1975.

The oil crisis of 1973 and the accompanying recession convinced governments that cuts in public expenditure were essential, and since social expenditure constituted such a high proportion of the total, it became the main victim of retrenchment. High social expenditure was seen as one of the main causes of the economic problems. Several factors contributed to the intensification of retrenchment throughout most of the 1980s: the election of conservative governments promising to 'roll back the state', especially Reagan in the United States and Thatcher in Britain, the rejection of Keynesian economic theories in favour of monetarism, and a further period of recession in the early 1980s. Recession in the first half of the 1990s, and the attempts in Europe to meet the conditions for entry into the European Monetary Union, meant renewed attempts to curb social expenditure. It should be emphasised, however, that the desired reductions in social expenditure were not realised. Policies of retrenchment achieved only a slowing down in the rate of growth of government spending on welfare.

Curtailing the role of the state

During the 1980s, there was a growing disenchantment with the state, and this has persisted into the 1990s. The most obvious changes have occurred in Central and Eastern Europe with the overthrow of totalitarian states, but the loss of faith in the state has been a worldwide phenomenon. Salamon and Anheier (1994, p. 113) write of 'widespread loss of confidence in the state'. Among the causes of the disenchantment were the numerous instances of corruption, but more important, in the long term, was a loss of faith in the capacity of government to solve economic and social problems and adequately meet people's needs. Nowhere was this more apparent than in the area of health and welfare services. The general agreement that the balance of advantage lay with state provision was increasingly challenged. Evers (1993, p. 3) claims that 'the concept of dominant state-centred welfare has corroded and lost its hegemony'. State services were criticised for being too centralised, too bureaucratic, too remote, too unresponsive to people's needs and too dominated by professionals and administrators. In many discussions of reducing state involvement in welfare, it is *direct provision* of welfare that receives most attention, although it is quite possible to reduce state provision while retaining or even increasing the state's financial and regulatory roles.

In the minds of governments, however, the most serious drawback of heavy state involvement in health and welfare was the huge expense that this entailed. Although governments' responses to what are perceived as the excessive costs of state welfare exhibit considerable variety in points of detail and in the severity of the action taken, there is a broad similarity in the aims being pursued: the restraint of public expenditure which may involve reducing levels of service and encouraging alternative forms of provision; administrative restructuring combined with new forms of public sector management and decentralisation. These issues will form the basis of the remainder of this chapter.

Curbing public expenditure

At the most general level all governments have taken action to reduce or control deficits by setting global norms. This may take three forms:

1. Stating an upper limit for the deficit as a proportion of GDP.
2. Setting an upper limit for public expenditure as a proportion of GDP.
3. Setting an upper limit for public sector borrowing.

Within these global norms particular areas of government activity are the subject of expenditure restraint, sometimes in the form of across-the-board cuts, but much more usually on a selective basis.

A study by the OECD (1985) examined the annual growth rates of social expenditure as a percentage of GDP in twenty countries. The report compared the annual growth rates of social expenditure in the period 1960 to 1975 with the rates between 1975 and 1981. What is clearly demonstrated is that social expenditure continued to grow but at a much slower rate after 1975. By far the biggest change occurred in The Netherlands with a decrease of 8.8 percentage points, followed by Australia with a reduction of 7.2 percentage points and Canada with a fall of 6.2 per cent. The lowest cuts in the growth rates, just over 1 per cent, occurred in France and Belgium.

Reductions of over 4 per cent were recorded in the UK and the USA. It should perhaps be noted that Reagan did not come into power until 1981 and the full effects of Thatcherism were still to be felt in Britain. The average reduction in the rate of growth in social expenditure for all OECD countries was 3.8 per cent.

A more recent OECD study (1994) makes the following statement:

> All countries are now confronted by increasing demands on their social policy expenditures while, at the same time, they face growing resource constraints and, often, budget deficits. And the current recession has underscored the serious financial pressures affecting systems of social protection. . . . The result, a dilemma which is of major concern in many countries, has led to a rethinking of the objectives and of the financing of all public policies, and social policies in particular.
>
> (p. 7)

This study extends the social expenditure figures to 1990. It demonstrates a continuing increase in expenditure, but again with lower rates of growth than were achieved in the 1970s. Extreme caution is necessary in interpreting these figures for two reasons: (i) the definitions of different categories of expenditure and of GDP vary as do the methods of collection; (ii) the OECD definition of social expenditure is very narrow, including health and all forms of income maintenance programmes, but excluding education and personal social services. The analysis is divided into two groups: European Community (EC)[2] countries and countries outside the EC. In the latter group the average total growth of social expenditure as a percentage of GDP between 1980 and 1990 was 2.95 per cent, but this overall figure conceals considerable variation with Norway showing a 7.3 per cent increase and Sweden, at the other extreme, showing a marginal increase of 0.87 per cent. The OECD figures for EC countries are provisional estimates only; they indicate an average increase of 0.09 per cent. For firmer figures, a publication of the European Commission (1995) gives an average increase of 1.1 per cent. All of this increase is accounted for by the first five years of the decade, since there was a decline of 0.7 per cent between 1985 and 1990. During the whole of the decade social expenditure as a proportion of GDP fell in Belgium, Germany, Ireland and Luxembourg. Even after three years of recession, when spending on unemployment compensation necessarily rose, social expenditure as a proportion of GDP was still lower in Belgium, Germany and Luxembourg in 1993 than it had been in 1980. The EC countries did less well than the other OECD countries during the 1980s, because the recession had more serious consequences there and governments took more stringent action. It has to be remembered, however, that Western Europe includes most of the high-spending welfare states, with social expenditure in Denmark, Finland, France, Germany, The Netherlands, Norway and Sweden all exceeding 30 per cent of GDP in 1993.

The early 1990s witnessed a rise in social expenditure and renewed efforts to curb it. The European Commission (1995) gives some of the reasons:

> Slow economic growth, the persistence of high unemployment, an ageing population, the problems of controlling growth of health expenditure, all impose strong pressure on systems of social protection and their financing. . . . The financial restraints have been particularly evident in recent years because of the recession of the early 1990s and the prevailing concern of policy to reduce budget deficits and limit public expenditure growth in order to contain inflationary pressure, to avoid imposing excessive costs on businesses.
>
> (pp. 3 and 7)

Government after government declared a series of austerity measures from the mid-1970s onwards. The calls for financial prudence and cuts in social expenditure were particularly evident in the early and mid-1980s, and equally draconian measures were introduced in the period from about 1993 onwards. These affected most West European countries, Australia, New Zealand, Japan, and the United States, though some European governments have been forced to modify their plans by union opposition, strikes and demonstrations. Conflict in France in 1995 and 1996 was particularly bitter and drawn-out. Nevertheless, although concessions were made, the social security budget was cut. These cuts were in addition to the cuts in the 1980s.

It would be impossible to describe in detail the many attempts in all countries to reduce or contain social expenditure. The discussion will be limited, therefore, to the more significant changes. Since the impact of cuts is cumulative, those imposed in the 1980s will be considered first, followed by more recent measures. Because of major concerns about the growing costs of retirement pensions and alarmist talk of 'the impending demographic time-bomb' (European Commission, 1995, p. 13), retirement pensions will be treated separately. The final section will be an assessment of the attempts to curb expenditure, considering the degree to which they have been achieved and their impact.

The 1980s

The UK under Thatcher and the USA under Reagan led the way in the early 1980s in anti-state rhetoric, attempts to roll back the state and a determination to curb social expenditure. Both leaders were adherents of the New Right sharing its antipathy towards the welfare state. In relation to Britain, Walker (1993, p. 68) says:

> The overriding factor in the active promotion of a shift in the welfare mix in the UK was the ideological change represented by the election of the first Thatcher government in 1979 . . . the gradual evolution of pluralism in the personal social services was overtaken by the Conservative Government's radical political agenda and, in particular, the policy of residualizing public sector provision.
>
> (p. 69)

One-nation conservatism was abandoned in favour of a market-based system which resulted in a more deeply divided society and greater inequality. During the 1980s just about every social service underwent restructuring of a very fundamental kind. The cuts in expenditure were not evenly spread, and among the services hardest hit was housing: public expenditure on housing declined by 28 per cent in real terms between 1981 and 1991. The restructuring began in 1980 when the government introduced two Social Security Acts. Among the changes introduced by this legislation, the more important were:

1. The benefits to strikers were reduced.
2. The earnings-related supplements to unemployment, sickness and widows' benefits were abolished (from January 1982).
3. Short-term benefits were increased by 5% less than the estimated rate of inflation.
4. The link between average earnings and pensions was broken, so in future pensions would be uprated only in relation to prices, resulting in lower increases.

5. The availability of exceptional needs payments and exceptional circumstances additions was reduced.

The major reform of the social security system occurred between 1986 and 1988. The Act of 1986 is a long document, but four of its major features merit special comment: exceptional needs payments were replaced by loans; housing benefit was made much more difficult to obtain; benefits under the state earnings-related pension scheme were reduced; there was a considerable increase in means tests.

Thatcher's commitment to New Right ideology was matched by Reagan. O'Connor (1998) says:

> Reagan's election victory was a watershed in American history because it signalled the end of the New Deal order. . . . From the presidency of Franklin Delano Roosevelt through the administration of Jimmy Carter, government intervention in the economy, downward redistribution of income, and government spending for social provision were considered national priorities. . . . As, arguably, the most ideological president in modern American history, Reagan expedited the eclipse of the New Deal through a concerted and relentless critique of big government.
>
> (p. 38)

O'Connor (1998) examines three major pieces of welfare retrenchment legislation: the Omnibus Budget Reconciliation Act of 1981 (OBRA); the Social Security Amendments of 1983; the Family Support Act of 1988. OBRA affected just about every social programme. O'Connor cites evidence from Bawden and Palmer (1984) whose calculations are based on a comparison of expenditure under OBRA and the projected expenditure from the pre-Reagan period. Among the hardest-hit were the mainstays of programmes for the poor and unemployed: expenditure on Aid For Families With Dependent Children (AFDC) was cut by 14.3 per cent; the food stamps programme suffered a 13.8 per cent reduction; and unemployment insurance was pruned by 17.4 per cent. Social security was less severely treated with a cut of 4.6 per cent. Medicaid and Medicare expenditures were also cut by 2.8 per cent and 6.8 per cent respectively. OBRA removed 500,000 families from the Medicaid rolls. Student loans, compensatory education and employment and training services were severely curtailed. The Social Security Amendments of 1983 were mainly concerned with taxation in relation to benefits, although detailed rule changes also reduced certain entitlements. The main effect of the Family Support Act was to strengthen the workfare[3] provisions of OBRA.

Action in the 1982, 1983 and 1984 budgets involved almost a 10 per cent cut in social programmes, as compared with prior policies. Medicare and Medicaid suffered cumulative expenditure reductions between 1982 and 1985 of 5 per cent and 4.5 per cent respectively (Bawden and Palmer, 1984). The reductions in housing expenditure were extremely severe: the 1984 budget proposed a 94 per cent cut in the level of new budget authority for housing. According to Hartman (1983, p. 1) 'the intention of the Reagan administration was virtually to end all programs that directly add, through construction and substantial rehabilitation, to the stock of housing available to lower-income households'. Bawden and Palmer (1984, p. 177) describe the views and policies of President Reagan as 'a coherent ideological attack on the principles that have governed social policy in this country for the last half century'.

The UK and the United States during the 1980s were dominated by governments who took their inspiration from the New Right. It should not be assumed, however, that governments of the left did not follow similar, if less extreme, policies of retrenchment. The case of France under the socialist presidency of Mitterand is an interesting example. Ashford (1985, p. 578) claims that 'within a few months the Mitterrand government had gone on a spending spree of unprecedented proportions'. The budget deficit in 1981 was in excess of 200 billion francs, the social security budget alone having a deficit of 16 billion francs. In 1982 Mitterrand was forced to reverse these policies and a stringent austerity programme was introduced, including higher taxes and 'paring 10 billion francs in benefits from unemployment plans (mainly by cutting out certain categories of eligibility altogether, putting restrictions on the rights of those looking for their first jobs and stretching out pre-benefit delay periods for those eligible)' (Ross, 1987, p. 205). The 1986 elections produced a conservative majority in the Assembly with M. Chirac as prime minister. Chirac imposed more stringent spending cuts and increased privatisation.

In New Zealand the Labour Government, in power from 1984 until 1990, presided over a programme of economic and social restructuring which was pure New Right, embracing the free-market model, restricting social provision and introducing a system of charges. The reforms, pushed through by Finance Minister Douglas, outdid anything attempted by Mrs Thatcher and Ronald Reagan. Douglas has since left the Labour Party to form a new right-wing party. The current Labour leadership has expressed regret at having moved so far to the right in its acceptance, when in power, of neo-liberal ideology and policies.

Australia's neo-conservative government led by Fraser gave way in 1983 to a Labour Government with a less extreme attitude to public expenditure. In the budget of 1986, however, the Australian Government announced an austerity programme involving fairly substantial cuts in public expenditure on health, education and social security. These cuts, however, were a response to economic difficulties rather than a sign that the government was moving towards neo-liberal economic and social policies.

Considered together, the five countries discussed represent most of the measures taken in response to the economic difficulties of the 1980s. It is now time to draw these together and relate them to similar changes in other countries.

The most direct method of reducing costs is simply to reduce the benefits payable. We have seen that this occurred in Australia, France, New Zealand, the UK and the United States. Similar action was also taken in The Netherlands, one of the high-spending welfare states. All social insurance benefits were cut in both amount and duration in 1984. Another European example is Germany. In what was then West Germany, the 1982 Budget reduced maternity allowances, children's allowances and unemployment benefits. Moving to the other side of the Atlantic, a Conservative Government took up office in Canada in 1984. Banting (1995) observes:

> During its first term in office, the government's social policy was relatively muted, but this tentativeness faded with its reelection in 1988. The Conservatives dropped plans for expansion of child care, reduced unemployment benefits, clawed back some pensions from upper-income recipients, restructured child benefits, froze transfers to the provinces for health care and postsecondary education, and restrained the rate of growth in its support for provincial social assistance programs.
>
> (p. 288)

Benefit cuts also occurred in some of the South American countries – they were particularly fierce in Chile under Pinochet's military government.

Equivalent to reducing benefits – at least in its effect on recipients – is freezing them or increasing them by less than the rate of inflation. For three successive years in Britain child benefits were frozen in the late 1980s. The Danish government froze the indexation of welfare benefits for the whole of 1982, and automatic indexation of other benefits was suspended between 1982 and 1985. In Belgium indexation was suspended in 1984, 1985 and 1987. Greece and Luxembourg followed the same course in 1983 and 1984 respectively. In the UK the indexation of long-term benefits by reference to wages or prices, depending on which of them gave rise to the largest increase, was abandoned in favour of indexation to prices alone. These examples come from a report on social protection from the European Commission (1993) which also says that 'in The Netherlands, the automatic indexation of benefits was suspended altogether for most of the 1980s' (p. 34). Changes in indexation procedures, involving a reduction in the real value of benefits, occurred in most West European countries at some time during the 1980s and also in Australia, New Zealand and the United States.

An effective method of reducing public expenditure is to raise eligibility criteria so that fewer people qualify for the service or benefit. During the 1980s most welfare states followed this course. It would not be profitable to detail all the changes since they are numerous and technical. Greater use of income or means tests or lowering the cut-off point, is, however, an obvious way to reduce the number of recipients. Many countries followed this course in the 1980s, but for two good examples we can return to the United States and Britain. The restructuring of social security in Britain involved a considerable expansion of means-testing. Bennett (1987) sums up this change of emphasis:

> Under the Social Security Act, means-tested benefits becomes the fulcrum of the social security system. There is a shift in the centre of gravity of the benefits system away from benefit as of right towards benefits requiring a test of income. (p. 125)

The United States went further than other countries in restricting eligibility during the 1980s. Palmer and Sawhill (1984) make the following comment:

> Lower-tier safety net programs were generally cut by imposing tighter income eligibility limits and offsetting benefits more fully for earnings and other sources of income. The result has been to exclude

many of the working poor and near-poor from government programs
. . . to greatly reduce benefits for others, and to target a higher
percentage of the reduced funds on the poor.

(p. 13)

As a consequence of these changes an estimated 400,000 to 500,000
lost AFDC eligibility, and for most of these families loss of AFDC
eligibility also entailed loss of Medicaid benefits. About one million
or more people no longer qualified for Food Stamps.

Another strategy is the transfer of costs to the recipients of services and benefits. This can be achieved by introducing or increasing
waiting days before benefit is paid, as was done in The Netherlands
and Denmark, for example. A similar effect is achieved by means of
charges and cost-sharing arrangements. Prescription charges in
Britain provide a notable example of this, having increased by 1,525
per cent between 1979 and 1990. Similar examples of the increased
use of charges can be found. In West Germany, for example, there
were increases in charges – notably in the health insurance system.
Charges for prescriptions and dentures were introduced under legislation of 1977. In 1981/82 both of these were increased and charges
were introduced for spectacles, medical appliances and hospital care.
In the United States cost-sharing has long been a feature of the
American Medicare and Medicaid systems, but the patients' share
increased during the 1980s.

The 1990s
The recession in the early 1990s led to increases in expenditure for
two main reasons: (i) increased unemployment and contractual obligations to pay unemployment benefits and (ii) declining or static
GDP. This in no way lessened governments' determination to curb
expenditure, and increases were relatively modest, although larger
than had been achieved in the 1980s. Between 1990 and 1993
expenditure on social protection in the European Union rose by 2.5
per cent of GDP. Expenditure on health care which had been
growing at 3.5 per cent a year between 1985 and 1990 expanded by
only 2 per cent a year between 1990 and 1993. The European
Commission (1995) says that 'In a number of countries, including
Italy and Portugal, where national health services were being developed over this period, the fall in the relative importance of public
spending was substantial'. The report adds that this trend 'was
particularly the case in the period 1990 to 1993, reflecting the

budgetary constraints which prevailed over this period' (p. 108). On a wider front, the OECD (1994) reports some success in restraining the growth of health expenditure through cost-shifting, contracts, competition and a performance-related approach to reimbursing physicians and hospitals.

Particular financial pressure on the countries of the European Union arises from the movement towards the European Monetary Union which lays down stringent criteria for admission to the system. Budget deficits have to be kept below 3 per cent of GDP and the public debt has to amount to no more than 60 per cent of GDP. All fifteen governments are busily making cuts to try to meet these criteria, and the savage pruning of welfare spending is an important part of this process (for once, tabloid language is probably appropriate). The pressure has been steadily increasing since the signing of the Maastricht Treaty in 1991, but has been particularly intense since 1993/94. In the United States, the pressure for curbing expenditure comes from three sources: the landslide victory of the Republicans in the Congressional elections in late 1994; Clinton's own election promise to 'end welfare as we know it'; the undertaking to balance the budget by 2002 (Republicans) or 2005 (Clinton) combined with tax-cutting policies. Australia and New Zealand suffered from the world recession between 1990 and 1993 and between 1990 and 1996 New Zealand had a cost-cutting government. In Central and Eastern Europe the problems have stemmed from a very rapid shift to market economies, high rates of unemployment, rising poverty and greater inequality.

The proposed remedies have been extensions or modifications of those adopted in the 1980s. There have been further reductions in benefits by various means. In Germany, for example, there were cuts in unemployment benefits on several occasions from 1994 onwards, and in 1996 sickness benefit was reduced from 100 percent of average earnings to 80 per cent, and there were cuts in social assistance payments. These changes were accomplished in the face of union opposition, although the demonstrations were smaller and less disruptive than in France over pension and other benefit changes in 1995 and 1996. Action in France included an extended national strike, protesting as much about increased taxes and contributions as about reduced benefits. Although the strikers were able to extract considerable concessions from the Gaullist government, the social security budget was cut.

There were also protests in Belgium over the cuts in the 1996 budget and some unrest in Italy for the same reason. In Austria, the coalition Cabinet's failure to agree an austerity budget for 1996 led to a general election in 1995. There was a cabinet reshuffle in early 1997, the new government re-affirming its determination to continue the cuts in welfare begun in 1994. Most other European nations sought to contain their social security budgets. Even Sweden, which had departed from the general trend in the 1980s, was forced to implement austerity measures from 1991 onwards. Sick pay was reduced by 20 per cent after 90 days, a five-day waiting period for unemployment benefits was introduced and income replacement rates were reduced (Stephens, 1996, p. 48). In 1995 child allowances were reduced for the first time since their introduction in 1948, and other welfare benefits were reduced from 80 per cent of average earnings to 75 per cent. Stephens (1996) in a study of changes in Denmark, Finland, Norway and Sweden made the following comment about the early 1990s:

> In all four countries, significant rollbacks were resisted until a severe and apparently long term employment crisis hit. This meant that demands on the welfare state rose while the intake of social security contributions fell, making prevailing entitlements unaffordable. Thus replacement rates were cut, waiting days introduced, qualifying conditions increased, and services cut. Moreover, the degree of cutting reflects the depth and duration of the employment crisis, with Finland and Denmark cutting the most and Norway very little.
>
> (p. 55)

Although strenuous efforts are being made to curb social expenditure, the resources available for welfare expenditure in Western Europe far outstrip those available in Central and Eastern Europe and the states of the former Soviet Union. Nevertheless, when unemployment benefits were introduced, in 1989 in Hungary and in 1990–91 in most other countries, they were 'fairly generous by international standards, with fairly long periods of entitlement to benefits and reasonably high income replacement rates for those who qualified for them' (Standing, 1996, p. 236). Economic problems, including rising rates of unemployment and inflation and rapid economic restructuring, combined with pressure from international financial institutions, especially the International Monetary Fund and the World Bank, led to rapid retrenchment. The result was reduced rates of benefit, much stricter eligibility criteria, and reduced periods of entitlement. Standing (1996, pp. 236–7) claims that 'by 1994, across the region only a minority of the unemployed were receiving unemployment benefits'. The percentages ranged from less than 10 per cent in Croatia and Ukraine and 13 per cent in Russia to 45 per cent in the Czech Republic and 48 per cent in Poland. The situation was exacerbated by the withdrawal of the welfare services associated with places of employment.

In the United States, Reagan's anti-welfare measures were consolidated but not greatly extended by Bush and as O'Connor (1998) comments:

> The move from Bush to Bill Clinton has not brought about a liberal counterrevolution in welfare policy. In fact, the exact opposite has occurred, with Democrats demonstrating that they too can get tough on welfare. With a campaign promise to 'end welfare as we know it', Clinton's election unleashed a plethora of reform bills that both mirror and extend Reagan's critique of welfare.
>
> (p. 57)

The most severe cuts affected AFDC which was to be replaced, along with other principal safety net programmes, by a single block grant to states which are given greater discretion to design their own welfare programmes. Under the new arrangements AFDC recipients are to be restricted to two years' benefits after which they will be required to work or join a work/training programme: there will also be a lifetime limit of five years' benefits in total. States are allowed to deny further benefits to women who have additional children while on AFDC, and mothers under the age of eighteen will be required to live with an adult. Extra savings will come from greater stringency in the food stamps programme. Although the cuts in the first half of the 1980s resulted in reductions in the rate of growth of health expenditure, rises in the cost of Medicaid and Medicare gathered pace in 1986, with the increases in the costs of Medicaid giving greatest cause for concern. This rapid increase in Medicaid costs came about largely through the indefatigable efforts of Representative Henry A. Waxman and his supporters who secured extensions in the categories and contingencies covered by Medicaid. It should be noted, too, that the fastest growing item of Medicaid expenditure was subsidising the Medicare programme. Clinton has promised reductions of $127 billion and $54 billion over ten years in Medicare and Medicaid expenditure respectively. Clinton had constant fiscal battles with Congress, and in 1995 and 1996 the Federal government was shut down for weeks at a time because the Republican Congress refused to sanction the President's budget.

The conservative National Party that formed the government in New Zealand after 1990, went even further than its Labour predecessor in implementing neo-liberal economic and social policies. The policies included widespread cuts to welfare benefits. In the election of December 1996, when New Zealand used a system of proportional representation for the first time, no party secured an overall majority, but the National Party remains in power thanks to a coalition with The New Zealand First Party which has a Maori leader and depends on the support of the Maori population. As a condition of joining in a coalition with the National Party, the New Zealand First Leader, Mr Peters, insisted on a promise of higher spending on education, health, law and order and pensions.

There were also elections in Australia in 1996. The Labour Party was defeated, after thirteen years in office, by the conservative Liberal–National Party Coalition. All that has been proposed in relation to benefits is an increase in waiting times, and there seems little appetite for far-reaching welfare reforms at present. It is interesting that in 1984 New Zealand's welfare state was more extensive and generous than that of Australia, but as of the mid-1990s, according to Castles (1996, p. 106), 'social protection through social security rests on firmer foundations in Australia than in New Zealand, and, indeed, arguably, on firmer foundations than in any other English-speaking nation'. This was written, however, before the ousting of the Labour Government.

The European Commission (1995, p. 44) says that 'measures have been introduced in a number of Member States, and proposals have been made in others, to target expenditure more closely on those most in need of assistance'. Means-testing is perhaps the most obvious form of targeting, and in a study of all twenty-four OECD countries Gough *et al.* (1997, p. 40) conclude that 'means-tested social assistance schemes have in recent years acquired an increasing importance in the vast majority of industrialized countries'. Central and Eastern Europe was excluded from this analysis, but the trend towards much greater reliance on means-tested social assistance is equally apparent in these countries. In the UK the most recent extension of means-testing has been the replacement of unemployment benefit with the Job Seeker's Allowance (JSA). The new arrangements are complex, but the major change is that flat-rate benefits without a means test are paid only for the first six months of unemployment instead of twelve months. After six months, the payment of benefit is subject to a means test. In Australia, too, 'selectivism has been intensified, with an assets test imposed on age pensions, and the one non-income-tested benefit, the child allowance, becoming tested against both income and assets' (Castles, 1996, p. 44). Throughout the European Union income thresholds governing access to benefits have grown in significance. Family allowances in Germany, Italy, The Netherlands and Spain had already moved in this direction by 1995 and others were planning similar changes. In Central and Eastern Europe means-testing and other forms of targeting increased rapidly after 1990.

Tightening eligibility criteria is a particular form of targeting, ensuring that only the poorest or most disabled, for example, receive benefits. This has happened in the UK in relation to housing and sickness benefits. In April 1995 short-term sickness and longer-term invalidity benefits were amalgamated into an incapacity benefit and the medical criteria were made more stringent. In The Netherlands eligibility criteria for sickness and invalidity benefits were tightened in 1993 when regular medical examinations were introduced.

The transfer of costs to individuals, families and private industry begun in the 1980s continued into the 1990s. Cost sharing mechanisms were consolidated or extended, especially in health care. The OECD (1994) talked of economies to be made through cost-shifting which included 'asking private insurance employers and patients, or their relatives, to bear a greater share of, in particular, ambulatory care, medicines and certain types of long-term care'. The means of achieving the shift varied from 'the introduction of cost-sharing mechanisms for individual patients . . . to dropping particular services or medicines from existing coverage, to encouraging individuals or companies to purchase private health insurance' (p. 23). Prescription and other charges were imposed or increased. There were, for example, substantial increases in charges in Belgium in 1994. In the UK, the inexorable rise of prescription charges continued. We have seen how these charges increased by 1,525 per cent between 1979 and 1990: further increases in the 1990s brought this figure to 2,600 per cent by 1996. In Germany employers have for many years been responsible for the payment of sickness benefits and

The Netherlands and the UK followed suit in the 1990s. In 1994 in The Netherlands, employers became responsible for the first six weeks of benefit, but there are plans to extend this to fifty-two weeks. Employers in the UK had been required to cover the first eight weeks of sickness benefit since 1982, but in 1994 the period of employer responsibility was extended to twenty-eight weeks.

Retirement pensions

Retirement pensions feature prominently in concerns about growing public expenditure and attempts to control pension costs exhibit most of the methods used to reduce expenditure. Given this, it might be helpful to consider the action taken worldwide to ease what is perceived as 'the burden of pensions'. The problem stems partly from demographic factors: the rapidly increasing elderly population and falling fertility rates. The European Commission (1995) gives statistics relating to member states, but they apply with equal force in all advanced industrial countries. In the EU people over 65 constituted 15 per cent of the population in 1995 or 23 per cent of the population of working age. By 2005, people over 65 will constitute 26 per cent of those of working age. This percentage is projected to rise to 30 per cent in 2015 and to 35.5 per cent in 2025.

There is little that can be done in terms of social policy about demographic trends, but social policy initiatives in the 1980s have exacerbated the problem. The emphasis in that decade was on labour reduction strategies – taking as many elderly people as possible out of the labour market in the face of rising unemployment, especially among young people. Government and occupational schemes actively encouraged early retirement by offering pension enhancement. The statutory retirement age (the age of eligibility for public pensions) declined in many countries during the late 1970s and the 1980s. In Central and Eastern Europe the pensionable age had always been low by international standards, but it was expected that most people would go on working beyond the minimum pension age, largely because pensions were paid at very low levels. As far as Western Europe is concerned, the European Commission (1995) signals a switch in policy in the 1990s:

> In most member states, the emphasis of policy has switched during the first half of the 1990s from active encouragement of earlier retirement – including, in some cases, reducing pensionable age as

well as increasing income support for those no longer working – to containing the growth of expenditure on pensions.

(p. 30)

The most common approach to reducing the pensions bill has been to raise the age of retirement, thus reducing eligibility. In Germany, the pensionable age for men and women will be progressively raised to 65 from the present age of 63 for men and 60 for women. The equalisation of the retirement ages for men and women is a feature of many of the changes. Such changes are taking place in Greece, Portugal and the UK where common retirement ages of 65 are being implemented. In Italy, the present retirement age of 62 for men and 57 for women will be replaced by a flexible scheme allowing both men and women to retire at any time between the ages of 57 and 65. The 1997 pension reforms in Sweden also introduced flexible retirement ages with a minimum of 61, but with no limit on the number of extra years for which an insured person can contribute, all of which will qualify for additional pension. In France, the age of retirement remained at 60, but a longer contribution record was needed for full pension entitlement. Standing (1996, p. 240) says of Central and Eastern Europe that 'many governments have moved in the direction of raising pension ages incrementally, and a few have moved to reduce the gender differential, which was traditionally five years'. However, gender differentials remain in Poland and Hungary (both five years) and the Czech Republic (two years). In the United States the 1983 Social Security Amendments had the effect of increasing the age of retirement: by 2002 individuals would have to be 67 years old to receive full retirement benefits.

Some of the reduced expenditure resulting from raising the pensionable age will be realised only in the long term, since most of the changes are being implemented incrementally. Other means have been found to reduce the amounts payable. The European Commission (1995, p. 38) identifies 'a widespread tendency to reduce the scale of benefits paid, taking the form, in particular, of changing the basis on which pensions are based and/or uprated'. Sweden and Italy have switched from an incomes-based calculation to one based on contributions. France, Germany, Portugal and the UK have retained an income base, but changed it in such a way as to reduce payments. The UK changed the calculation of average income from the best twenty years to lifetime earnings in the State Earnings-Related Pension. At the same time the benefit was reduced from 25 per cent of average earnings to 20 per cent. Pensions in France will in future be based on average earnings in the best twenty-five years rather than ten and Portugal has moved from a calculation based on the best five of the last ten years to one based on the best ten of the last fifteen years. The Pensions Reform Act in Germany in 1992 linked pension adjustments with net rather than gross earnings. In Denmark and The Netherlands more account is now taken of the pensioner's or their partner's additional income in determining the amount payable. Finland has reduced the maximum amounts payable to public sector workers from 65 per cent of previous earnings to 60 per cent.

Finally there have also been moves to increase the importance of private pension arrangements. This trend has been most clearly exemplified in the UK which is 'the only EU state in which private schemes, including both company pensions and individual arrangements, can substitute for part of the statutory scheme rather than simply supplementing it' (European Commission, 1966, p. 16). The policy of encouraging private pensions takes two forms: making the State Earnings-Related Pension Scheme less attractive and subsidising personal pensions. A fresh subsidy came into effect in 1997. The countries of Central and Eastern Europe are under pressure from international financial institutions to privatise part of their pension schemes. Both Italy and Spain have introduced fiscal measures designed to encourage private pension schemes. As statutory pensions are eroded in the ways described above, private pensions become comparatively more attractive.

Assessment

This assessment will fall into two parts: (i) the success of the policies of retrenchment in reducing public expenditure and (ii) the effects of the retrenchment on living standards. The catalogue of cuts outlined in the previous section might lead to assumptions about massive reductions in public expenditure, but the overall impact on total government spending has been less than the rhetoric would lead one to suppose. The most that has been achieved is a slowing down in the rate of increase of expenditure. In the UK, for example, public expenditure in real terms rose by 32 per cent between 1981 and 1995. In 1995, social expenditure accounted for 62.8 per cent of total public expenditure which compares with 56 per cent in 1981, but there had been a fall from 64.6 per cent in 1994. Mrs Thatcher came to power in 1979 to roll back the state and reduce public expenditure. In the early years of her first administration she failed to do so, and indeed, until 1983, the reverse happened. In 1982 government expenditure as a proportion of GDP (known as General Government Expenditure or GGE) rose to 47 per cent, its highest level since 1975. This was followed by a continuous fall until 1988 when it reached its lowest level for twenty-two years. From 1988 to 1993 GGE rose. After a small fall in 1994, there was a further rise in 1995 when the GGE ratio of 43.4 per cent was not markedly different from its level in 1979. President Reagan had a similar experience. O'Connor (1998, p. 50) says that 'though Reagan was unable to reduce federal welfare spending outright in real terms, the administration was successful in slowing the growth rate of real non-defence federal spending'. What, then, prevented the achievement of lower levels of government expenditure in the UK and the USA? O'Connor (1998, p. 51) explains the failure in the United States as being 'due to a number of factors, such as the severe recession of the early eighties, increased medical costs, the growing elderly population, and the general intractability of entitlements'. Similar factors were at work in Europe, Australia and New Zealand. A good treatment of retrenchment in the United Kingdom under Thatcher and in the United States under Reagan is to be found in a closely-argued study by Pierson (1994). He argues that, although both governments were serious about retrenchment, they failed to meet their targets. While Pierson accepts the reasons put forward by O'Connor, he says that there are three more compelling *political* explanations which operated in both the UK and the USA and may be applicable to other welfare states. The first of these relates to the great popularity of the welfare state and the political risks associated with damaging any important parts of it. A second reason is the opposition to retrenchment of very powerful interest groups, including those who work in the various services as administrators or professionals: in many cases these groups are highly organised. The third reason is the failure of those seeking retrenchment of the welfare state to demonstrate that there are coherent alternatives that would do a better job.

One of the problems for governments wishing to make cuts was that plans sometimes had to be trimmed in the face of opposition from either representative assemblies or civil servants, or because of public disquiet such as that expressed so forcibly in France in 1996.

President Reagan was faced with a Democratic Congress which thwarted his most extreme plans, to the extent that the administration achieved only about half of the cuts in domestic expenditure that were being sought. President Clinton is faced with a Republican majority in Congress. His record is mixed: he vetoed two welfare reform bills on the grounds that their treatment of children was too harsh, but his own welfare policies are scarcely less severe. Mrs Thatcher, ever the pragmatist, was well aware of the unfavourable electoral consequences of cutting expenditure on health and education. In most of the countries of Western Europe there is a similar level of support for these services and 'attachment to the existing system of social support remains deeply entrenched in popular opinion' (European Commission, 1995, p. 7). There are, however, some services which command less public support. Mrs Thatcher, for example, felt able to reduce expenditure on social housing with impunity. What happened during her term of office was a shifting of priorities. One of the reasons for her inability to cut expenditure drastically was that savings in one area were matched by expenditure increases in others – particularly social security, law and order and defence. The increases in law and order and defence were policy choices; the increases in social security were not something she would have chosen. They were brought about by increased unemployment.

In most countries, one of the main reasons for the persistence of high levels of public expenditure, was a combination of recession and entitlements. Recession means increased unemployment and unemployed people are entitled to unemployment benefits, so that expenditure on social security grows as unemployment grows. The increased number of claimants may easily swamp the effects of reduced payments to individuals. This is essentially what happened in the recession of the early 1980s, and again in the recession of 1990 to 1995. This is illustrated by figures produced by the European Commission (1995) which show the annual percentage change in real expenditure on a range of social benefits in three periods: 1980–85; 1985–90; 1990–93. In the earlier period, expenditure on unemployment increased by an average of 9 per cent a year in the twelve nations of the European Community. In the middle period, there was an annual reduction of expenditure on unemployment compensation of 2.1 per cent. In the final period the average annual increase in the same countries was 13.9 per cent. The data in this publication covers only the period up to 1993, but the recession did not end in that year. A similar increase occurred in 1994. In 1995 and 1996 as the recession eased, unemployment fell very slightly in most countries. By the middle of 1997, however, unemployment had increased in Germany, France and Sweden and was proving stubbornly high in many other countries. The highest rate in the EU was in Finland (15%) followed by Belgium (13.7%), France (12.6%), Spain (12.5%), Italy (12.2%) and Germany (11.5%). Even in Sweden, a country traditionally with low levels of unemployment, the rate in mid-1997 was 9.1 per cent. In contrast to these countries with intractably high rates of unemployment, is Luxembourg with 3.7 per cent, Japan with 3.5 per cent and Norway with 3.4 per cent. The UK and the USA are also at the lower end of the range: 5.5 per cent and 4.8 per cent respectively.

Germany illustrates the problems of attempting to contain public expenditure in times of rising unemployment. In 1980 unemployment in Germany averaged 3.2 per cent. In 1990, the rate (excluding the new Länder) was 6.2 per cent. In 1993 the rate in the former West Germany was 7.3 per cent and 8.9 per cent including the new Länder. There was a slight fall in 1994, but in 1996 the rate began to rise substantially. By February 1997 the unemployment rate had reached its highest level for more than sixty years: 11.3 per cent. Between 1985 and 1990 expenditure on unemployment compensation declined by 1.4 per cent a year. Between 1990 and 1993 the average annual increase in the same expenditure was 15.9 per cent.

All unemployment figures have to be treated with some caution, but extra care has to be taken with some of the figures from Central and Eastern Europe, since data collection techniques are sometimes rudimentary. Standing (1996, p. 237) claims that unemployment rates in Central and Eastern Europe have been 'chronically under-recorded'. Slovenia has the highest unemployment rate in this region with 14 per cent in October 1996. This is followed by Poland (13.6% in December 1996), Slovakia (12% in October 1996), Bulgaria (11.1% in October 1996) and Hungary (10.1% in December 1996). The official unemployment rate in the Ukraine is stated as 1.4 per cent, but given that industrial output fell by 15.4 per cent in October 1996, this figure is difficult to credit. A little more credence might be accorded to the rate of 3.5 per cent in the Czech Republic.

It should not be assumed that the failure to reduce overall government expenditure has meant that the attempts to curb spending have had no impact on people's lives. If benefits are reduced, eligibility conditions tightened and costs passed on to users, the effects are considerable. We have already noted that more than 400,000 were denied AFDC by legislative action in the United States in the 1980s. The more recent Welfare Bill signed by Clinton, according to Alexander Cockburn (1996), 'will cast an additional 2.6 million people, including 1.1 million children, below the poverty line'. He adds that 'the cost in terms of malnutrition, homelessness and despair is incalculable'. Between 1979 and 1993 the proportion of the American population living below the poverty level increased from 11.7 per cent to 15.1 per cent – an additional 13.1 million. In the same period, the proportion of children below the age of six living below the poverty level increased from 18.1 per cent to 25.6 per cent.

An indication of the impact of welfare cuts is to be seen in New Zealand where food banks have grown in number during the 1990s. There are now 400 annually handling £9 million of food. Field (1996) quotes a food bank co-ordinator as saying: 'Families, people with children working in low-paid jobs, have to go cap in hand and ask for food. You cannot imagine how much dignity they shed, just to ask for food'. The welfare state in New Zealand has suffered from a continuous process of attrition since 1984. Although there have been promises of increased spending on education, health and pensions, the coalition government formed after the 1996 elections will find it difficult to reverse the trend

A report by the European Federation of National Organisations Working With the Homeless, published in 1993, said that over 2.5 million people had been identified from official records as being homeless in the European Community. However, the true number is probably double that. Germany has the highest number with 12.8 homeless people for every 1,000 population. High concentrations also occurred in the UK (12.2 per thousand) and France (11.1 per thousand). These high figures, however, may paradoxically reflect higher provision of services in these three countries, and low figures in other EC countries may merely indicate a lack of response. Carvel (1993) quotes the view of the President of the Federation that 'the figures demonstrate the sorry consequences of the decision by most, but not all, of European governments to reduce their investment in social housing and housing for low-income and single people in the 1980s'.

In the UK the poor have been hard hit by a series of cuts in eligibility for sickness, unemployment and housing benefits. There is growing evidence of low levels of living among those dependent on state benefits. Particularly worrying is the evidence of inadequate diets, and even malnutrition, among poor people (Dowler and Calvert, 1995; National Consumer Council, 1995; Kempson, 1996). In some areas, centres have been set up to distribute cheap or free food among poor people. Housing benefits have been seriously eroded over several years. The Social Security Advisory Committee (1988, pp. 26–7), commenting on the reduced entitlement imposed under the Social Security Act of 1986, claimed that the majority of households on housing benefit would receive less help with their rent and rates and that over one million claimants would 'lose entitlement altogether'. In the event, the government was forced to make concessions, introducing a transitional scheme to compensate recipients for any losses in excess of £2.50 a week. Changes to housing benefits in 1995 and 1996 reduced the entitlements of about 400,000 recipients.

Central and Eastern Europe has witnessed the withdrawal of guaranteed work, growing unemployment and greatly increased poverty for large sections of the population. These changes have been accompanied by reductions in unemployment and other benefits, making them harder to obtain and paying them for shorter periods. At the same time, social insurance is increasingly relying on higher employee contributions and reduced employer contributions. According to Standing (1996, p. 236) 'the results have been predictable and dismal'.

New public management and the contract state

The restructuring of the public sector has been a feature of the 1980s and the 1990s. Changes may be grouped together under the title of the new public management. The terms used to describe the resultant forms of the state vary: the 'enabling state' (Gilbert and Gilbert, 1989; Deakin and Walsh, 1996); the 'contract state' (Hambleton, 1994; Kirkpatrick and Lucio, 1996); the 'entrepreneurial state' (Osborne and Gaebler, 1992); the 'managerial state' (Clarke and Newman, 1997). The changes described below have far-reaching implications for the provision and delivery of health and welfare services.

The most significant shift is the introduction of markets or quasi-markets into the public sector in an attempt to 'transform the state, locally and centrally, into an "enabling organization", responsible for ensuring that public services are delivered, rather than producing them itself' (Deakin and Walsh, 1996, p. 33). The state becomes principally a purchaser/commissioner of services which are provided under contract by commercial or voluntary agencies. The move towards contracts and managed markets has a long history in the United States and began in Britain during the 1980s. Contracts are a growing feature of welfare provision in many countries. Australia and New Zealand have both moved in this direction as has Italy and, more tentatively, France. Even Germany and The Netherlands, with their traditionally strong and independent voluntary sectors, are beginning to move, albeit slowly and hesitantly, towards contracting. In Germany, for example, Bauer (1996, p. 8) describes the emergence of 'new social politics' in the following way: 'While third sector organisations traditionally became favoured as mostly privileged partners of the public sector, the latter now is shifting to new social politics. Their goal is the implementation of market principles by contracts and the demands for efficiency combined with quality assurance'. In relation to The Netherlands, Melief (1993, p. 85) argues that although contracting is relatively undeveloped in the Dutch welfare state, there are indications that 'the service organizations that offer personal services financed by the insurance system may find themselves developing into service contractors'. The aim of this transformation was said to be greater efficiency brought about by increased competition. The OECD (1994) indicates the considerable extension of contracting across many countries in health care:

> A . . . trend emerging from the structural reforms, observable in both tax-based and insurance-based health care systems, is the introduction or growing reliance upon contracts as a key mechanism by which to allocate funds among service providers. . . . Contracts have emerged as a central mechanism by which to encourage and inform providers and achieve an increase in their productivity . . . and increase the responsiveness of providers to the concerns of the purchasing body.
>
> (p. 23)

Among the desirable outcomes of contracting in both health and social care would be, it is claimed, more choice for consumers. There can be no guarantees that increased competition will lead to greater efficiency in welfare services. Assuming that it does lead to savings, will it simply mean reduced expenditure or will it mean doing more for the same level of expenditure?

On the other hand, Walsh *et al.* (1997) state:

> In spite of the presumed consistency in terms of global solutions to common problems, what is actually understood by contracting is highly variable: contracting means different things in different cultures.
>
> (p. 183)

In the United Kingdom, for example, contracts and specifications are very detailed, whereas in France they are very brief and loosely defined. This implies a different relationship between the purchasers (public agencies) and providers. Sweden demonstrates the different forms that contracts can take. Walsh *et al.* (1997) refer to Von Otter's work in which three forms of contracting are identified in Sweden: the mixed-market model; the public competition model; and the consumer choice or voucher model. There is an important distinction between the first two: in the mixed market model private sector providers may be selected, whereas in the public competition model the choice is restricted to public providers. In Italy, once a contract has been agreed, it remains in place with little or no change of providers. Different contractual forms imply different levels of competition, but in most instances the aim of contracting has been to increase the element of competition in the provision of public services.

Support for markets and competition in public services is to be found in the much-publicised book, *Reinventing Government* by Osborne and Gaebler (1992). The sub-title of the book, *How the Entrepreneurial Spirit is Transforming the Public Sector*, indicates its main thrust. The authors, borrowing a phrase from Savas (1987), argue that governments should be 'steering rather than rowing', which is a colourful way of describing the activities of the enabling state. Osborne and Gaebler claim that 'entrepreneurial governments have begun to shift to systems that separate policy decisions (steering) from service delivery (rowing)' (p. 35). The success stories related by Osborne and Gaebler are chosen to support their thesis; failures of entrepreneurial government are not mentioned.

What Osborne and Gaebler are urging is consistent with New Right ideology and public choice theory – not only that governments should do less, but also that the ethos and practices of the private sector should be incorporated into the public sector. What the public sector needs is a strong measure of managerialism. The language of the private sector is used: competition, markets, strategic management, performance indicators and targets. The *management* style typical of private enterprise is to replace the *administration* typical of the civil service. In the process citizens become first consumers or potential consumers, and then customers or potential customers. Ranson and Stewart (1994) criticise this development, stating that 'consumerism provides an incomplete and ultimately inadequate language for the public domain. Its emphasis is on the individual in receipt of a service, rather than on the citizen as an active participant in the polity' (p. 19). Nor can it be assumed that 'even the direct consumers of a public service ... will behave in the same way as in the market. The consumer will have different expectations and follow different patterns of behaviour because the public are citizens as well as customers' (p. 246). Quasi-markets produce quasi-citizens.

Another aspect of new public management is the hiving off into executive agencies of sections of the central administrative machinery. In Britain these are frequently described as next steps agencies. By the end of 1997 there will be about 150 agencies employing 75% of all civil servants (Horton and Jones, 1996). Although executive agencies work within the constraints of a framework document and performance targets, they are less constrained than traditional administrative departments, and they are clearly expected to become increasingly entrepreneurial. The next steps initiative leads to more fragmented government, and this trend is accentuated by a parallel one of decentralisation in many countries.

The changes described above are by no means restricted to Britain. Hood (1991, p. 3) claims that 'the rise of "new public management" ... over the last fifteen years is one of the most striking international trends in public administration'. The blurb to a book by Hughes (1994) states:

> Throughout the industrial world, the rigid, hierarchical, bureaucratic form of public administration, which has dominated for most of the twentieth century, is changing to flexible, market-based forms of public management. This new 'managerialism' represents not simply a minor change in management but a transformation of the role of government in society.

Hughes clearly thinks that the changes have mainly beneficial effects, and he would join with Osborne and Gaebler in applauding attempts to reduce the number of civil servants. Reducing the number of public servants can be seen in two lights: as a method of restricting the reach of government and as a method of curbing public expenditure. Because public services tend to be labour intensive, relatively small percentage cuts in staff can produce substantial savings. Japan, Belgium, Finland and New Zealand all used personnel ceilings and freezes during the 1980s. In the United States the numbers of federal, state and local employees were slightly reduced in 1981 and 1982, and although the reduction amounted to only 1.8 per cent, it nevertheless constituted a reversal of an almost continuously upward trend since 1960. The staff reductions coincided with an increase in contracting out and a consequent weakening of the public service trade unions. The Conservative government in Britain was especially active in attempting to reduce staffing levels. The prime minister appointed Sir Derek Rayner, managing director of a large and profitable chain of retail stores, to examine management efficiency in the public services. Rayner reported directly to the prime minister and was given wide discretion. In every area which Rayner examined, staff savings were recommended. In 1979 there were 742,000 civil servants. By January 1983 the number had fallen to 625,000. By April 1985 there had been a further reduction to 606,000; the total for 1988 was 590,000 and by December, 1996 there had been a further decline to 520,000. The United States has also made reductions in the number of civil servants during the 1990s and the governments elected in New Zealand and Australia in 1996 promised civil service cuts.

One way of reducing central government staffing levels is by decentralising, although any savings made may be compensated for by increases at the more local levels of government. Thus, while decentralisation does not of itself reduce public expenditure, it does reduce the responsibility of central government.

Decentralisation

Decentralisation does not necessarily reduce the scope and power of the state and promote participatory democracy; power is merely dispersed to a greater number of administrative units. The best that can be achieved may be the curtailment of the power of the *central* state. There is no guarantee that local or regional units will be any more committed to citizen empowerment than central authorities, and as Lorenz (1994a) argues, decentralisation may lead to the deeper entrenchment of clientelism as has happened in Italy: 'The Italian experience of decentralisation still tends to play into the hands of the old patronage system which is deeply ingrained as a pattern of dependence' (p. 32). Lorenz (1994a) also warns of the danger of laws purporting to facilitate decentralisation being subverted by vested interests. He cites Greece as an example of a country which passed decentralising legislation in 1982 and 1986, but where 'political power remains concentrated in the hands of central government and political parties' (p. 32).

Decentralisation to local units of government has been a major theme in Denmark, France, Germany, Italy, The Netherlands, Norway, Spain, Sweden, the United Kingdom and the United States. In Germany and The Netherlands the principle of subsidiarity underpins decentralisation. The process of decentralisation in Italy began in earnest with Law 833 in 1978 when responsibility for health and welfare services passed to over 8,000 communes which established local health units responsible for both health and social welfare services. France, historically one of the most highly centralised nations, also embarked in 1981/82 upon structural change with increased independence being granted to departmental and communal councils. The changes in the UK have been more mixed, with decentralisation in some policy areas and increased centralisation in others. There may be contrary trends even within the same area of provision. In education, for example, budgeting has been devolved to schools, but a centrally driven national curriculum has been imposed and national tests and league tables have been introduced. Mrs Thatcher and her ministers had an antipathy towards local government, and throughout the 1980s legislation and administrative action sought to control local government expenditure, reduce local government functions in education, housing and urban development and impose compulsory competitive tendering. At the same time the Greater London Council and the Metropolitan Councils were abolished. The Major governments of the 1990s were much less confrontational in their dealings with local government. The general trend in both Western and Central and Eastern Europe has been towards greater decentralisation, but there have been some moves in the opposite direction. For example, Denmark and The Netherlands, two highly decentralised countries, have made some tentative moves towards greater centralisation. However, Evans and Harding (1997, p. 28), drawing on Bennett (1990), distinguish between *decentralising* and *decentralised*. They assert that 'a decentralising France, for example, remains much more centralised, in absolute terms, than a centralising Denmark'. Japan provides an even better example than France of a country which, despite much talk and some action, remains highly centralised.

Decentralisation can occur at several levels and stages. The transfer of power from central to regional or, in a federal system, state authorities, may be accompanied by transfer from the regional to the local level, and from the local level to communities or neighbourhoods. There might also be a further stage in which autonomy is given to individual units or facilities – for example, schools, day and community centres. This implies decentralised management in which decisions, especially those affecting the allocation of resources, are taken at lower levels than is customary in bureaucratic organisations. In a discussion of decentralised or devolved management, Burns, Hambleton and Hoggett (1994) identify several forms of devolution, the most radical of which entails devolved units becoming almost independent

In federal countries there is, of course, always an additional tier of administration between national and local government. In Australia, Canada, Germany, India, Switzerland and the United States, for example, the powers of the sub-national units are written into the constitution, although the constitutional principles are often so general, that there is much room for interpretation. In the United States the role of the federal government had been expanding its scope ever since the New Deal, with particularly fast growth in the Great Society era of the 1960s and the early 1970s. President Reagan sought to reverse this trend and made much of what he called 'new federalism', which O'Connor (1998, p. 55) identifies as the Reagan administration's 'most important and long-lasting policy change, giving states a greater say in the allocation of federal welfare resources'. The main features of new federalism, given effect by a series of measures between 1981 and 1987, were the removal of federal regulations relating to state and local governments; the separation of functional and financial responsibility between the federal, state and local governments (sometimes referred to as 'dual federalism'); the transfer of some federal functions to states;

reduced federal grants; and the replacement of fifty-four specific categorical grants by nine block grants (O'Connor, 1998).

Regional government, a level between national and local government, has been firmly on the agenda within the European Union since the 1970s, but interest intensified during the 1980s and showed no signs of abating in the 1990s. There has long been talk of a Europe of the Regions and the Maastricht Treaty created a Committee of the Regions, with 222 members, in 1994. Regional governments have grown in stature during the 1980s and more especially during the 1990s. In some instances, regions have challenged national governments. In Italy, for example, Bossi of the Northern League has campaigned for secession of the North of Italy, and although such a change seems unlikely, the electoral success of the League in 1996 forced Prime Minister Prodi 'to adopt a strong dose of devolution' (Smart, 1996). In Belgium, with two regions, Canada with twelve regions, and Spain, with seventeen regions, sub-national institutions partially defuse potentially divisive language and cultural differences. However, regionalism has not satisfied the strong separatist movements in Quebec and Spain. Evans and Harding (1997, p. 27) claim that in Germany, 'the influence wielded over Länder decisions by the Federal authorities has been growing, not declining, over the last thirty years'. This may be true over the longer term, but Smart (1996) claims that in recent years the Federal government has become 'accustomed to bowing to the assertive politicians at the helm in the powerful German Länder'.

France established twenty-two directly elected regional councils in 1982 and extended their powers in 1983 and 1986. These were interposed between the national government and the departmental and municipal councils. Le Galès and John (1997) claim, however, that the French regions have not been a success: they 'remain as unimportant political actors and relatively weak institutions in the French administrative system' (p. 52). The problem is that the regions were given little power and inadequate resources and were faced with the growing power and budgetary strength of the departments and municipalities, particularly in the area of social policy. Le Galès and John (1997) say that the revival of regionalism in the UK may be jeopardised if note is not taken of the French experience. The Labour Government elected in 1997 held referendums on Scottish and Welsh devolution. The results were positive, and Scotland will have a parliament with the power to raise tax and there will be a

Welsh Assembly without tax-raising powers. In England, Regional Chambers are to be set up with the possibility of transforming these into elected regional authorities where there is sufficient popular support for the idea.

Osborne and Gaebler (1992), as one would expect, are enthusiastic supporters of all forms of decentralisation. They argue that the developments in information technology have rendered centralised institutions redundant, and made decentralisation both essential and much more easily achievable:

> Today information is virtually limitless, communication between remote locations is instantaneous, many public employees are well educated, and conditions change with blinding speed. There is no time to wait for information to go up the chain of command and decisions to come down.
>
> (p. 250)

The authors distinguish between traditional and entrepreneurial leaders: the former respond to a fiscal crisis by increasing bureaucracy and centralisation; the latter 'instinctively reach for the decentralized approach' (p. 251). The advantages claimed for decentralisation are considerable: greater flexibility and responsiveness; increased operational effectiveness; an enlarged willingness and capacity to innovate; 'higher morale, more commitment and greater productivity' (p. 253).

Osborne and Gaebler cannot conceive of any potential drawbacks to decentralisation. The possible connection between decentralisation and clientelism is not considered. The dangers of fragmentation and the associated problems of co-ordination are likewise ignored, as is the possible descent into parochialism. To be fair, however, Osborne and Gaebler recognise that certain policy areas may be more effectively administered at federal level: international trade; macro-economic policy; much environmental and regulatory policy; anti-poverty policy; social insurance programmes; services requiring costly investment (e.g. health care).

Frequently, in debates about mixed economies of welfare, decentralisation is linked with ideas about participation and empowerment; indeed Osborne and Gaebler (1992) make this link. The thrust of the argument is that people feel more able to participate in smaller local communities. It has already been noted, however, that decentralisation does not lead automatically to user, citizen or community empowerment. Even if decentralisation is accompanied by the transfer of responsibility for the provision of public services from the state to alternative suppliers, user-led services will not simply emerge. Transfer from an impervious central bureaucracy to an equally impervious local one does not increase empowerment. The problem is how to ensure that users have a say, that goes beyond mere consultation, in stating their needs, in deciding what kinds and levels of service best meet those needs, and in determining how the services shall be provided and by whom. The involvement of users in policy-making, service provision and even the management of facilities and services all need to be carefully considered. Decentralisation may certainly contribute to the achievement of these aims, leading to increased empowerment. Empowerment is very much in vogue, but frequently support for it is no more than lip-service, lacking any real substance. The truth is that empowerment is not easily achieved, which is not to say that it should not be attempted. However, simply not recognising the difficulties, assuming that wishes will be transformed into reality, is not a sensible way forward.

The case for and against state involvement in welfare

The New Right's views of the role of the state were outlined earlier in the chapter. Their case against extensive state involvement in welfare is an expansion and refinement of those arguments coupled with a range of moral/ethical prescriptions. Green (1996), Director of the Health and Welfare Unit at the Institute of Economic Affairs, emphasises what he regards as the moral case against the welfare state:

> The welfare problem is not primarily financial but moral. The difficulty is not so much that the welfare state cannot be afforded, but that welfare programmes have tended to impair human character, above all by undermining the older ethos of 'community without politics'.
>
> (p. ix)

Green believes that the welfare state impairs human character by making welfare services less effective in what he considers to be their 'central task of bringing out the best in people who are temporarily down on their luck' (p. ix). Whether the long-term unemployed in times of recession or the chronically sick would accept that their condition could be described as being 'temporarily down on their luck' is, I think, questionable. A second impairment of human character is that the welfare state reduces opportunities for altruism and mutual aid. This seems to fly in the face of the evidence that increasing state welfare has by no means been accompanied by a decline in voluntary action and that the last three decades have witnessed a quite remarkable upsurge in self-help or mutual aid. Titmuss (1970) argues that the public social services enlarge our freedom by allowing for the expression of altruism. This could also be said of the informal and voluntary sectors, both of which involve gift relationships, but the distinguishing feature of statutory services is that they generalise altruism, allowing us to behave altruistically towards *strangers*; Titmuss refers to this as 'anonymous helpfulness' (1970, p. 212). This rather metaphysical point is expressed in the following quotation:

> The ways in which society organises and structures its social institutions – and particularly its health and welfare systems – can encourage or discourage the altruistic in man; such systems . . . can allow the 'theme of the gift' – of generosity towards strangers – to spread among and between social groups and generations. This is an aspect of freedom in the twentieth century which, compared with the emphasis on material acquisitiveness, is insufficiently recognised.
>
> (1970, p. 225)

The Institute of Economic Affairs has also helped to popularise the notions of an underclass and the dependency culture (Murray *et al.*, 1990, Murray, 1994). Both of these concepts (although, using other terminology, they have a long history) became particularly prominent in the United States from the Reagan era onwards. Probably the most influential writer in this area is Charles Murray, a right-wing American political scientist who once advocated 'scrapping the entire federal welfare and income-support structure for working-aged persons, including AFDC, Medicaid, Food Stamps, Unemployment Insurance, Worker's Compensation, subsidized housing, disability insurance and the rest' (1984, p. 227). Marsland, a conservative British writer, criticises the welfare state because

> it does enormous harm to its supposed prime beneficiaries – the vulnerable, the disadvantaged and the unfortunate. By generating

dependency it makes normal, capable people who happen to be in temporary difficulty, a fractious, subjugated underclass of welfare dependants. The welfare state thus cripples the enterprising, self-reliant spirit of individual men and women and lays a depth-charge of explosive resentment under the foundations of a free society.

(1996, p. 186)

Several points need to be made about this emotive statement. First, it is based on precious little evidence. Second, it is revealing how 'vulnerable, disadvantaged and unfortunate' people, in the first sentence, become people 'who happen to be in temporary difficulty' in the second. Third, it turns on its head the Fabian argument, most ably expressed by Titmuss (1968; 1970), that the welfare state is a force for social integration.

Dean and Taylor-Gooby (1992), in a report of an empirical study of dependency, reject the New Right's interpretation of dependency. The results of their research indicate that

social security claimants are not part of an underclass characterised by a distinctive dependency culture, but that such claimants subscribe by and large to mainstream norms, values and lifeways. . . . Reforms to the British social security system introduced in the 1980s were in many ways counterproductive. Certainly they have not reduced state dependency and they have worked against the grain of social change and popular expectations.

(p. 124)

In this respect the reforms may be said to have failed, but Dean and Taylor-Gooby postulate that the reforms may not have failed at all in that 'it could be argued that the government has succeeded in constituting state dependency as uniquely problematic' (p. 124). Dean and Taylor-Gooby argue that dependency, indeed interdependency, is a universal human condition, and that there are many different forms of dependency: for example, workers are dependent upon employers and *vice versa*; entrepreneurs are dependent upon capital markets and on the customers who buy their products; there are interdependencies in families and other social groups.

As we have seen, Hayek and other New Right theorists see the state as the potential enemy of liberty. Liberty may therefore be seen as the absence of government intervention. However, Hayek clearly acknowledges that rights and agreements have to be enforced by law. Only libertarian anarchists would define freedom as the total absence of restraint: certainly Green, Hayek, Marsland and Murray would not define liberty in this way. However, they do hold that the state should do only what is necessary to enforce contracts, agreements and uphold the rule of law. In the welfare field the more moderate free market liberals (Murray would not be included in that category) would accept that the state should provide minimum services. Goodin (1988) observes, however, that when the New Right talk about minima, they mean that the minimum amounts they specify should constitute the maximum amounts available. Goodin says:

> Among those who would roll back the welfare state, there seems to be no reasoned rationale for rolling it back to the safety net and then stopping. There is no reason, in principle, to suppose that the same arguments offered for rolling it back to the safety net will not later be used to justify rolling it right back through the safety net.
>
> (1988, p. 17)

There has been a long-running debate about the relationship between liberty and equality. The New Right argue that the search for equality of outcome through state action is doomed to failure and bound to lead to infringements of rights and personal liberty. In marked contrast, one of the justifications of the welfare state used by the Fabians and others is the contribution which it supposedly makes to equality. Their argument is that liberty and equality are not incompatible, and both are unachievable in an unregulated market economy. Government intervention is both necessary and desirable to ensure that public purposes are pursued and that needs are met. The state rather than being the enemy of freedom and the potential violator of rights is the only institution capable of promoting the freedom of all and protecting everyone's rights. For theorists of a Fabian persuasion, as for other socialists, equality and freedom are interdependent. Freedom without some measure of equality is meaningless. Economic subordination is as objectionable as political subordination, and since unchecked markets produce gross inequality, not only in income and wealth but also in status and power, they also reduce freedom. As Weale (1983) points out:

> The accumulation of resources in private hands, which may be used for controlling the conduct of others, in principle poses as great a threat to individual liberty as government power. For this reason there is no general inference to be drawn to the effect that the protection of individual liberty requires *laissez-faire*.
>
> (p. 57)

Weale also provides an interesting perspective on the relationship between economic security and liberty, indicating at the same time the need for government involvement. The central idea is that of autonomy, of which Weale writes:

> There is one overriding imperative to which government action ought to be subject in the field of social policy, and that is the principle that the government should secure the conditions of equal autonomy for all. . . . This principle of autonomy asserts that all persons are entitled to respect as deliberative and purposive agents capable of formulating their own projects, and that as part of this respect there is a governmental obligation to bring into being or preserve the conditions in which this autonomy can be realised.
>
> (1983, p. 42)

Autonomous action is the product of deliberation in which the individual makes choices from among a range of options. There will be constraints, but these should not be so confining as to deprive the individual of autonomy. Economic deprivations result in a loss of autonomy, because alternatives are absent or strictly limited. Economic security, then, is necessary if the principle of autonomy is to be observed, and this implies that it is the state's responsibility to provide a comprehensive system of income maintenance. Furthermore, if people are to make full use of their autonomy, they need to acquire basic social and intellectual skills. Weale concludes that the state therefore has a responsibility to provide 'high-quality mass education up to the standard school-leaving age, with the aim of equipping all children with the cultural resources necessary for them to become autonomous social agents'. It might be possible to construct a similar case in relation to other social services – health and personal social services, for example – although Weale does not do so.

The principle of autonomy guarantees only that minimum needs will be met. Distribution above the minimum, in Weale's analysis, relies on a contractarian argument. The most widely known modern variant of the contractarian perspective is that developed by Rawls (1972). The theory begins with an imaginary original position in which men and women are equally free and rational. They are also equally ignorant about their own and others' abilities and about the positions they are likely to occupy in any future society. Rawls refers to this as 'the veil of ignorance'. The next step in the argument is to ask what distribution of resources and roles would men and women in the original position choose. Rawls claims that two principles would govern people's choices: (i) that rights and duties would be equally distributed and (ii) 'social and economic inequalities . . . are just only if they result in compensating benefits for everyone, and in particular for the least advantaged members of society' (p. 14). This second principle, called the difference principle by Rawls, obviously has distributional implications. People's decisions behind the veil of ignorance would depend upon their level of risk aversion: the more averse they are to take risks (e.g. the risk that their abilities will land them at the bottom end of society), the more they will favour an egalitarian distribution of resources.

Another aspect of the equality debate is that the state can ensure wider and more even coverage than either the voluntary or the commercial sector. By definition, it is the one institution which covers the whole of the nation. There is never, of course, complete uniformity of provision: there will be urban/rural, class, gender, age, ethnic and religious divisions. There may be even more variation when states are federal or highly decentralised. Nevertheless, state health insurance or income maintenance schemes, for example, have at least the capacity to offer the same or broadly similar terms to all citizens, which is very different from the actuarial basis of commercial insurance. On the other hand, the increasing emphasis on earnings-related benefits may result in the extension of income inequalities into the benefit system. A further consideration is that voluntary and commercial agencies may be more subject than states to variations in income, and they are also less permanent.

Goodin (1988, p. 51), however, claims that it is a mistake to use social equality as 'the most fundamental justification of the welfare state'. He believes that a more successful defence of the welfare state can be mounted if the welfare state is viewed as having more limited aims. He claims that 'the essential function of the welfare state is to prevent the exploitation of vulnerable members of society' (p. ix). Goodin believes that welfare states may be justified in going beyond the minimal purpose of meeting basic needs, but that the best defence against the attacks on welfare by the New Right are arguments about protecting those who are not in a position to protect themselves:

> There is an especially compelling and interestingly different ethical case to be made for having at least a minimal welfare state. There may well be reasons for moving beyond the minimal welfare state

thus justified. But those will be *other* reasons, quite distinct from the reasons that can be offered to justify the minimal welfare state. They are not necessarily any worse, or less compelling, for that. It is important, however, to realize that they are distinct.

(1988, p. 20)

Another argument used by the New Right is that the welfare state is inefficient. The case they make has several strands.

● The payment of benefits is a disincentive to work and save. The disincentive to work is said to come about in two ways. The high rates of tax required to pay for a welfare state mean that people keep less of any extra income, and they may decide that extra effort is simply not worth it. The evidence is, to say the least, equivocal. Higher rates of tax may discourage some people from working hard, but this may be more than outweighed by those who work harder to ensure that their take-home pay remains the same. The second disincentive to earn comes about more directly. If people can receive in benefits almost as much as they can earn through work, they are likely to choose not to work. The evidence here is also weak. Benefits are usually very low – lower than all but the very lowest earnings, and the benefit system treats voluntary unemployment punitively. Nor is it apparent that people will choose not to work. There are very strong social pressures impelling people towards work and work is an important source of self respect and social identity. Disincentives to save arise, it is claimed, in a similar way: benefits discourage people from saving to meet the contingencies of sickness, unemployment and retirement.

● Public services are not subject to the disciplines of the market, and are therefore wasteful. This is particularly true if they are monopolies. Lack of competition gives no incentive to reduce costs, and there is no direct link between performance, revenue and costs. Nor do the producers have any incentive to develop entrepreneurial flair and innovate. If services are provided at zero-cost to consumers, they have no incentive to ration their use. The assumptions here are that the only incentive to providing a good cost-efficient service is the promise of greater profits. Effectively meeting need and notions of public service may be sufficient to ensure efficiency.

● We have already looked at public choice theorists who would agree with the strictures noted above, but they would also point to the tendency for bureaucrats to maximise both their budgets and the size and scope of their bureaux. This, together with pressure group politics (the politics of excessive expectation), gives rise to big government which inevitably overreaches itself, leading to policy failure.

● Social expenditure diverts resources from productive use in commerce and industry into non-productive social welfare. This argument is by no means new, but it is interesting to note that among the most powerful arguments for increased social expenditure since the nineteenth century has been the contribution that services make to productivity. This is most obviously the case in health care and education; it is not an unreasonable claim that a healthier, more educated labour force is likely to be more productive. Social security maintains people as effective consumers during times of recession. The OECD (1994, p. 12) disagrees with this part of the New Right's analysis: 'Non-inflationary growth of output and jobs, and political and social stability are enhanced by the role of social expenditures as investments in society'.

In very general terms, the New Right believes that the welfare state damages capitalism and that the two are therefore incompatible. This was not the view of the architects of welfare states after the Second World War. Beveridge and Keynes were persuaded that state services were essential to the smooth running of the capitalist system, not least because they helped to maintain social and political stability. As we have seen, Marxists also see the welfare state as contributing to the long-term aims of capitalism by legitimating class power and capital accumulation.

It would be a mistake, however, to assume that criticisms of state welfare are limited to politically committed groups of right and left. Criticism also came from consumers. Walker (1993, pp. 74–5), for example, says that 'disillusionment with certain aspects of the social services set in gradually and, during the 1980s has become more outspoken'. Walker identifies grassroots criticism and pressure from users, carers, feminists and ethnic minority groups. These criticisms were mainly about the quality and nature of state services, as opposed to more generalised criticism of the principles upon which the welfare state is based.

Conclusion

Since the mid-1970s there has been a sustained attempt to reappraise the role of the state in general terms and in welfare specifically. This debate has given rise to a variety of terms in an attempt to encapsulate the changes: the most appropriate of these terms, from a mixed economy perspective, are the 'enabling state' and the 'contract state'. Both terms imply a reduction in the state's role as a direct provider of services. The enabling state is one which is responsible for creating and maintaining the conditions in which needs can be met by non-state agencies: the contracting state implies a particular form of relationship between public agencies as purchasers and independent providers.

There are three closely related overarching issues arising from these changes. The first concerns the role of the state in planning, finance and regulation. The second concerns the relationship between the state and the citizen. The third concerns the relationship between the state and the commercial, voluntary and informal sectors.

The state is in a position to take an overall view of the direction of social policy and to set priorities for its future development. This necessarily involves a degree of planning which allows the individual priorities of voluntary and commercial providers to be co-ordinated or regulated to serve public policies or purposes.

The failures of the system of five-year national plans in Central and Eastern Europe and the Soviet Union have given planning a bad name, and the undoubted serious deficiencies of centralised economic planning are used as an argument against all planning. Decentralised planning which is democratically controlled and participative in nature, as proposed by Walker (1984), for example, has much to commend it. Another approach is suggested by market socialists, Estrin and Winter (1989, p. 116), who recommend indicative planning: 'a decentralized, and preferably democratic, process of consultation and discussion concerned exclusively with plan construction and elaboration'. Such plans would not include prescribed methods of implementation, which would be left to negotiation among individual agents. The French system is cited as an example of this form of planning.

Planning of a mainly indicative kind is present in most welfare states, its most common location being either local or regional. Plans exist in a variety of policy areas: health, personal social services, housing and urban development and labour market policies. In some cases, plans drawn up locally have to be approved at national level. This is the case, for example, in the British system of community care. Local authorities have to produce rolling three-year community care plans which have to be approved by the Department of Health. As systems in many countries become more fragmented and decentralised, the need for planning, to bring about a greater degree of integration and coherence, becomes increasingly apparent.

One advantage of plans is that they can be questioned and evaluated, and those responsible for drawing them up and implementing them can be held accountable. Plans will also include assessments of needs, rather than demands, and strategies for meeting them. They can also consider environmental issues, although this is one area where the centralised economic plans in Central and Eastern Europe and the Soviet Union failed so woefully. The sole aim of these plans was to maximise and rationalise production, and other issues were not addressed. This emphasises once again the need for planning to be flexible, decentralised and participative.

In so far as planning includes the setting of priorities, it also involves regulation. This is an area of intense debate in many countries. Since the early 1980s, there has been a general sentiment in government circles in favour of de-regulation. In some ways, however, mixed economies of welfare may require not less but more regulation. In the next chapter, there is some discussion of managed and regulated markets and managed competition, in which governments make and enforce the rules and manage the markets. In transferring welfare provision to profit-oriented firms public agencies have to guard against exploitation and the erosion of standards. Contracts for care represent additional forms of regulation. There are several problems associated with regulation: (i) it is time-consuming and costly; (ii) it is difficult to police and evasion is always a possibility; (iii) it is difficult to devise and apply appropriate sanctions; (iv) it is difficult to achieve a balance between too little and too much regulation. Too little regulation may give providers a virtually free hand and provide inadequate protection for service users, whereas too much regulation may be stultifying and pose a threat to the independence of providers. As will be seen in Chapter 4, this last point is of particular significance for voluntary organisations.

Chapter 4 will also demonstrate the importance of statutory funding of the voluntary sector either through grants or contracts, and the increasing use of contracts means that both commercial and voluntary providers depend heavily on public finance. It is necessary to stress that the use of non-government agencies for provision does not automatically reduce public expenditure, although the impetus towards mixed economies may in part be the expectation of savings.

The second overarching issue is the effect of the changing nature of the state on its relationships with citizens. Earlier in this chapter we saw how new public management sought to redefine citizens as customers or consumers. This is justified on the grounds of choice, the expectation of higher quality and the customer's right to complain about poor service. There are some grounds for arguing that public agencies can learn from the private sector in terms of their relationships with service-users, but the wholesale importation of market principles into the public sector has drawbacks, not the least of which is the reduced emphasis on citizenship and its associated rights. It is worth recalling Ranson and Stewart's (1994) argument that the emphasis in consumerism 'is on the individual in receipt of a service, rather than on the citizen as an active participant in the polity' (p. 19).

In the 1970s public services were much exercised by participation. The language has changed, so that the term 'empowerment' is now very much in vogue. It is a term that is very difficult to define with any degree of precision, a problem compounded by the different meanings attached to it by different groups. It is most commonly used in relation to service users. The aim is to create user-led or needs-led services in which users have a say in stating their needs, in deciding what kinds and levels of service best meet those needs and in determining how the services will be provided and by whom. The problem is that services continue to be resources-led and user involvement does not go much beyond consultation. In times of resource constraint, it is difficult to see how service provision could be anything other than resources-led, but within these limits, the views of users could be paramount.

But empowerment will not just happen, and it may be more difficult to achieve than is sometimes supposed. A pre-requisite is the creation of structures to facilitate empowerment, but even more important is attitudinal change in which professionals, bureaucrats and politicians surrender some of their power. The simplistic assumption that empowerment will result automatically from a transfer of responsibility for the provision of health and welfare services to alternative suppliers cannot be sustained. Markets and voluntary organisations exhibit a middle-class and racial bias and they are little more successful than the state in the involvement of users.

The third overarching issue – the relationship of the state to the other three sectors – brings us back to the main focus of this book. Mixed economies of welfare are concerned with the inter-relationships and balance between the state, commercial under-takings, the voluntary sector and the informal sector in producing and distributing health and welfare services among citizens. This chapter has considered some of the criticisms of state welfare and some of its strengths and this has been set within a discussion of different views of the state, the changing ideas over time about the appropriate level of state intervention, and governments' attempts since the mid-1970s to cut social expenditure and curtail the role of the state. In the next three chapters the commercial, voluntary and informal sectors will be subjected to a similar analysis, and we will then be in a position to re-assess some of the arguments reviewed in this chapter. It was appropriate to start with the state because the debate surrounding the other three sectors is frequently conducted in the context of a re-assessment of the nature and roles of the state. The debate concerning the state–market interface has received most attention and this is the focus of the next chapter.

Notes

1. A good account of the different forms of feminism may be found in Dale and Foster (1986) and in George and Wilding (1994).
2. Austria, Finland and Sweden were not members of the European Community in 1990. The term European Community was still being used in 1990. It was replaced by the term European Union in 1993.
3. Workfare is a system that makes benefits conditional upon recipients accepting work or training. The work provided is usually of low status.

CHAPTER 3

THE COMMERCIAL SECTOR AND SOCIAL WELFARE

Introduction

The welfare state was never intended to replace private markets completely. Indeed, some would claim that it was specifically designed to facilitate capital accumulation through the creation of a disciplined, educated and healthy labour force, the provision of infrastructural services and the maintenance of demand, and to provide legitimacy for the capitalist system. Goodin (1988, pp. 160–1) argues that the 'true justification of the welfare state' is its role 'in safeguarding the preconditions of the market'. The welfare state therefore implies state intervention in market relationships; in some instances it was thought sufficient to modify the free play of market forces, in other instances partial or substantial replacement of the market occurred, but there were no examples of commercial provision being completely ousted. Flora (1985) sums the position up in the following way:

> The development of the Western welfare state is not to be understood as a step on the road towards socialism. It should be interpreted instead as a complementary process in the evolution of a relatively coherent tripartite structure consisting of: capitalist market economy, democratic mass polity, and welfare state.
>
> (p. 12)

This calls to mind the distinction made in the postwar debate about the welfare state in West Germany between a 'social market economy' (supported by the Christian Democratic Party) and a 'socialist

market economy' (supported by the Social Democratic Party). Both
accept the need for a market economy, but the Social Democrats
accord a much more important role to the state in modifying the
effects of market forces.

The balance between the commercial and public sectors varies
from one country to another, but there are also considerable variations within countries as between one service and another, and even
between different subdivisions of a single service. It is plain that
private markets in the social services are much more prominent in
the United States than they are in Britain and they are more
significant in Britain than in Sweden. One can postulate three
possible positions in relation to service provision:

1. Private markets alongside the statutory system which remains the
   main provider. Education is in this position in most Western
   European countries.
2. Private markets as the main provider, but with a substantial role
   left for the state; housing in most countries is probably a good
   example of this position, although the complex arrangements of
   housing allowances, rebates, vouchers and subsidies obscure
   market/public sector divisions.
3. Private markets as the main provider with a residual role left for
   the state; for example, housing and, to a lesser extent, health in
   the United States.

However, this categorisation oversimplifies the position in a
number of ways. First, it deals only with provision and ignores the
important role of the state in regulating and subsidising commercial
suppliers. In practice, the inter-relationships are infinitely more
complex and less clear-cut than the threefold division implies.
Second, the categorisation fails to acknowledge the difficulties of
deciding precisely where the dividing line between public and private
activity lies. This is further complicated by the incorporation of
private-market practices into public-sector services: charges, the
insurance principle and competition might be thought of in this way.
Third, and probably the most serious limitation of the categorisation,
is that it takes into account only the public sector–private market
relationships; the presence of a vigorous voluntary or non-profit
sector means three sets of two-way relationships and an overall relationship involving all three sectors.

Market theory and ideology

The nature of markets

Stated simply, markets are a means of bringing together buyers and sellers for purposes of voluntary exchange. The items involved in this exchange may be raw materials, agricultural produce, manufactured goods, labour or capital.

Markets consist of networks of dealings in which the outcomes are determined by the apparently unco-ordinated actions of large numbers of individuals and firms. The classical view is that prices are determined by the relationship between supply and demand. The equilibrium price is that at which demand and supply are identical. In conditions of perfect competition, no single buyer or seller controls enough of the market to be able to affect prices by his or her own actions, so that large numbers of competing separate firms, seeking to maximise their profits, adjust their outputs to the known market price. When the equilibrium position is reached, no participant can improve his or her position without someone else losing; perfect competition, therefore, ensures the most efficient allocation of resources. Any interference with perfect competition will lead to a loss of efficiency and is therefore to be deprecated: trade unions (except as friendly societies), cartels, monopolies and monopsonies (a single or dominant buyer) are equally condemned.

The neo-classical approach to markets is criticised by economists of the Austrian school for being too static and taking too little account of entrepreneurship. The Austrians place less emphasis on prices and more on competition, and argue that the market is characterised by disequilibrium. The competitive process can be expected to produce a number of monopolies (a reward for competing successfully) but, provided that competition is unhindered, these will be relatively short-lived.

A variant of the neo-classical approach to markets is provided by economists who talk about contestability rather than competition (see Ham below). Contestability is a concept developed by Baumol *et al.* (1982). The crucial distinguishing characteristics of perfect contestability are the complete absence of any barriers to market entry and exit, and perfect information in the possession of both providers and customers. In the extreme case, entry to the market would be entirely costless. Forder *et al.* (1996) explain the theoretical advantages of perfect contestability:

> In a perfectly contestable market, incumbent providers are compelled by the threat of market entry to produce at minimum cost (productive efficiency), and to set prices at marginal cost (allocative efficiency), except in some natural monopoly cases. If they do not, new providers can (costlessly) enter the market, slightly undercut the incumbent's price and take away their business.
>
> (p. 204)

It should perhaps be noted that this quotation refers to *perfect* contestability which may be as unattainable as *perfect* competition. Ham (1996), in relation to the British Health Service, employs a more realistically achievable form of contestability, and writes about contestability *rather than* competition: he describes contestability as 'the middle way between planning and competition'. He states:

> In a contestable health service, the emphasis is placed on co-operation and co-ordination but with the option of moving to alternative providers if other means of improving performance do not work. This provides the incentive to ensure the efficient use of public resources while at the same time enabling services to be properly co-ordinated. Contestability assumes that government as regulator will continue to oversee the financing and provision of health care at a national level but that there will be considerable local freedom in determining the shape of service delivery.
>
> (p. 10)

Neo-classical economic theorists are firmly committed to free markets. They believe that unfettered markets, in which individuals pursue their own self-interest, lead to the best results for society as a whole. As we have seen, some of the other commentators who have examined markets recognise the potentially damaging effects of unrestricted markets, arguing that markets should be subject to regulation and that some goods should be removed from the operation of the market altogether. The extent and degree of market regulation vary from one country to another, as does the range of goods left to the market.

The idea of managed markets gained great publicity at the time of the Clinton health proposals from about 1993 onwards, but the theories were developed several years earlier. The main proponent of managed competition is Enthoven (1985; 1993) who acted as advisor to Mrs Thatcher in her reforms of the British National

Health Service in 1990 and provided the theoretical framework for the National Health Care Reform Task Force established in the United States in 1993. The system proposed by Enthoven relies on private insurance with providers forming themselves into units integrating insurance and direct health care services. These insurance-controlled units would either employ health professionals (as in health maintenance organisations at present) or contract with groups of independent professionals (as in preferred provider organisations at present). A crucial element of the proposals is to encourage greater cost-consciousness among consumers who would be required to pay, at least in part, for the annual premium, with exceptions for those on very low incomes. Consumers would be required to enrol in one of the insurance-controlled health care plans. Agencies would be established on a regional basis to act as intermediaries between providers and consumers and to help consumers by offering comparative information about competing plans. Enthoven calls these agencies health insurance purchasing co-operatives. There are already schemes of this nature in California and Florida. Green (1997) supports the introduction of a suitably adapted system in Britain; he describes the scheme as a 'good compromise that meets the main objections put by critics of market competition whilst simultaneously allowing scope for the emergence of a competitive system' (p. 49).

A point to be borne in mind is that private markets may take several forms. The most familiar is direct payment for goods and services, but this is less common in social services than it is in other transactions, and an insurance-based private market system may be seen as an acceptable alternative to a direct payment system. Private insurance cover is most likely to be used for high-cost services where public provision is non-existent or judged to be inferior. Outside the Medicaid and Medicare systems, health care provision in the United States (especially hospital care) is financed in this way.

In social and health care areas, markets are often considerably modified by the use of subsidies, allowances, vouchers and regulation. In the health insurance systems of Western Europe, for example, practitioners are virtually private providers, paid by patients whose costs are wholly or partly reimbursed, but the payments received by practitioners are set by government. As already noted, the position in housing is similar with largely private suppliers regulated by government and the market modified by the payment of producer or consumer subsidies.

The arguments concerning the public–private mix in welfare are conducted at several levels, ranging from the comparison of inter-sectoral costs to the purely ideological. It is not always easy to separate the different levels as the descriptive merges into the prescriptive. Even the most pragmatic arguments concerned with technicalities have an ideological element. We will now turn to the arguments which are grouped under three broad headings: efficiency; choice, freedom and rights; equity and equality.

Efficiency

The pressure on resources for social welfare has brought the issues of efficiency and effectiveness to the forefront of the social policy debate. The debate is still hampered by problems of definition and measurement, despite the attempts being made to devise acceptable social indicators. This is not the place to pursue this point; suffice it to say that efficiency and effectiveness are very closely related, but they are not synonymous. A very clear definition of what they term *social* efficiency is provided by Knapp *et al.* (1994). Interestingly, they argue that efficiency is little concerned with equity:

> By socially efficient we mean provision which minimises the cost of achieving a given quality of service (or maximises the user benefits or outcomes from a given cost), and which, via allocative efficiency, increases the range of choice. Efficiency will not necessarily produce an equitable allocation of resources. That is one which is fair by the criteria of social justice.
>
> (p. 149)

Effectiveness, however, is concerned primarily with the degree to which needs are being met. It may also involve more difficult-to-measure elements such as user involvement in need assessment and service planning and evaluation.

Those who contend that market provision is more efficient than public provision argue their case on three fronts: comparisons of intersectoral costs, more general arguments about the benefits arising from competition, and claims that public provision has features that render it inefficient. We will examine the arguments in each of these areas in turn.

There have been many comparisons of intersectoral costs princi-pally in the United States, but also in Britain. An interesting British study reported by Judge and Knapp (1985) compares the private and local authority costs of providing residential accommodation for elderly people. Judge and Knapp (1985, p. 139) conclude that 'private residential homes in England and Wales are less costly and might represent better value for money than their non-profit counterparts in the public and voluntary sectors'. A drawback of this study, acknowledged by the authors, is that it takes no account of output – it was assumed that the services provided and their quality were similar in the two sets of institutions. Several reasons were advanced for the difference in costs, the most important of which was 'the traditional virtues of small business enterprises'. These 'virtues' include the heavy involvement of the owners and their families in the business, often working very long hours. This allows for-profit homes to employ very few people, who are usually paid less than trade-union negotiated wages. Keeping staff to a minimum and paying them low wages very obviously reduces costs, but the question arises as to how far this can be pushed without reducing the quality of the service. Furthermore, if family members work very long hours, their own efficiency may eventually suffer. A British study of services for people with learning disabilities by Cambridge and Brown (1997) has this to say about reduced costs:

> Insofar as a mixed market has offered cheaper services, these have been bought at the expense of the conditions of service of the workforce. Reductions in pay and conditions have to offset a reduction in the profit margin. Badly paid staff, with few rights and job insecurity, are not the best advocates for other relatively powerless people.
>
> (pp. 32–3)

One of the implications of this work is that facilities requiring a great deal of capital investment and relying on highly paid skilled labour do not lend themselves to operation by small business enterprises: a district general hospital, for example, is a very different proposition from a small residential home. It should be noted that Judge and Knapp urge caution in the interpretation of their findings: 'We emphatically do not mean to suggest that all service delivery agencies in the public domain . . . should be handed over to small businessmen' (p. 149). In many instances, they recognise, this would be impractical. Nevertheless, as we shall see, in the intervening twelve years this is precisely what has happened. It should also be noted that Biggs (1986), in a study of residential care for older people, produced quite different results which showed that independent facilities were in fact more rather than less expensive than those in the public sector.

Contradictory results are also a feature of much of the American research focusing in the main on health care in hospitals and nursing homes. Most emphasis has been on comparing non-profit and for-profit facilities. In relation to hospitals, there are as many studies indicating lower costs in for-profit establishments as there are indicating higher costs. To some extent this confusion is the result of using different units of measurement. It is generally agreed that for-profit hospitals have higher daily treatment costs, but it is equally well-documented that stays are shorter, bringing down the cost per admission. Marmor *et al.* (1987, p. 230) state that 'investigations of the hospital industry have found only small, inconsistent differences in reported costs of proprietary and nonprofit facilities'. Even when costs per admission are used the results reveal discrepancies with some showing a cost advantage favouring for-profit hospitals, some showing the advantage lying with non-profits and the remainder showing little or no difference. Marmor claims that the evidence relating to nursing homes is less equivocal with the majority of studies showing for-profit homes to be cheaper. However, Marmor makes three further points which have a significant bearing on quality and costs. First, he maintains that there is consistent evidence 'that for-profit facilities are disproportionately represented among institutions offering the very lowest quality care'. Second, he claims that cost differences are less apparent when physicians control the delivery of care. When this is the case, for-profit facilities are less able to push for cost reduction (either through greater efficiency gains or reductions in quality). Third, he says that physician control does not appear to affect the willingness and ability of for-profit establishments to avoid unprofitable patients:

> Providers of medical care can avoid unprofitable patients in three ways. First, facilities can simply be located away from low-income areas. Second, they can choose not to provide services used dispro-portionately by the uninsured or underinsured. Third, they can actively screen and discourage admission by those unable to pay for care. This screening could be accomplished by requiring a means test prior to admission or by not offering sliding fee scales for patients unable to cover fully the cost of care.
>
> (1987, p. 231)

Marmor cites evidence that all three of these strategies are employed more often by for-profit providers than by public or non-profit providers.

Evidence that reduced costs may be bought at the expense of quality in for-profit enterprises can be found in some work looking at compulsory competitive tendering in the British health service. Milne (1987) identified savings of one-third or more when services are contracted out to commercial operators, but found that in a majority of contracts reductions in total expenditure resulted from changes in specification – a reduced amount of work being done and a lower level of service provided. Moreover, managers sometimes took the opportunity to reallocate work, so that nurses, for example, might be required to carry out work formerly done by ancillary staff.

There are serious conceptual and methodological difficulties in comparing intersectoral costs. Not the least of these difficulties is that of relating cost to quality which requires some means of measuring quality. There is much talk of quality at the present time, but Pollitt (1993, p. 162) claims the term quality 'has come to be used in a bewilderingly promiscuous way'. The problem is that quality is difficult to define and even more difficult to measure. Nor is it simply that quality in human services is difficult to define; it is defined differently by people who occupy different positions, each of whom may have a different agenda. Pollitt (1993) writes: '. . . analysis soon reveals that different groups define quality differently, adopt different approaches to its improvement, and wield greater or lesser leverage in the struggle to determine which definitions, methods and measurements will be adopted in its pursuit' (p. 161).

The same problem occurs when attempting to evaluate neo-liberal claims that perfect competition in free markets guarantees the most efficient allocation of resources. Producers, seeking to maximise their profits, compete with each other for a bigger share of the market. There is an incentive to reduce costs to a minimum and to improve the quality of the product. Producers who can achieve neither will eventually be forced to close down. The comfortable assumption is that the best interests of everyone are served by all market participants pursuing their own self-interest. Public services, by contrast, are said to be inefficient, inflexible and unresponsive. Important theoretical backing for the radical right's ideas about the inefficiency of public provision came from adherents of the public choice school (Downs, 1957, 1967; Buchanan and Tullock, 1962;

Niskanen, 1971, 1978), who sought to apply economic theory to the behaviour of governments. More particularly, they argued that the methods employed in the analysis of markets could be applied to the public sector. The notion of disinterested public service was said to be a myth and the behaviour of bureaucrats was just as self-interested as the behaviour of individuals in the market. The difference was that bureaucrats were not subject to the discipline of the market and the necessity of making a profit.[1] Public agencies are hidebound, unimaginative and resistant to innovation. Novak (1991, p. 106) claims that competitive markets, in contrast to government, encourage innovation:

> In a market system things move; wealth grows; opportunities open; breakthroughs are made; new groups rise to wealth. Practical intelligence assesses existing arrangements in order to invent others, to offer new services, to meet unmet needs, to discover better ways. The inventiveness encouraged by market systems may be their most important characteristic.

Another advantage claimed for markets is that they are an effective way of processing and transmitting information in the form of prices. If the supply of a particular product, material or service is insufficient to meet demand, its price will rise; if, on the other hand, supply exceeds demand, the price will fall. A higher price is a signal to current and potential producers that there are profits to be made, and this will be an incentive to increase output. A lower price will have the opposite effect. Estrin and Le Grand (1989, p. 3) stress the importance of the conjunction of information and incentives: 'When they [markets] work well, they are an excellent way of processing information, while simultaneously providing incentives to act upon it.'

Gray (1992) also stresses the importance of information and incentives, and claims that the market is immeasurably superior to central planning in both respects. As evidence of this, Gray cites the economic failure in the former Soviet Union and in the former communist states of Central and Eastern Europe. According to Gray, the failure of central planning is partly to be explained by 'the absence of the benign incentives provided by the disciplines of market competition and the presence of incentives to mismanagement and mal-investment' (p. 6).

Gray, however, emphasises the epistemic problems facing central economic planners – problems stemming from the limitations of human knowledge. Without the information provided by prices, central planners are at a grave disadvantage. The work of Hayek (1976), Polanyi (1951) and Shackle (1972) is used by Gray to substantiate this claim. According to Hayek, it is not simply a lack of knowledge on the part of planners that creates problems, but the nature of the knowledge possessed by those making economic decisions. Frequently this knowledge is intuitive and local, and it is constantly changing. Such knowledge is not available to central planning agencies, and it can never be made available. Polanyi makes a similar point when he writes of tacit and local knowledge, much of which remains unarticulated and may not be capable of articulation. Shackle's main argument is that the future is entirely unpredictable, and central planners are therefore reduced to guessing. This is no less true of participants in markets, but the consequences of wrong guesses are less far-reaching than are errors in central plans.

Many of the advantages claimed for markets are conditional in nature. For example, some of the efficiency advantages claimed for markets are conditional upon competition. The greatest advantages, it is claimed, occur when there is perfect competition in which many suppliers compete for the custom of knowledgeable consumers. For a variety of reasons, however, market failure may result from imperfect competition. The development of monopolies, in which a single supplier or a very small group of suppliers controls the entire market, is the most obvious example of imperfect competition. When there are only a few producers, cartels to regulate output or prices may be formed. Market imperfections also arise when there is a single or small group of purchasers.

There are several instances of 'natural monopolies' when it would be wasteful or prohibitively expensive to duplicate units of production – gas, water supply and electricity distribution come into this category, although recent privatisations in Britain and elsewhere indicate that public provision is not considered the only answer to potential monopolies in public services. It is not entirely clear, however, whether private monopolies are to be preferred to public. Local monopolies may also arise, even when there is a large number of suppliers nationally, if mobility problems and the cost of travel render the use of alternative facilities impractical. Parents, for example, may very well believe that a primary school fifteen miles away from where they live is better than the one down the road, but they may also believe that fifteen miles is too far for a young child to travel.

However, the claimed advantages of competitive and contestable markets may begin to diminish well before monopolies emerge. In a study of social care markets, for example, Wistow *et al.* (1994) found that there were too few suppliers:

> It was a widely held view among the people we interviewed in local authorities that there is no sizeable, vibrant non-statutory sector ready and willing to take on a larger service-providing role, particularly in relation to domiciliary, day and respite care. Today's private and voluntary sectors, they argued, are unable to supply sufficient quantities of services of the requisite standard to replace local authority provision.
>
> (p. 101)

Not only were there too few suppliers, but those that did exist were underdeveloped, and 'private agencies had neither the skills nor the inclination to diversify from residential care' (p. 102). Furthermore, the full benefits of *perfect* contestability depend upon the absence of barriers to market entry or exit. A later report of the same study (Forder *et al.*, 1996) identified considerable barriers to both entry and exit. Too few and underdeveloped suppliers were themselves restraints, but in addition, incumbents frequently had cost advantages. Entry to the market was by no means costless, and potential providers were hampered by resource constraints – especially an adequate supply of cheap labour. There were also barriers to exit. These included: (i) non-recoverable or sunk costs which continue even when production ceases; (ii) user vulnerability and commitment to care; (iii) product differentiation with providers committed to a market niche and where changing the product is likely to be costly.

Perfect competition and contestability also require knowledgeable consumers, and, in the vast majority of transactions, people do have the necessary knowledge to enable them to make reasonable decisions about which goods and services to buy from among those available. However, there are certain very technical or professional services which most people have to take on trust, although independent advice services, consumer protection agencies and legislation help to reduce the danger of exploitation. Many studies indicate that consumers of social services are not particularly discriminating. On the whole they tend to express satisfaction with services even when expert opinion and the application of a variety of criteria indicate a number of inadequacies. Browne (1984), in an interesting American study, examined children's day-care facilities provided under a variety of different auspices. She found that consumers did not exercise 'a high level of discrimination'. She comments:

> One of the theoretical advantages of the mixed economy of day care derives from competition among providers seeking to attract well-informed consumers. To the extent that consumers lack the knowledge, skill and, perhaps inclination to discriminate among day care provisions of different quality, the mixed economy of care operates with a low degree of internal regulation.
>
> (p. 330)

Shaw (1995, p. 145), in discussing the problems associated with interpreting user surveys, notes that 'there is ample evidence high satisfaction levels can co-exist with high problems or poor service'. This is not to suggest that parents and other social service consumers are unintelligent – it is more related to a lack of experience of alternatives and a desire not to appear ungrateful. The Browne study asked parents already using day care. A study of the decision-making process and the availability of alternatives might have revealed rather more discrimination. Another possibility is that parents have to take what they can get when there is an overall shortage of places, and they are thankful to have found somewhere. There is, however, a difference between a service such as day care, which is relatively easy for lay people to evaluate, and a more complex and technical service such as health care. We will return to the problems of making choices in social and health care in the next section of the chapter.

A further source of market failure is the problem of externalities. Levacic (1991, p. 36) says that 'externalities occur when the actions of one economic agent affect the welfare of others in a way that is not reflected in market prices.' There are external costs and external benefits. An example of the former is pollution from productive processes, and an example of an external benefit might be the benefit to a rural community of keeping an uneconomic railway line open. Prices reflect only the costs and benefits to those directly involved in the transaction. The market, by ignoring external costs and benefits, tends to overvalue goods which incur external costs and undervalue goods which confer external benefits. This leads to over-production of the former and under-production of the latter.

Another form of externality is concerned with public goods which confer general benefits from which people cannot be excluded – defence, law and order and public health are the most obvious examples. If a private individual or company were to spend money on a public good they would be faced with 'free riders' – people benefiting from facilities to which they had made no contribution. This is one of the reasons why responsibility for the provision of such services often falls upon public authorities. It is worth noting, however, that the growth of private security firms and the opening of private penal institutions in the United States and the United Kingdom indicates that markets may arise even in the most unpromising areas.

An assumption underlying the private-market case is that the sum total of individual purchasing decisions will result in a sufficient quantity of the goods being produced to satisfy 'social' requirements. The goods in question are sometimes referred to as merit goods, the most notable examples being education and health services. The point here is the existence of externalities which occur when the purchase of a benefit by an individual also results in benefits to others. Purchasers will consider only their individual gain. Education is an example of a service which confers benefits upon society at large over and above those conferred upon the individual. Another example is preventative health services, which may stop the spread of infectious diseases.

Economic theories of markets depend upon assumptions about rational behaviour with providers attempting to maximise profits and consumers attempting to maximise satisfactions/benefits. The study by Forder *et al.* (1996) which was referred to earlier questions the assumption of rational economic behaviour by potential entrants to the social care market. According to classical theory, the rational potential provider could anticipate that existing providers would respond to new entrants by reducing output and price. This is the only way in which the profitability of all (albeit reduced) could be ensured. Assured by this expectation, the rational decision would be to set up the business. But this is very abstract and the authors say that 'many other considerations are relevant . . . and these may take us further away from the view that markets induce efficient behaviour'. One such consideration is that people thinking of entering the market may not conform to the textbook model of the perfectly rational individual. Such a person may conclude that the incumbents are firmly entrenched and will resist pressures to reduce output and prices, inflicting considerable damage on new entrants. If this is the assessment of the potential provider, he/she may decide not to enter the market.

The behaviour of the consumer of social or health care may not be judged rational in the strict economic sense, but decisions to consume, or to refrain from doing so, are not taken solely on the basis of economic rationality. A whole host of considerations enter into the decision, and the overriding factor is what appears rational to the individual concerned. For example, it may be economically rational for a frail elderly person to live with her/his adult children, but this may be unacceptable to both parties for a variety of reasons. An interesting slant on the optimal rationality thesis is provided by communitarian socio-economists. Burkitt and Ashton (1996) explain the communitarian position:

> There is no assumption in communitarian economics that people act rationally, or that they pursue only or largely self-interest. Instead, they are perceived to be moral beings stimulated by moral consider-ations. . . . Communitarian socioeconomists are less deterministic than those of the neoclassical school. Their interactive analysis allows for the possibility of greater flexibility and fluidity in market activity, shape and scope than is allowed for by the individualistic optimal rationality of a neoclassical model.
>
> (pp. 6 and 7)

Etzioni (1988) argues that individuals acting alone are not neces-sarily capable of maximising their own personal advantage; collective decision-making is both more rational and more efficient because 'those involved together can compensate for the cognitive, experi-ence and knowledge limitations of each individual in the group' (Burkitt and Ashton, p. 7). Furthermore, people who are sick, those who are physically or mentally frail or young children may not be in the best position to take hard-headed economically rational deci-sions. This last point connects with the challenge mounted by Titmuss (1967) to the assumption made by those who support market provision that social services in kind, particularly medical care, have no characteristics which differentiate them from goods in the private market. Titmuss identified thirteen ways in which medical care differed from goods normally purchased in the open market. All of them are related in some way to uncertainty and unpredictability and the vulnerability of consumers.[2]

Many of those who advocate market provision of welfare services are, of course, fully aware of the market imperfections briefly touched upon above. Their response would be that the imperfections could be rectified or modified and that even imperfect markets are superior to public provision. As Friedman and Friedman (1980, pp. 263–4) say:

> Perfection is not of the world. There will always be shoddy products, quacks, con artists. But on the whole, market competition, when it is permitted to work, protects the consumer better than do the alternative government mechanisms that have been increasingly superimposed on the market.

The supporters of commercial provision, then, are claiming that the state system is less efficient than the market system. One of the problems is, of course, that if you apply the criteria of the private market to the public system, then obviously the latter may be found wanting. Public provision, it is argued, is inefficient because it lacks the discipline of the marketplace. Bureaucrats have no incentive to reduce costs because they are not constrained to make profits. Consumers have no incentive to restrict demand when goods or services are provided at zero cost or are heavily subsidised. In this situation demand invariably outstrips supply, and in the absence of rationing by price, other forms of rationing have to be adopted (waiting lists and queues, for example). It must be understood, however, that third-party payments (by government or insurance companies) to private providers do not put any pressure on consumers to reduce demand. Unless some form of cost-sharing is introduced, the consumer still receives the service at zero cost. Furthermore, the public system has its own checks and balances: notably political accountability and the possibility of participation. Neither of these is as fully developed or as effective as it might be, but at least the potential is there.

In this section we have looked at the claim that private market provision is more efficient than public provision. The conclusion must be that the case is not proven. In some respects markets perform well, but in others they fall down. Some of the arguments favouring markets are highly theoretical and their relevance to the real world of health and welfare is questionable. There is a general acceptance that efficiency and cost are important and that public authorities have to be accountable for the way public funds are used.

Very often the claims made by supporters and opponents of markets in welfare are based on ideology rather than empirical evidence. If this is true of efficiency issues, it applies with even greater force to choice and freedom and rights and to issues of equity and equality.

Choice, freedom and rights

The debate between Titmuss and Lees in the early and mid-1960s was primarily an argument about choice in welfare. Lees claimed that the ballot box was the only choice open to most welfare consumers. This was unsatisfactory since the ballot box allowed choice only between rival programmes or packages of measures. The vote was too insensitive an instrument for registering choices between specific services. Lees argued that the only way in which consumers could express their preferences was through participation in private markets.

Titmuss's response was to ask: choice for whom? Presumably for those who could afford to pay. Markets respond to demand rather than need, and demand is effective only if it is backed up by the ability to pay. Choice might very well be enlarged for those with sufficient income, but it would be correspondingly reduced for poor people. Furthermore, some social service clients are in no position to make choices – mentally handicapped people, those with psychogeriatric problems and deprived children, for example. But choice is also restricted for people who do not fall into these especially vulnerable groups. It is restricted first of all by lack of knowledge or, more precisely perhaps, by inequalities of knowledge. Most people believe that the teacher, the social worker, the health visitor or the doctor knows best. How do people make choices between competing neurologists when they have no experience on which to base their choice? How do people know whether they are receiving good care or bad care? The truth of the matter is that consumers do not make choices, professionals do. It is the general practitioner, for example, who controls access to hospital and specialist services, and it is the consultant who controls the use of hospital resources. Private markets are unlikely to alter this situation significantly – working-class consumers, in particular, are not going to be more inclined to question a professional's judgement simply because a service is being paid for.

Titmuss argued that markets in health care would not promote choice because of lack of knowledge among consumers. While lack of knowledge is particularly obvious in medical care, it also affects other areas of social provision, as Glennerster (1992, pp. 20–1) points out:

> Where a producer is making a standard product that can be tested comparisons are possible. What characterises most social services is their highly personal nature, and this makes simple, widely available measures of quality difficult to produce. . . . Individual consumers thus face a more difficult prospect operating in these kinds of market than the everyday high street shop. The reasons all have to do with limited and uncertain information.

Green (1997) takes issue with this view which he says is far too paternalistic. He makes three points. First, he turns the argument about uncertainty on its head, arguing that the competitive process is best able to deal with uncertainty about who the best suppliers are, what the charges are likely to be and what consumers know or want. Second, he asserts that it is only through being required to exercise choice that consumers become more knowledgeable and more discriminating. He outlines the implications of this:

> Consequently, well informed consumers are not a *pre*-condition for a market, without which a market cannot work. A vital function of competition is to *allow* consumers to become well informed by giving rise to the comparisons on which judgements can be based. To argue that a competitive market is not possible because consumers are not *already* well informed in practice leads to the continuance of monopoly, which puts them in an even weaker position.
>
> (1997, p. 43)

Third, Green says that the argument that consumers do not have the knowledge to choose is partly based on a failure to distinguish between the expertise possessed by consultants in a particular medical specialty and knowledge about a particular patient's own case. Once an illness has been contracted, the patient has the incentive to acquire the necessary knowledge to understand his/her particular condition.

Green possibly understates the difference in knowledge and the difficulties of altering that position. Even if the patient does understand his/her condition, it does not necessarily equip him/her with the capacity to work the market. This is particularly true in the case of medical specialisms. In general practice there is usually some community knowledge about different practitioners, and choices can be made on the basis of an individual's or family's circumstances. For example, a family with young children or a single elderly person may choose on the doctors' reputations in dealing with young or older age groups, or their willingness to undertake home visits. With specialists, the problem of making choices is much more intractable, particularly in conditions which are relatively rare. In these circumstances, there may be no community knowledge: it is precious little use seeking the advice of a neighbour or friend about choosing between consultants who are completely unknown to them.

The New Right equate freedom in the marketplace with freedom in a general sense. By freedom they usually mean freedom from government intervention. Friedman and Friedman (1980) maintain that 'economic freedom is an essential requisite for political freedom' because it reduces the scope and extent of political power and disperses it among a greater variety of individuals, groups and institutions (p. 21). Hutton (1997) describes what he calls the absurdities of this interpretation:

> The vocabulary of Western liberalism – of freedom, choice, independence and even morality – has been recast to denote thoughts consistent only with competitive economic individualism. Freedom is the freedom to buy and sell; choice, the right to exercise choice in markets; independence is independence from the state; moral conduct, the exercise of individual choice. With the words reprogrammed to have these meanings, any questions that use them have their answers prefigured. Enlarging freedom means enlarging economic freedom; maximising choice means maximising the operation of markets. No public institution can be independent because it is government-owned and financed and the state is collectivist; to be independent therefore implies an institution to be private.
>
> (p. 18)

Individual freedom depends on the ability to participate in markets, but what of those who are excluded through lack of resources? Political freedom must have a hollow sound to those who cannot pay school fees or doctors' bills or who can afford only substandard accommodation. The freedom to do without essential services is a freedom that most people would happily forego. Freedom is more than an absence of government intervention. Indeed, government intervention is essential to the freedom of the poor, the unemployed, the chronically sick, deprived children and the homeless.

It is worth noting at this point that the same faith in markets and their association with political freedom can be observed in many of the former communist countries of Central and Eastern Europe. Orosz (1995) says of Hungary, for example:

> The years 1990 and 1991 were characterised by wild illusions concerning the speed and feasibility of the introduction of a market economy. The view that had evolved over previous decades – that the market economy necessarily entails political democracy – was unassailable. It was also believed that the market would solve the grave inefficiencies in the field of welfare. However, privatisation has not proved to be a universal panacea, and expectations related to the market have considerably diminished.
>
> (p. 94)

The same views were also expressed in many of the other countries of Central and Eastern Europe, and as in Hungary, the disillusion may now be setting in.

The classical liberal view of freedom is merely the absence of coercion or constraint. Gray (1992) rejects this negative formulation of freedom which is, he says, 'a dead end' (p. 21). There is nothing *intrinsically* valuable about the absence of coercion, and 'the value of negative liberty must therefore be theorised in terms of its contribution to something other than itself, which does possess intrinsic value' (p. 22). Gray concludes that the chief value of negative liberty is to be found in the contribution it makes to the positive liberty of autonomy, which he defines as:

> the condition in which a person can be at least part author of his life, in that he has before him a range of worthwhile options, in respect of which his choices are not fettered by coercion and with regard to which he possesses the capacities and resources presupposed by a reasonable measure of success in his self-chosen path among these options.
>
> (p. 22)

In a later publication on communitarian liberalism, Gray (1996, p. 17) claims that 'market exchange makes no inherent contribution to autonomy'. Autonomy is a local virtue rather than a universal one and it is dependent 'on a strong network of reciprocal obligations' (p. 18). Despite Gray's reservations, writers from a wide variety of political perspectives are agreed that autonomy is of immense value in a society, and that markets make a major contribution to it. Miller

(1990, p. 46) puts the point most strongly, stating that, when freedom is defined positively as self-determination, then markets are 'a practically indispensable means of ensuring that people make autonomous choices about matters such as work and consumption'. There would be less agreement about the most appropriate scope of markets, about the need for regulation and about the range of welfare provision thought necessary to enable people to exercise their autonomy.

We saw in Chapter 2 that the principle of autonomy can be used to justify state provision of at least a basic minimum. The argument used there was that autonomy is not guaranteed by markets, and if autonomy were to be used as central principle the government had a responsibility to ensure that the necessary conditions were in place. This argument has some connection with Esping-Andersen's (1990) notions of commodification and de-commodification – concepts which are helpful in explaining variations in market provision, and which have considerable implications for autonomy. The work highlights two key welfare state variables: commodification/de-commodification and social stratification.

Esping-Andersen recognises the central importance of social citizenship in welfare states, but argues that the concept is better understood when it is tied in with the granting of inalienable social rights unrelated to performance which 'will entail a de-commodification of the status of individuals vis-à-vis the market' (p. 21). In addition, it is necessary to consider how status as a citizen relates to class position.

The spread of industrial capitalism and its attendant markets meant that people's survival depended entirely on the sale of their labour, and their welfare became a function simply of the cash nexus. People became commodities. However, 'the introduction of modern social rights implies a loosening of the pure commodity status. De-commodification occurs when a service is rendered as a matter of right , and when a person can maintain a livelihood without reliance on the market' (pp. 20–1). Market dependence is the central issue, and de-commodification is the means by which the dominance of market relations is weakened and autonomy strengthened. It should be noted that contemporary welfare states are unequally de-commodifying; dependence on markets varies considerably from one country to another.

Esping-Andersen contends that the mere existence of benefit

systems does not guarantee de-commodification. The forms in which the benefits are delivered and the rules of entitlement are also important. Thus, in residual welfare states, predominantly based on assistance as opposed to insurance, the receipt of very low levels of benefits is dependent upon needs and means tests; the system debases those who use it. The result, according to Esping-Andersen, is 'actually to strengthen the market since all but those who fail in the market will be encouraged to contract private-sector welfare' (p. 22). Insurance-based systems render benefits dependent upon contributions and work status, and their de-commodifying potential is thus reduced. Similarly, universal systems of the Beveridge type offer only limited de-commodification because benefits tend to be meagre.

There is a strong tendency for welfare states to cluster by regime-types. Esping-Andersen identifies three clusters: the liberal welfare state; the conservative corporatist welfare state; the social democratic welfare state. The liberal welfare state provides modest benefits, with a heavy reliance on means tests and the deliberate imposition of stigma as a deterrent to the 'workshy'. De-commodification is minimal and market provision is extensive. A dual system of welfare develops, with poorer people dependent on state benefits and the better-off buying services on the private market. Esping-Andersen cites Australia, Canada, Japan,[3] Switzerland and the United States as examples of this model. The conservative corporatist model includes Austria, Belgium, France, Germany and Italy. There is a reliance on state insurance schemes, with benefits related to class and status. The social democratic regimes, including Denmark, Finland, The Netherlands, Norway and Sweden, provide high-quality services on a universal basis, with rights enjoyed by all social classes. Esping-Andersen says that this model 'crowds out the market' (p. 28). The United Kingdom is described as a welfare state in transition from a social democratic past to a liberal future.

Esping-Andersen examines the potential of these clusters of welfare state regimes for de-commodification which, it will be recalled, is concerned with freeing people from dependence on the market: the greater the de-commodification, the less the significance of markets. Esping-Andersen devises a set of criteria for measuring de-commodification and for ranking welfare states according to the amount of de-commodification they allow. In an attempt to capture the degree of market independence for the average worker, the scoring system is applied to pensions, unemployment benefits and sickness benefits. One of the weaknesses of the analysis is that it concentrates on income transfers, and takes no account of direct services in kind which might also serve to reduce dependence on the market. There is a rough correspondence between welfare state regimes and the degree of de-commodification. Thus, liberal regimes in Australia, Canada and the United States have low de-commodification scores. At the other extreme, the social democratic regimes of The Netherlands, Denmark, Norway and Sweden (in ascending order) have the highest levels of de-commodification. Austria, France, Germany and Italy, all conservative corporatist regimes, come somewhere in the middle of the de-commodification rankings. There are, however, some discrepancies. For example, Switzerland, characterised as liberal, has a higher score than social democratic Finland; Belgium (conservative corporatist) has a score equal to The Netherlands (social democratic); Japan (liberal) comes eleventh out of eighteen nations. The Central and Eastern European countries are not included in Esping-Andersen's analysis. This exclusion is not surprising, given that the book was published in 1990 and was concerned with welfare capitalism. However, Deacon *et al.* (1992) demonstrate that the models do have some relevance for the former communist countries. The great uncertainty in Central and Eastern Europe – only a relatively short time after considerable political and economic upheaval – makes prediction hazardous. Another problem is the lack of the necessary data. Deacon (1992), while recognising that entirely new forms of welfare may emerge in Central and Eastern Europe, believes that variants of the models in North America and Western Europe are the most likely outcome.

Esping-Andersen's analysis is useful in directing our attention to market dependence. The implications of this are almost the direct opposite of the arguments of Miller (1990) that markets facilitate autonomy. An implication to be drawn from Esping-Andersen is that social rights which release people from market dependence is one way of promoting autonomy or positive freedom. Miller (1989) also argues, on the other hand, that markets may be supported on the grounds that they promote greater freedom to choose the products that one wishes to buy and the supplier one wishes to patronise. They also allow some choice as to the type of work one does and the place in which one does it. On the other hand, markets discriminate against those without the financial capacity to participate effectively in market transactions. We return to the question posed earlier: 'Choice for whom?'.

The argument about choice, freedom and rights has necessarily raised issues of equity and equality. We will now examine these in rather more detail.

Equity and equality

Equality and equity are not, of course, synonymous: equity is concerned with distributional fairness or justice, whereas equality is concerned with giving people the same opportunities and the same access to resources and services. In order to produce equality of outcome, people who start from unequal positions must be allocated different quantities of resources. Equality may not be thought equitable because fairness and justice are seen as requiring unequal rewards for unequal skill and effort.

A distinction has already been made between efficiency and effectiveness; efficiency being connected with costs and outputs, effectiveness more concerned with the degree to which needs are met. Equity and equality are sometimes seen as being in opposition to the principle of efficiency. It is quite feasible to argue, though, that equity, equality and efficiency are all served when need is adopted as the main distributive principle, that is when services are provided effectively. Distribution according to need may result in the most efficient use of resources, because each unit of resource received by those with low command over resources produces more welfare than the same unit received by someone who is relatively well-off. Nevertheless, the demands of equality, equity and efficiency may not always coincide, and when they are in conflict, choices have to be made.

Gray (1996) adopts a communitarian approach to equity. He argues that both neo-liberalism and social democracy fail to see equity in its cultural context by conceiving it in 'simple global terms, as libertarian rights or in a principle of equality' (p. 44). By contrast, Gray believes that norms of fairness must be local and contextual rather than universal and global. Equity should reflect shared local understandings. This adds complexity to the notion of fairness, because there will be conflicting claims that have to be settled by collective decisions. Gray's analysis is firmly rooted in communitarianism and rests on a belief in local communities and in their capacity to re-energise traditional family and community values. If one goes beyond local communities, then rights and equality assume greater importance. Communtarianism emphasises duties and responsibilities rather than rights. Gray's basis in communitarian liberalism, partly explains his focus on shared local understandings. He extends this notion to distributional questions which, he claims should take account of 'shared understandings of need, merit and desert' (p. 55).

The use of the term 'need' poses a number of conceptual problems. It is more difficult to define and measure than demand, which is measured by a customer's ability and willingness to pay the price. There is also the problem of whose needs we are talking about (individuals, families, groups or whole communities) and whose definition of needs is to be accepted. It has to be remembered, too, that needs are relative, varying from culture to culture and over time, and that they are to a considerable extent socially determined. But although the concept of need is beset with problems of interpretation and measurement, its use in social policy is remarkably persistent. At a simple, practical level, it does make sense to talk about people's housing, health, educational and financial needs, and it does make sense to talk of the needs of elderly and disabled people or deprived children.

It is frequently claimed that markets are impersonal and morally neutral. As Miller (1990, p. 72) says, 'much liberal thinking in recent years has been dominated by the principle of neutrality.' He defines an institution or practice as neutral 'when, as far as can reasonably be foreseen, it does not favour any particular conception of the good at the expense of others' (p. 77). Miller claims that markets act neutrally with regard to people's conceptions of the good which are based on the possession, use and exchange of commodities, but that they are less able to deal neutrally with conceptions of the good which extend beyond the private enjoyment of commodities. Notions of the good life that include community and fellowship ideals, for example, are not treated neutrally, and Miller, a market socialist who favours workplace co-operatives, says that markets actively discriminate against co-operative work relations.

The labour market is certainly not neutral: it discriminates on grounds of age, disability, gender and race. Nor is credit, especially mortgages for house purchase, equally available. Even if markets are morally neutral in theory, they are not neutral in their operation or effects. The OECD (1994, p. 12) says 'that policy interventions are necessary both to correct market failure and to promote their smooth functioning particularly in the provision of personal services and intangible investments in human potential'. They explain the argument more fully:

> Unrestrained market forces, in their normal selection process, exclude some individuals from the fruits of competition and from the main stream of society. Social policies pursue the goal of improving well-being through various forms of correction to market processes. Some provide protection against risks such as the loss of income because of unemployment or marital breakdown, and against the consequences of illness or injury, while others alleviate the effects of other misfortunes and the resulting personal hardship.
>
> (p. 12)

This can be illustrated by contrasting need, however imprecisely defined, with alternative distributive principles such as desert and demand. The allocation of social service resources according to need results in a greater degree of equality than either of the alternatives. In most welfare states the principles of need and desert co-exist. The British Poor Law distinction between the deserving and the undeserving poor never entirely disappeared, despite the sheer prejudice surrounding the notion and the difficulties of definition and measurement. Had welfare states unequivocally embraced the principle of need they would have achieved a much greater degree of equality than is presently the case. However, there is every reason to believe that a purely private-market system would result in greater inequalities. Private markets respond to demand; if you cannot pay the price, you do not receive the service. Since people's initial resources vary, some will be able to purchase more than others so that scarce resources will go disproportionately to those who can pay the most. The poor and disadvantaged are the losers.

The answer to the dilemma, according to the neo-liberal economists, is not to provide people with services in kind, but to give them the means of purchasing services from the private market. Ideally, this should be in the form of cash, perhaps through a system of reverse income tax, but vouchers might be used to ensure that the extra resources are spent on specific services. Vouchers will be looked at in a little more detail later, but for the moment it should be noted that, as compared with cash benefits, they deny choice, which is one of the main advantages claimed for private markets. However, marketeers' attitudes towards redistribution are ambivalent, since the market system depends upon unequal rewards. In terms of practical politics, the British government under Thatcher, and the Reagan government in the United States, accepted what they saw as the need for inequality. In relation to Britain, Walker (1990) claims that the greater inequality experienced during the 1980s did not just happen through drift or as the unintended consequences of policies. Inequality was used as a deliberate strategy:

> In sum then, as a conscious act of public policy, the Thatcher administration implemented and sustained throughout the 1980s a radical strategy aimed at widening already substantial inequalities in income and wealth.
>
> (Walker, 1990, p. 41)

This is not to suggest that growing inequalities are solely the result of increased emphasis on markets: there is a whole range of factors implicated in the shift. Nevertheless, marketisation was an integral component of the overall strategy. It is clear that inequalities are an essential feature of markets which could indicate that certain basic services, in which a degree of equality might be thought desirable, should either be provided on non-market lines or that markets in health and social care should be regulated. Britain and the United States experienced growing inequality in the 1980s and early 1990s, and this is partly attributable to reduced state provision and greater reliance on markets or their deregulation. Piven and Cloward (1993) calculate that between 1977 and 1992 the poorest decile of the American population lost 20.3 per cent of its post-tax income while the income of the top 1 per cent increased by 135.7 per cent. The implementation of free market liberal policies in Australia (Watts, 1990), Canada (Riches, 1990) and New Zealand (Shirley, 1990) had similar consequences. Food banks in Canada, New Zealand and Britain recall pre-war soup kitchens and serve as an indictment of free market approaches to welfare.

In Central and Eastern Europe, markets in health and welfare came into being as a consequence of political unrest and the overthrow of what had become unpopular regimes (Dahrendorf, 1990; Glenny, 1990). Deacon (Deacon *et al.*, 1992) says:

> The revolutions of 1989 were clearly at least partly motivated by the wish of significant sections of the population to join in the fruits of western capitalist consumerism. A more or less rapid introduction of

market mechanisms with a pluralization of forms of property is an inevitable outcome of these social changes.

(p. 9)

Deacon sees these changes as having two effects upon social policy: 'a shift in the pattern of social inequality from those based on bureaucratic privilege to those based on market relations', and 'an incursion of market relations directly into the welfare sphere' (pp. 9–10). However, a paper by Szalai and Orosz (1992), indicates that the changes in Hungary have been less far-reaching than the rhetoric would suggest, and that the erosion of the old regime, and the institutions associated with it, began well before 1989. A much more recent assessment by Standing (1996), which extends to the whole of Central and Eastern Europe, shows how conflicting demands were resolved in favour of markets:

After the burst of euphoria around 1989, there was a widespread desire for market freedoms coupled with strong state guarantees of income security. This combination was never feasible or likely to be pursued by governments struggling for domestic and international legitimacy. External pressures to create a specific type of neo-liberal market economy were strong, and adverse distributional outcomes were presented as the short-term pain for long-term gain.

(p. 251)

Inequality is not a major concern of those proposing commercial provision of social services. They assume that most people will be able to afford adequate provision either out of income or through private insurance arrangements. The latter is regarded as particularly significant in health care. Private insurance companies, however, do not accept poor risks such as elderly people, the chronic sick or people with a poor work record. Such people would become the responsibility of a poor-quality residual state system. To say the least, this is socially divisive.

Markets in health and welfare may create greater inequality in a variety of ways:

1. By excluding poor and disadvantaged people from its benefits.
2. By creating a two-tier service.
3. By affecting the distribution of services and enabling more prosperous areas to attract better and more resources.

There are ways of tempering these features of markets. For example, income-related cash benefits or service-specific vouchers could be paid to those who would otherwise be unable to participate in markets except on the most disadvantageous of terms. Positive discrimination in favour of deprived areas or communities is a strategy tried in most countries. Improved and more accessible sources of advice and information would also help, as would tighter consumer protection legislation. Regulation by statutory agencies – monitoring commercial providers and setting minimum standards – may reduce the possibility of exploitation, although regulation is extraordinarily difficult to enforce and can be costly.

Government support of the private market sector in health and welfare may take several forms. Financial support is the most obvious and easily measurable form of encouragement, but governments may be equally important in promoting a system of values which sustains market provision and denigrates public provision. Such a strategy might include the emphasis on an enterprise culture, the promotion of a self-centred 'get-rich-quick' philosophy combined with a crude form of materialism which implies that personal worth is to be judged in terms of income and wealth. Financial backing may be offered in several ways:

1. Tax relief on the contributions to private pension schemes, mortgage repayments, private health insurance or school fees.
2. Certain costs being borne by the state; in the UK, for example, most of the costs of training doctors, nurses, teachers and social workers are met out of public expenditure with the private sector contributing very little.
3. Various forms of partnership.
4. Direct payment of fees for the use of private facilities.
5. The use of vouchers.
6. Systems of reimbursement which may cover costs and include an element of profit.
7. Contracting out in which the government enters into specific contracts with commercial suppliers to provide a particular service at a particular cost.

Contracting out leads directly into a consideration of quasi-markets.

Quasi-markets

There is a growing literature on quasi-markets, particularly in

Britain and the United States, but also from several European countries (Evers and Svetlik, 1993; Johnson, 1995) and from Australia and New Zealand (Domberger and Hall, 1996). Limitations of space prevent an extensive treatment here. All that will be attempted is an outline of the main features of quasi-markets, but readers with a particular interest in this area may wish to follow up some of the references. We will start with a straightforward definition offered by Bartlett (1991):

> In general terms, the quasi-markets revolution involves a process of separation of state finance from state provision of welfare services, alongside the introduction of competition in the provision of services between independent agencies. These agencies may be under private or public ownership, and may have profit or not-for-profit objectives, but are no longer to be under exclusive public control. The agencies involved are to operate systems of service delivery that involve the extension of public choice and competition between private, voluntary or public suppliers within a framework of rules and funding set out by the state.
>
> (p. 2)

Quasi-markets operate in the production and delivery of public services. They arise when finance and provision are split. Thus state agencies cease to be the sole providers of services: they become enablers, commissioners and purchasers. They remain responsible for seeing that services in sufficient quantity and of sufficient quality are provided, but provision is by independent suppliers who may be either commercial or voluntary and in some instances providing arms of the public authority. The idea is for the providing agencies to compete for contracts, one of the main objectives behind quasi-markets being to introduce the discipline of competition into public services. Competition is expected to induce efficiency, increase choice and empower users. Contracts specify what is to be provided, how much of it is to be provided and for whom it is to be provided. Crucially, it includes an agreed price, and there are likely to be a number of quality standards laid down. Arrangements for monitoring and evaluation may also be specified.

Some of the arguments about markets in general also apply to quasi-markets, so that efficiency, choice and freedom and equity issues are all relevant. Some of them have even greater force in quasi-markets. Competition, for example, is restricted by several factors. We noted that Forder *et al.* (1996) found that in social care there was an insufficiency of suppliers and barriers to market entry and exit. There is also a strong tendency for purchasers to use known suppliers and for the contracts of incumbents to be renewed, sometimes over many years. Furthermore, there are important equity considerations in some services which may necessitate reining back competition. This has been the case in the British National Health Service in which 'equity concerns have led to attempts to curb market mechanisms' (Cutler and Waine, 1997, p. 20). Competition gains are likely to be modest therefore, and even those that are achieved may be more than counterbalanced by very high transaction costs in negotiating, managing and monitoring contracts. Costs will also be incurred if purchasers feel forced to intervene to overcome some of the structural and informational imperfections of the market.

This brief look at quasi-markets has almost certainly oversimplified what is a very complex debate. In particular, it has talked about quasi-markets as though they were completely undifferentiated, whereas quasi-markets in different service areas exhibit quite different characteristics. Cutler and Waine (1997), for example, point out some important differences between quasi-markets in health and education. A wider range of quasi-markets is to be found in Le Grand and Bartlett (1993) and Bartlett *et al.* (1994).

The expanding role of private markets in health and welfare

There has been a significant growth in private market provision of health and welfare services over the last twenty years. Stoesz and Midgley (1991, p. 38), in a study of the radical right, state that:

> Within democratic-capitalist states, the commercialization of human services has proceeded rapidly during the last two decades. Proprietary firms have exploited markets in nursing care, hospital management, health maintenance organizations, child day care, and even corrections.

Evidence of the widespread nature of this shift can be found in papers on Australia, Canada, New Zealand, the United Kingdom and the United States (Taylor, 1990). Huber (1996), Goodman and Peng (1996) and Standing (1996) provide evidence relating to Latin

America, East Asia and Central and Eastern Europe respectively. Johnson (1995) looks at the influence of private markets in health and welfare in nine countries spread across Western Europe, North America and Central and Eastern Europe. The details of the changes in each country and their extent do, of course, differ very considerably. In the United States markets have always played a prominent role, especially in health care, and they continue to do so. At the other extreme, private health and welfare markets have never been a major feature of Scandinavian welfare states, and although there have been some changes in this direction, private market provision is relatively undeveloped. The most far-reaching changes have probably occurred in Chile followed by Argentina, New Zealand and Britain. The movement towards markets in Central and Eastern Europe, also represents a big break with the immediate past, although unofficial, often illegal, markets in health care existed during the communist era. The best known of these unofficial arrangements was the 'gratitude money'[4] paid by patients to their doctors in Hungary.

During the last twenty years, the term 'privatisation' has come into use in several different contexts. One use of the term is to describe the sale of public assets – the transfer of nationalised industries to private ownership. Within the social service field privatisation refers to a greater reliance on private markets and on the informal and voluntary sectors in the provision and financing of welfare; it may also imply a reduction in the regulatory role of the state. In this chapter we are concerned with the commercial sector, and our attention now turns to the ways in which private provision – the buying and selling of goods and services – has come to play a more prominent role in the welfare state.

But before we look at the more detailed changes, it should be noted that alternative welfare state strategies might serve to encourage or hinder the development of a vigorous commercial sector within mixed economies of welfare. Although it was written some time ago, Kohl's (1981) analysis of public expenditure trends is still useful. Kohl distinguished between public consumption expenditure (expenditure on direct service provision) and transfer expenditures (for the redistribution of cash incomes). Two basic patterns can be discerned: the Scandinavian pattern, followed by Denmark, Finland, Norway, Sweden, Britain and Ireland, which emphasises direct service provision, and the continental pattern, followed by most other countries in Western Europe, but especially Belgium, Italy, France, The Netherlands and Luxembourg, which emphasises transfer expenditure. Kohl related these patterns to two different approaches to social policy:

> The Continental pattern emphasises the redistribution of cash income relegating final consumption decisions to individual preferences. While this may be an effective way to achieve income maintenance or greater income equality, cash transfers encourage reliance on the market provision of social services and thereby reinforce private modes of producing and delivering such services. . . . The Scandinavian pattern, on the other hand, favors the public provision of services whereby collective choice more directly shapes the structure of supply and the mode of control.
>
> (pp. 313–4)

This helps to explain why the radical right prefers cash benefits rather than services in kind and why they prefer subsidising consumers rather than suppliers.

As part of the drive towards privatisation, purely commercial arrangements have come to play a more significant role in welfare provision and finance in recent years. The mechanisms of the shift of emphasis towards markets may include the following:

1. A general expansion of commercial facilities and services through the usual market processes.
2. The sale of assets (e.g. council houses in Britain and the sale of hospitals and schools).
3. Contracting out either entire services or parts of a service.
4. A reduction in public funding through cost-sharing, charges or reduced subsidies.
5. Fiscal and other financial measures, such as vouchers, designed to promote private provision.
6. The use of more stringent eligibility criteria for the receipt of statutory benefits or services.
7. Deregulation: freeing markets from government intervention and supervision.

Changes of this kind have occurred in nearly all welfare states, although Denmark, Finland, Norway and Sweden have experienced relatively minor modifications. It is tempting to ascribe the changes to centre-right or right-wing governments, and certainly during the early and mid-1980s, such governments were in power in Britain, Canada, Denmark, The Netherlands, the United States and West Germany. On the other hand, Denmark did not experience great ideologically inspired change, and the most market-inspired developments outside South America occurred in New Zealand under a social democratic government. Markets are also popular in Central and Eastern Europe, some of which have social democratic or reformed communist governments which appear to be more firmly neo-liberal than many regimes in Western Europe. Central and Eastern Europe went from state dominance to neo-liberalism without an intervening period of Keynesianism.

The expansion of commercial facilities has been most marked in health care and in residential accommodation, especially for elderly people. Private facilities in health care increased almost everywhere. For example, Standing (1996) says of Central and Eastern Europe that 'commercial private clinics and private access to better facilities have been spreading, while resources devoted to the public health care system have been curtailed' (p. 245). The development in Central and Eastern Europe has been slow, because few people have the necessary resources and the private insurance industry is undeveloped. The private sector in health is small in Sweden for quite different reasons: a highly developed state sector and social democratic notions concerning equity. Nevertheless, the 1980s saw some growth of private medicine in Sweden, the advantage being speedier care rather than better care. The Swedish developments have mainly been very small scale and in units similar to Health Maintenance Organisations in the United States. One such unit opened a hospital in the late 1980s, but less than 6,000 people have any form of private health insurance (Olsson Hort and Cohn, 1995).

It is generally acknowledged that the United States has easily the biggest private sector in health provision in the world, both in terms of total expenditure and as a proportion of all health expenditure. What is less often recognised, however, is that in 1991 the government accounted for 43.9 per cent of all health care spending (European Commission, 1994) and that 54 per cent of the funding for hospitals comes from government (Salamon, 1992). However, government expenditure as a proportion of total health spending is very much higher in European Union countries: the lowest proportion occurred in Portugal (61.7 per cent) and the highest in Luxembourg (91.4 per cent). In the United Kingdom 83.3 per cent of total expenditure was government expenditure; this was higher than the EU average of 78 per cent.

In the United States non-profit hospitals are the major providers of hospital care. The for-profit sector is small by comparison: in 1989 for-profit hospitals constituted 17 per cent of all hospitals with 11 per cent of the total number of beds. This may seem insignificant, but the trajectory of growth has to be considered. Between 1980 and 1989 the for-profit share of hospitals increased by 28 per cent; its share of beds went up by 41 per cent; and its share of expenditure grew by 156 per cent. The main expansion was in short-term specialty hospitals (Salamon, 1992). Nursing home provision in the United States has long been dominated by for-profit providers, in 1987 owning 75 per cent of the establishments and providing 71 per cent of the beds. The main surge of nursing home expansion in the private sector occurred in the 1970s following the introduction of Medicare and Medicaid programmes which promised new and lucrative sources of income. These sources of income became much more stretched in the 1980s as measures were taken to curb the quickly rising costs of Medicaid. Nevertheless, in the early 1980s Laming (1985, p. 18) was still able to write:

> The growth of the nursing home business in the United States has been spectacular. I had contact with one nursing home chain which in 1984 acquired or opened new homes at the rate of one every five days, and some of those homes had 200 or more beds.

Laming quotes the report of a Senate Committee, published in 1983, which found that 'the average return on equity for Texas nursing homes was 33.8 per cent, a rate higher than oil, banks and fast food franchises' (p. 19). Salamon (1992) identifies similarly rapid expansion in the clinic and home health field: 'between 1977 and 1987 the number of for-profit outpatient clinics and related health service establishments increased by 270 per cent, the number of people they employed increased 433 per cent and the revenues they received increased by 493 per cent (p. 65).

The core of the American health care system is its basis in private insurance. There are several problems associated with these arrangements, the most serious being the large numbers without any health cover. The Henry J. Kaiser Family Foundation (1994, p. 2) provides evidence that the number of people under 65 without health insurance on any one day rose from 32.6 million in 1988 to 37.1 million in

1993, an increase of almost five million people in five years. It should be noted that there would be much larger numbers lacking insurance at some time during the year: the Kaiser Foundation estimates that 51.3 million people fell into this category in 1993, and a third of these (18.2 million) were without health insurance for the entire year. There would be still more with inadequate insurance. It should be emphasised that these figures do not include those using Medicaid and Medicare. More recent figures quoted by Phillips (1996) indicate that the number of uninsured continued to rise, exceeding 40 million on any one day in 1996 (p. 70).

Medicaid and Medicare, introduced in 1965, represented a major extension in government responsibility for health care. Medicare was designed for older people who contributed to the scheme during their working lives. Medicaid was specifically aimed at poor people, but it is used by many among the non-poor. There has been widespread concern about the rapidly escalating costs of Medicaid which covered 12.2 per cent of the population in 1993 (Summer and Shapiro, 1994). We saw in Chapter 2 that attempts have been made to cut the cost of Medicaid and Medicare by successive American administrations. This takes three forms: (i) increasing the proportion of deductibles and co-payments, ensuring that patients bear a part of the cost (ii) reducing the amounts reimbursed to providers (iii) specifying maximum costs for treating particular illnesses through a procedure known as diagnosis related groups (DRGs). The gradual erosion of Medicare benefits has meant that elderly people now have to find approximately 50 per cent of medical bills out of their own pockets or supplementary insurance.

The lower rates of reimbursement and the other restrictions have led to a reluctance on the part of some for-profit hospitals to willingly accept Medicaid patients. Currie (1990) demonstrates that this is part of a more general problem:

> In the face of increased needs and simultaneous cost-cutting pressures, many hospitals now routinely practise what's often called 'wallet diagnosis'; it is the patient's insurance status, rather than medical condition, that determines what kind of care they will receive or indeed whether they will receive care at all. The process is dramatically illustrated by the sharp rise in 'patient dumping' in the 1980s.
> (p. 311)

During the 1980s there was a rapid rise of new forms of health service provision in the United States. The most prominent of these were Health Maintenance Organisations (HMOs): prepaid group schemes which usually offer a full range of medical services for a fixed annual fee or monthly sum: in 1996 there were 58 million subscribers. In some cases doctors are employees of the HMO, in others they are under contract to an HMO. Originally, most HMOs were non-profit agencies, but this has changed so that now the majority are for-profit enterprises, and the operation of some of them is giving cause for concern. Phillips (1996), for example, says that there is widespread unease about the cost-cutting programmes of some HMOs which are thought to be unduly restricting the care available to subscribers. According to Phillips (1996, p. 71) some HMOs operate 'gag rules' which 'forbid doctors . . . from telling patients about treatments that the plan's managers regard as too expensive. Another form of gag is designed to prevent doctors criticising the HMO. Another initiative has resulted in Preferred Provider Organisations which negotiate contracts with an insurance company which pays discounted fees-for-service directly to the provider. The commercial insurance companies have moved into these managed forms of care, so that vertical integration takes place: one organisation providing both insurance and medical care. As Navarro (1994) says:

> The insurance companies already control large areas of health services delivery, through HMOs, preferred provider organizations, and other forms of prepaid group practice. Eighty-two percent of the delivery system is now under some form of managed care, contracted by, controlled by, and/or influenced by insurance companies.
>
> (p. 209)

One of the advantages claimed for free markets is the way in which they simultaneously enlarge choice and empower consumers. It is quite clear that neither advantage accrues to health service consumers in the United States. The power lies with the huge insurance companies and the large health care corporations.

Considerable space has been devoted to health care in the United States, because it is probably the best example of an important human service dominated by markets. The example tells us something about the operation of markets in the health and welfare field, and may serve as a warning to those countries contemplating a greater role for markets in their own health services.

The National Health Service (NHS) in the UK is organised along quite different principles from the American system of health care. The NHS is still essentially a public system, financed mainly from taxation. However, it is useful to consider changes during the last twenty years towards a more market-oriented system.

Among the earliest initiatives was the contracting out of non-clinical NHS services. After 1983, health authorities were *required* to put services out to competitive tender. Many of the contracts were won by in-house bids, and there was some dissatisfaction with the quality of some services. More recently other services have been contracted out or sold off to private operators (e.g. computing and information technology). The Conservative governments of the 1980s and 1990s were concerned to encourage private practice within and outside of the NHS.

In 1979 there were 150 independent acute hospitals in the United Kingdom, with 6,671 beds overall. By December 1993, the number of hospitals had increased to 224, with 11,391 beds. This proved to be a peak, however, because in 1995 and 1996 the number of beds in independent hospitals fell slightly to 11,098 beds in 221 units by 1996.

Private practice *within* the NHS centres around the once controversial issue of pay beds. Since the NHS and Community Care Act there has been a rapid expansion of pay beds, with some of the hospital trusts refurbishing areas of their buildings and setting up private patient units. According to the *Fitzhugh Directory* (Brindle, 1996) more than fifty trusts each made more than £1 million in 1995 and seven of these made more than £5 million. By 1995 the NHS had become the largest single provider of private care in the UK, income from private patients increasing from £83 million in 1988 which represented 11.2 per cent of the total market to £230 million, representing 15.1 per cent of the total market, in 1995.

Partnership arrangements are also a way in which the NHS can generate income from private health care. Partnerships have been given a boost by the development of the Private Finance Initiative (PFI) launched in 1992. Every regional office now has a PFI specialist in post whose job is to advise on and promote partnerships. In return for a long lease of a ward or unit or of adjacent land on which to build private facilities, a private operator will invest capital and make regular, fixed payments to the health authority. Usually the independent partner will buy ancillary services from the health authority. So far, however, development has been slow.

The reforms implemented under the NHS and Community Care Act of 1990 were expected to have the effect of encouraging private health care. Individual hospitals, while remaining in the NHS, have been given the opportunity to become independent of the district health authorities by forming self-governing Hospital Trusts, controlling their own funds and appointing their own staff. The trusts are expected to compete for contracts with private and conventional NHS hospitals, and they have been encouraged to enter into joint arrangements with private companies and to extend contracting out by means of competitive tendering. At the same time, the slimmed-down district health authorities, in securing services for their populations, were encouraged to shop around for the best deal and to make use of private facilities wherever this seemed appropriate. It is interesting to note that many other countries in the EU are making tentative moves in the direction of contracting (European Commission, 1995).

Much of the development of private medicine has been associated with an expansion of private medical insurance. Taking the figures relating to the three major provident insurers, the number of subscribers more than doubled between 1979 and 1990, increasing from 1.3 million to 2.7 million. The number of people insured almost doubled in the same period, increasing from 2.8 million to 5.4 million. The Department of Health, using data from all private insurers, says that 1990 was a peak year for private insurance with 6.7 million people covered. Between 1990 and 1995 there was a 14 per cent fall in the number covered to 5.7 million. The recession, combined with increased claims and higher medical bills, has brought an end to the years of very rapid expansion. Greatly reduced profitability between 1990 and 1993 has discouraged potential new entrants among insurance companies, and those already operating in this area are imposing 'stringent new rules for medical treatment' under which 'subscribers must now get approval from their insurers before starting treatment.' (Ferriman, 1992). The number of subscribers is now virtually static.

The spectacular growth of private nursing homes in the United States was followed a decade later in the UK. Until 1987 the figures for nursing home places combined private and voluntary provision: in 1980 the combined total was 26,900, and by 1986 this had risen to 47,900. The figures for later years indicate where the main expansion had taken place: in 1995, private nursing homes provided 191,000 places, compared with 17,000 in voluntary homes. This meant that 73 per cent of nursing home places were provided by the private sector, as compared with 6.5 per cent provided by the voluntary sector and 20.5 per cent provided by the public sector.

Nursing homes are one form of residential provision. Although in the UK there is separate registration for nursing homes and for accommodation without nursing attention, the forms overlap in the provision of care for frail elderly people. The growth in UK non-nursing residential accommodation matched that of nursing homes in the 1980s and early 1990s. In 1980, local authorities owned 45.8 per cent of all residential homes for older people and provided 62.7 per cent of the places; the private sector owned 34.7 per cent of the homes, contributing 17.4 per cent of the places, and the voluntary sector owned 19.5 per cent of the homes, and provided 19.9 per cent of the places. By 1995 the picture had changed dramatically: local authorities owned only 17 per cent of the homes, providing 26.8 per cent of the places; private homes constituted 67.75 per cent of the total, providing 55.7 per cent of the places, and the voluntary sector owned 15.2 per cent of the homes, contributing 17.5 per cent of the places. Between 1980 and 1995 the number of places in local authority residential homes fell by almost 40 per cent, while the number of places in private homes more than quadrupled.

Most countries have a private element in their residential provision. In the United States the private sector is the major provider of residential care for older people and it has a substantial presence in child welfare institutions. The private residential care sector is also dominant in Canada and Japan. In Scandinavia, Germany and The Netherlands, however, the private sector is relatively small; in Germany and The Netherlands the voluntary sector is a major provider of residential care. Initially, residential homes tended to be small family businesses, but a noticeable trend, especially in the UK and the United States, has been the entry into this market of large companies with diverse interests. Another recent development has been the diversification of residential care providers into day care and domiciliary care (e.g. meals-on-wheels).

In the UK, the rapid development of private residential and nursing homes could not have occurred in the absence a massive state subsidy in the form of income support payments. In 1979 the Department of Health and Social Security (DHSS) contributed £10 million to the fees paid by residents in private and voluntary homes, but by 1991 the bill had risen to almost £1.9 billion. Given the overwhelming dominance of private homes within the independent sector, the vast bulk of this money must have gone to private operators. Those running the homes frequently claimed that the amounts were inadequate, and residents in some instances were being asked to make up the difference between benefits and fees, and sometimes to pay for extras, which could include medical dressings, diabetic diets, nursing care during illness, chiropody and physiotherapy. The system was discontinued in 1993, when responsibility for financing residential care passed to local authorities.

An OECD study (1993) describes the subsidy to cover residential costs as a quasi-voucher. I am not at all convinced that the term quasi-voucher is particularly helpful. It is simply a consumer subsidy (as opposed to a producer subsidy). However, the OECD study claims that the UK scheme had the effect of quickly diversifying provision, but that it was very costly and distorted the market in favour of residential care, because the alternatives received no subsidy. The same study looked at housing vouchers in the United States. The study says:

> The American housing voucher programme is regarded as an unequivocal success. Designed to help low income earners facing the worst housing conditions and the greatest rent burden, it has reached the target population as well or better than the supply side or rent supplement alternatives, and has done so at lower administrative cost and with greater real income benefits to the recipients. Total outlays under the programme have been tightly controlled, its scope is being expanded, and fears that subsidies would end up in landlords' pockets through rent increases have not materialised.
>
> (p. 50)

Consumers' views are not reported. A quite different view of the provision of social housing in the United States is to be found in Currie (1990).

Vouchers are seen by their proponents as helpful in encouraging private providers and in promoting competition, but being product-specific, they are less effective in this respect than cash transfers. The use of vouchers and quasi-vouchers is becoming more widespread. For example, in the United States voucher schemes have been introduced in several states in relation to education and training, and food stamps are a direct form of voucher. The purpose behind these developments is identified by O'Connor (1998, p. 53) who says that 'the White House created incentives for parents to purchase child-care in the private market by increasing tax credits and demand-side vouchers'. Education vouchers are also used in Sweden and quasi-vouchers are extensively used in Australia (see Lyons, 1995). A recent experiment in the UK involved the use of vouchers in nursery education, with a view to their more general introduction at a later date. As in most voucher schemes, consumers could add money of their own. The scheme was not notably successful, the Labour opposition describing it as a 'bureaucratic nightmare'. Furthermore, the objectives of increasing private provision and facilitating greater consumer choice did not materialise: indeed, in order to benefit from the vouchers, ordinary schools began to take children of four.

Neo-liberals regard vouchers as infinitely superior to direct state provision, but only as a second-best alternative to cash benefits. They may be prepared to accept vouchers as an interim measure before the introduction of full market provision. An alternative to cash benefits, favoured by neo-liberals, are what are known as tax expenditures. Such measures, rather than paying direct cash benefits, achieve a similar effect by not deducting tax for certain items of expenditure in the first place. Unlike cash benefits, however, tax expenditures allow governments greater discretion to manipulate the tax system to reduce or increase redistribution and to reward particular patterns of expenditure. Thus private pension provision may be encouraged by allowing tax relief on contributions. Tax relief on mortgage repayments may be used to encourage house purchase.[5] The tax expenditure system consists of tax allowances (e.g. for children); tax reliefs (e.g. on pension contributions) and tax exemptions (e.g. on certain disability and housing benefits). Sandford (1993, p. 20) in a review of tax reforms in six countries states that 'tax reform was part of a wider movement to push back the boundaries of the state and revert to free markets'. This quotation appears in a paper comparing tax expenditures in Denmark and the United Kingdom (Kvist and Sinfield, 1997). They explain the basis of Sandford's analysis: 'Many tax expenditures were removed to widen the tax base while the reduction in tax rates also reduced the cost of those tax expenditures which remained' (p. 250). Kvist and Sinfield say that the evidence from Denmark and the UK is equivocal in that there have been reductions in tax expenditures in some areas and increases in others. Those readers wishing to know more about this complex topic may care to refer to Kvist and Sinfield or to a 14-country study by the OECD (1996).

At several points in this chapter we have referred to charges and co-payments, but this material needs to be brought together and expanded. Obviously, if charges are introduced or increased in the public sector, the comparative cost of using the private sector is reduced. In the UK, for example, massively increased prescription charges, the introduction of ophthalmic and dental consultation charges, increased public sector rents and increased charges for meals-on-wheels and home helps all had the effect of increasing the attractiveness of the private market sector. Increasing co-payments in the American health care system, with consumers meeting a higher proportion of the costs, have already been referred to. A similar change has occurred in France. Huard, Mossé and Roustang (1995, p. 75) say that 'the proportion of costs borne by the patient, after having diminished during the 1970s, has not stopped increasing since'. Castles (1996, p. 109) says that during the 1980s 'New Zealand made user charges a major component of its once universal health care system'. Belgium has also increased charges as the European Commission (1995, p. 110) indicates: 'In order to expand finance, charges were increased significantly in 1994, continuing the policy of imposing a greater share of the cost of care on patients'.

In this section we have been concerned with the buying and selling of services. Although occupational welfare, which we consider next, is based on different principles, it is most appropriately dealt with in a chapter on markets.

Occupational welfare

One of Titmuss's three social divisions of welfare was occupational welfare. In spite of the fact that Titmuss identified this form of welfare in 1956, surprisingly limited attention has been paid to it since. It is particularly important to take it into account when comparing welfare states internationally, because the importance of occupational or workplace welfare varies considerably from country to country.

Occupational welfare schemes can be initiated by employers, trade unions and professional associations or by both jointly. The incentive for employers to initiate schemes is that they may help in the recruitment and retention of staff, although this applies more in times of labour shortage. Health insurance is advantageous to an employer because it allows employees to choose times for treatment which are least disruptive of their work. Trade unions have a long tradition of offering friendly benefits to members. This may partly be a matter of solidarity, but it may also be seen as a way of attracting members.

Examples of extensive systems of occupational welfare were to be found in the countries of Central and Eastern Europe (including the former republics of the Soviet Union) *before* 1990. Current examples include Communist China, Japan and the United States. A brief comment about each might be instructive.

Enterprises in Central and East European countries operated an extensive range of social benefits: these included pensions, health services and even housing and education. Standing (1996) says:

> . . . the distribution of benefits was heavily focused on enterprises, which in the main were huge industrial combines with many thousands of workers. . . . What emerged were 'company towns', in which one or two giant enterprises dominated not just the industrial landscape but the range and level of social, cultural and educational services in the community. Entitlement was based on one's role and duration of employment in the enterprise.
>
> (p. 228)

Since 1990, many enterprises have discontinued or cut down their welfare activities in order to compete more effectively in European and international markets.

China, still recognisably communist, continues to rely heavily on occupational welfare, despite the government's efforts to reduce the cost to industry. Leung (1994) indicates the important role of workplace welfare: 'For more than three decades after the establishment of the People's Republic of China, government commitment to occupational welfare was unanimously conceived as a superior feature of socialism and was never challenged or even in doubt' (p. 349). Traditionally, it was the large state-owned enterprises that provided the most extensive and generous welfare benefits which included: comprehensive social security programmes; medical care (including hospitals); subsidies on food, clothing, housing and transport; schools; libraries; cultural and recreational facilities. Outside the state-owned enterprises benefits were much more restricted. The rising cost of pensions and other forms of social protection and of health care have led the government to search for reforms. The costs to enterprises are believed to be hampering their economic performance and work units are now being expected to contribute to pensions and medical care.

It is interesting to note the similarities between Japan, the former communist countries of Central and Eastern Europe and China. As in the other two areas, occupational welfare in Japan is mainly the preserve of larger companies and 'company towns' are one result. The range of benefits provided by the big companies in Japan is similar to those provided in Central and Eastern Europe and China: pensions and other social security benefits; housing; health services; education; cultural and recreational facilities. A further similarity is the pressure, with relatively minor effects at present, to reduce occupational provision to improve global competitiveness, particularly from the Pacific rim.

Esping-Andersen (1997), however, also notes similarities between Japan and the United States:

> If we turn to market-provided welfare, the Japanese regime is similar to the American. The huge fabric of company provided social benefits that one finds in Japan has its obvious roots in the residualism of public provision. Bargained welfare filled the empty void of the welfare state, and once it took hold and expanded it probably had a dampening effect on popular demand for an improved welfare *state*.
>
> (p. 184)

Occupational pension and health cover in the United States expanded rapidly during the years following the Second World War. There was a relative shortage of labour, and the labour unions, having despaired of Congress ever agreeing to the introduction of national health insurance or the extension of social security, began to press for occupational cover. The administration encouraged this development, realising that it would head off demands for more radical programmes. The United States is as clear a case as Japan of occupational welfare being used as an *alternative* to state provision. Once again, it is the bigger corporations which more often provide benefits. Navarro (1994, p. 207), for example, claims that 'one-third of small businesses do not provide any health benefits coverage to their employees and their dependents'. This is because for many small employers 'current premiums are prohibitively high'. The same pressures to be competitive have resulted in substantial reductions in occupational welfare since the late 1980s. Esping-Andersen (1996, p. 8) shows that the occupational coverage of medical care and retirement have 'declined dramatically during the past decade'. The proportion of the population whose health insurance coverage was employment-related declined from 62 per cent in 1988 to 58 per cent in 1992 and 57.2 per cent in 1993 and it was still falling (Summer and Shapiro, 1994, pp. 4–5). It is disturbing that the number of uninsured people continues to rise even in a long-term boom, but Phillips (1996, p. 70) says that 'many companies have replaced full-time employees with part-timers and contract workers who do not get medical insurance benefits'.

Pensions are without doubt the most common of the occupational benefits. They are to be found in all industrial countries, although the relationship between occupational and state pensions varies considerably. Coverage of occupational pension schemes is usually uneven, with male workers receiving more benefits than females, and non-manual workers more than manual.

Pensions in Britain have been surrounded in controversy in the 1990s. The origins of the controversy occurred in 1988 when employees were given direct subsidies to transfer from either the State Earnings-Related Pension Scheme (the second-tier public scheme) or their occupational scheme to a private pension. In the event, about 6 million people transferred, about 1.5 million from occupational schemes and the remainder from the State Earnings-Related Pension Scheme. It is estimated that as many as 1 million of those transferring may be worse off as a consequence. There has been much criticism of private pension providers (mainly insurance companies) for their sales methods and for misinforming potential customers transferring from other schemes. In the middle of all this there was the Maxwell scandal when it transpired that the owner of the *Daily Mirror* had misappropriated money from the employees' pension funds. The government was forced to introduce more effective regulation of the private pensions industry.

The European Commission (1996, p. 16) says that the 'UK is the only EU state in which private pension schemes, including both company schemes and individual arrangements, can substitute for part of the statutory scheme rather than simply supplementing it'. The Commission report says that the UK's experience illustrates 'two fundamental truths about privatisation':

> If the government has an overall policy on social protection in which the private sector is expected to play a significant role, the sector must be regulated to ensure that it discharges its responsibilities, and

the greater the responsibilities the greater the regulation. Secondly market forces cannot be relied upon to entice the private sector to play as large a role as the government might desire and it usually has to turn to fiscal incentives or direct subsidies.

(p. 17)

This is by way of a warning to Italy and Spain who are attempting to encourage the growth of private pensions.

The Labour Government in the UK is considering proposals to boost occupational pension schemes by compelling all employees to contribute to private occupational pensions. This would involve people building up personal pension funds, the amount of pension depending on the investment performance of the provider. This would replace the present pay-as-you-go system of financing pensions in which present contributors pay for present pensions. Entirely private pensions (stakeholder pensions) will also be available, principally for those who are unable to join an occupational scheme. This plan, which is purely exploratory at present, follows the arrangements in Australia and Singapore. Although compulsory, these pensions are essentially private in form. It is interesting to note that Sweden is experimenting with individual accounts, but within a state scheme. The World Bank (1994) has given its blessing to pensions consisting of minimum flat-rate state pensions (preferably means-tested) with the bulk of pensions coming from funded private pensions. This has added to the pressure on Central and East European countries to adopt this pattern.

Day care is another important occupational benefit, and in the absence of publicly provided facilities, employers may find it advantageous to offer workplace day care for young children. This may be particularly significant for those with a predominantly female workforce. In the UK, which has very few public facilities, a group of industrialists have formed a group entitled Employers for Childcare. Another commercial organisation, launched in America and Canada in 1985 but established in the UK in 1997, is Work/Family Directions which sells its services to companies, offering advice to both employers and employees about work–child care relationships.

So far we have concentrated on employer-based schemes, but occupational welfare also includes services provided by trade unions. At one time trade unions offered a wide range of friendly benefits, but this role declined as unions became more involved in negotiating over working conditions and pay with employers, and as statutory benefits became more generally available. In Sweden and Denmark, however, trade unions play an active role in the administration of unemployment insurance. Ginsburg (1992) describes the Swedish system:

> The unemployment insurance benefit (UIB) system is a clear exception to the universalism and direct public sector provision generally characteristic of the Swedish welfare state. UIB is administered by voluntary societies under the control of the trade unions, and financed by government, trade union and employer contributions.
>
> (p. 41)

Trade unions in Denmark are similarly involved in the administration of unemployment insurance (Toft, 1996). In Germany, social insurance is delegated to a mass of semi-autonomous institutions in which the unions participate. In the UK and the United States, the unions are not at all involved in the administration of social insurance, although instances can be found of trade union involvement in occupational welfare in both countries. The powerful Teamsters labour union, for example, handles the health and pensions schemes for the whole of the road transport industry in the United States. In the UK, the miners' unions have traditionally been extensively involved in welfare provision, and trade unions have been known to assist members to purchase private health insurance.

Before leaving the topic of occupational welfare, some of its potential drawbacks must be considered. There are some very clear equity issues, in that welfare depends upon work status. When welfare is dependent upon employment, the unemployed are excluded, as are many of those in part-time work and all of those in casual work; self-employed people are also outside of the occupational welfare system. China is an interesting example. Employment in state-owned enterprises is at present permanent (meaning for the whole of an employee's working life). Work outside of the state firms is increasingly on a fixed term contract basis. The distinction is an important one, because permanent employees make no contribution to pension and other benefits, whereas contract workers are required to contribute 3 per cent of their wages to a pension fund and work units pay a contribution equivalent to 15 per cent of the payroll. The Chinese government wishes to extend the contributory system to the whole of the economy, but the political consequences of withdrawing free benefits of long standing may be serious (Leung, 1994). As has been noted in Japan and the United States it is also an advantage to work in a large company. It is pertinent to note that in many economies most of the new jobs that are being created are in small businesses which receive direct encouragement from governments.

Another drawback is the effect of occupational benefits on mobility, leading to labour market inflexibilities, at a time when other influences are working in the opposite direction. This may be less of a problem in Japan where lifetime involvement with a company is still quite common. Lifetime involvement and the certainty of employment and old-age benefits, while undoubtedly attractive, also has the less appealing connotation of the pervasive influence of the company in employees' lives. For example, the company may take precedence over family, and employees may have to demonstrate unswerving loyalty to their employers.

Employers looking for ways of cutting costs, in an effort to become more competitive or in times of recession, may regard welfare benefits as an easy target. In conditions of labour surplus occupational welfare may decline, only to expand again if a labour shortage develops. This makes occupational welfare less stable and less predictable than statutory provision.

Conclusion

Over the last decade, markets have enjoyed a great deal of favourable publicity. Even committed socialists have come to accept the value of markets, and the countries of Central and Eastern Europe and the former Soviet Union have also now embraced the market system. Barry (1991, p. 231) claims that 'One of the most striking features of the development of social science over the last decade has been the re-establishment of the intellectual respectability of the decentralized market exchange system as a social institution.' Later in the same paper he says that 'The market at the moment is on the threshold of a new era of intellectual popularity.' He attributes this not merely to changes in fashion, but to 'the observed failures of alternative social and economic arrangements' (p. 241).

Taylor (1990, p. 5) takes an entirely different view of the apparent popularity of markets. He suggests that 'It may be the international growth of consumerism as such which has achieved "popularity" rather than the fact that such consumerism is presently being fed, in many western societies, by "deregulated" free market institutions.' This echoes Deacon's (Deacon *et al.*, 1992, p. 9) comment, referred to earlier in the chapter, that the 1989 revolutions in Central and Eastern Europe were 'partly motivated by the wish of significant sections of the population to join in the fruits of western capitalist consumerism'.

A significant feature of the greater emphasis on markets has been the degree to which public institutions have accepted market ideology and incorporated it into the processes of public policy making. Citizens have become customers, and market testing, competition and performance indicators have permeated the public sector. Similarly, as we shall see in the next chapter, voluntary organisations are also affected by the market. If they have to compete for contracts with commercial enterprises, they are obliged to take on some of the features of those with whom they compete. The question arises of how far the purposes of a mixed economy of welfare are served by the dominance across all sectors of a market ethos. Hutton (1997) challenges this dominance:

> Different ethical values apart from the market ethic must be protected; trust, fairness and the acceptance of obligations should not be seen as tiresome obstacles to the creation of economic efficiency, but as central to it. Human values need to be incorporated into the core of market processes not merely to produce a kinder, more tolerant society – fundamental though that is – but to enable the market economy to function better.
>
> (p. 13)

Choice for consumers is another claimed benefit of a market-led system. The argument throughout this chapter has been that markets may extend choice for those with the means of participating but reduce it for those excluded from full participation. Neo-liberals claim that markets are empowering, but markets also have the capacity to disempower. As Walker (1993) notes:

> Having a range of theoretical alternatives will not make the consumer sovereign if she cannot exercise effective choice. Moreover, a financial transaction does not necessarily mean the bestowal on the purchaser of either influence or control over the provider. . . . In other words, the private sector exercises equivalent power over users to public providers but it does not necessarily carry the same responsibility.
>
> (p. 80)

But the major debate is no longer about the relative merits of a market system as compared with a centrally planned system. The major questions now revolve around such issues as the most appropriate size and scope of the market, the degree of regulation that is thought to be desirable and the degree to which government ought to intervene to enhance certain groups' ability to participate in the market and modify market outcomes. Is there still a case for keeping certain services out of markets altogether? These are by no means new concerns in social policy, but they have gained particular significance in the light of recent changes in both western capitalist countries and in Central and Eastern Europe.

Having examined the for-profit sector, attention now switches to a group of organisations (the voluntary sector) in which the profit motive is absent.

Notes

1. For an overview of public choice theory see McLean (1987). A critical analysis of the theory is provided by Dunleavy (1991).
2. I am fully aware that this analysis was published by Titmuss over thirty years ago, but it is still extremely relevant and I am aware of no better treatment in more recent years.
3. In a more recent work (1997) Esping-Andersen discusses the Japanese welfare state in more detail. He concludes that at present the Japanese system is an amalgam of the conservative 'Bismarckian' regime and liberal residualism.
4. Could be either cash or goods (e.g. farm or garden produce). The system was in general use throughout Hungary.
5. It is instructive to note that the value of mortgage tax relief has been eroded by successive budgets in the UK, and the present Labour Government has signalled its intention to abolish it altogether.

CHAPTER 4

THE VOLUNTARY SECTOR AND SOCIAL WELFARE

Introduction

In this chapter attention switches to the voluntary sector. There are three major links with the previous chapter. The first is that voluntary organisations have become in an increasing number of countries participants in quasi-markets, perhaps competing with commercial providers. A second link arises from some blurring at the margins between large voluntary organisations and commercial operators; the language and practices of the market have invaded the voluntary sector. Third, the greater prominence given to both voluntary organisations and private market suppliers is part of the more general policy of reducing state provision and relying more on the other three sectors.

The use of voluntary organisations as providers of health and welfare services has a long history in most countries, and it is surprising that until recently the role of the voluntary sector in social policy was virtually ignored by academics and politicians alike. Kuhnle and Selle (1992, p. 1) refer to the lack of emphasis in the social policy literature: 'Theoretical and empirical studies of the place and role of voluntary organizations have been almost completely absent in the extensive literature over the last twenty years on the historical development of welfare states.' This echoes similar sentiments expressed by other authors. Gidron, Kramer and Salamon (1992, pp. 2–3) for example, claim that 'because it has been overlooked for so long in scholarly research and public debate, the private, non-profit sector is one of the least understood components of modern society.'

Although there is certainly some truth in these observations, the position is rapidly changing. There are now four scholarly journals published in English devoted entirely to voluntary sector studies, and the editors of one these have described their field as 'one of the most energetically innovative areas of study' in social science (Anheier and Knapp, 1990, p. 7). Kramer *et al.* (1993, p. 1) write: 'During the years since the mid-1970s there has been a tremendous upsurge of public interest in North America and Western Europe in the role of voluntary non-profit organizations as an alternative to government in the provision of quasi-public services.' Nor has the 'upsurge' been restricted to Western Europe and North America: it has been a truly worldwide development, encompassing countries with quite different histories and cultures and at different stages of development.

Academic interest in the voluntary sector has burgeoned. Every year more scholarly books and articles appear. Anheier and Seibel (1990, p. 3) estimated that there were over 200 researchers in forty different countries engaged in this area. This figure will now have been augmented by scholars in Central and Eastern Europe and in the developing countries. In the United States the *Independent Sector* (1993) identified thirty-five academic centres and programmes 'focusing on the study of philanthropy, voluntarism, and not-for-profit activity'; thirteen of these were newly established. This richness is not matched elsewhere, but most developed countries have several centres specialising in this field, and similar centres are being established in Central and Eastern Europe and in developing countries. The position is summed up by Hodgkinson and McCarthy (1992, p. 2): 'What began as a trickle of scholarly interest in the early 1980s has grown to genuinely global dimensions.'

Terminology and definitions

Readers may very well have noticed the varying terminology used so far in this chapter. It is now time to clarify terms and definitions. In the United Kingdom, Scandinavia, and sometimes in Italy, the terms used are 'voluntary organisations' and the 'voluntary sector'. The word 'voluntary' does not refer to the characteristics of the personnel, who may very well be paid; it refers rather to the manner in which the organisations were set up and the voluntary nature of membership or other forms of involvement. The common practice in the United States is to make a very broad distinction between the public and the private sectors and then to sub-divide the private sector into non-profit and for-profit organisations. The non-profit sector corresponds to the voluntary sector; the term 'non-profit' is suited to the American situation because 'the organizations are defined primarily in terms of their eligibility for exemption from federal income taxes on grounds that they are not principally profit-seeking' (Gidron *et al.*, 1992, p. 3). This does not mean that profits or surpluses are not made; the crucial distinctions are that profit maximisation is not the prime purpose of non-profit organisations and profits are not distributed among shareholders as they would be in a for-profit enterprise.

Because American scholars have pioneered research into the sector, the term non-profit has gained some acceptance in other countries. Gidron *et al.* (1992), Kramer *et al.* (1993) and Seibel (1992) reject the terms voluntary sector and non-profit sector in favour of a term which is widely used in Europe, and sometimes in the United States: the third sector. Seibel (1992, p. 206) prefers this term 'for both pragmatic and theoretical reasons'. He argues that analytically the term 'assumes a "third" type of organization, with a different style of organizational behavior as compared with private business or state bureaucracy.' The term, in my view, has one serious, and possibly fatal, flaw. It rests on the assumption that there are only three sectors, and ignores the informal sector. This is one of the shortcomings of much of the American work in this area.

The least acceptable of the terms in current usage are the terms non-governmental sector and non-governmental organisations. They are far too general to be of much use. They are sometimes used in developing countries – especially by the United Nations development agencies. A reasonable interpretation of the term could be to include all organisations outside government – an amalgam of the private market, voluntary and informal sectors.

Finally, the French use a much broader term, *économie sociale,* which includes co-operatives, savings and credit banks, mutual societies and associations. Archambault (1993, p. 1) refers to the sector's 'internal balkanization into distinct sub-components – a consequence of both the different legal treatments afforded to non-profit organizations, and the distinct political and religious orientations of major subsectors.' It is the associations which correspond most closely to voluntary or non-profit organisations elsewhere, and it is these which are most heavily involved in health and welfare provision.

The terminology is confusing and presents problems for those interested in cross-national comparisons. Salamon (1992) argues that all of the terms are misleading because they 'emphasize one aspect of the reality represented by these organizations at the expense of overlooking or downplaying other aspects' (p. 4). To further confuse matters, the terms are frequently used interchangeably even within a single piece of work. The need to avoid becoming entangled in a sterile semantic debate demands a bold approach. In this chapter the terms voluntary sector and voluntary organisations will be used except when talking specifically about the United States or quoting directly from authors who use one of the alternatives.

Before looking at definitions, a brief comment on the use of the word sector might be instructive. There are two points to be made. The first is that the term implies a degree of coherence that may not be present. As we shall see, one of the distinguishing characteristics of the voluntary sector is its great diversity. The second point is that the term sector implies a clear distinction between the spheres so categorised and that organisations can be unequivocally assigned to one sector or another. Some authors, however (DiMaggio and Powell, 1983; Taylor and Hoggett, 1994; 6, 1994) have talked about institutional or organisational isomorphism – the process by which organisations become more like either their funders or their competitors. In relation to Western Europe, 6 (1994, p. 401) makes the following comment:

> In the process of taking on new responsibilities, these organisations themselves have been transformed. Made accountable to state purchasers, and thereby, to the political process of policy-making, they have had to take on some of the characteristics traditionally associated with state bureaucracies. Encouraged or even required to compete with one another, and to respond to market forces, they have had to take on features of behaviour once thought to be characteristic of for-profit firms.

The question, though, is not simply whether voluntary organisations have been 'squeezed by the state and then lured into the market' (Taylor and Hoggett, 1994, p. 125). A supplementary question is whether the voluntary sector, in spite of these changes, remains sufficiently different to justify its designation as a distinctive entity. My contention is that it does, but this may become clearer once we have looked more closely at definitions.

Since the purpose of this chapter is to consider the role of the voluntary sector in health and welfare services, we need to know the kind of organisations we have in mind. I propose to adopt the definition developed by Salamon and Anheier (1992) in connection with the Johns Hopkins Comparative Nonprofit Sector Project. Although recognising the respective strengths of different types of definition, they reject legal, financial/economic and functional definitions in favour of a structural/operational definition. They identify five key distinguishing features of the organisations that comprise the voluntary sector:

- **Formal.** There must be some form of organisational and institutional structure. This excludes 'purely *ad hoc*, informal, and temporary gatherings of people. . . . Otherwise the concept of the nonprofit sector becomes far too amorphous and ephemeral to grasp and examine.'
- **Private.** There must be institutional separation from government. This does not preclude either working collaboratively with government or the receipt of substantial government funding.
- **Non-profit-distributing.** The emphasis here is on the *non-distribution* of profits. It does not mean that surpluses cannot be made, but the maximising of profits is not the primary purpose of the organisation.
- **Self-governing.** The organisation decides its own constitution, administrative structure and practices, policy and activities.
- **Voluntary.** There must be 'some meaningful degree of voluntary participation, either in the actual conduct of the agency's activities or in the management of its affairs.' (Salamon and Anheier, 1992, pp. 11–12).[1]

Definitions carry the danger of assuming conformity where none exists, or at the very least of masking diversity, but it should be apparent that the definition proposed by Salamon and Anheier is broad enough to include an enormous variety of voluntary organisations. The variety even within a single country is vast, but it becomes even more bewildering in an international context. There are variations in size, geographical coverage,[2] purposes, scope and range of functions, organisational and managerial structure, sources of finance and relationships with each other and with government. A controversial recommendation by Knight (1993) seeks to formalise these differences by dividing the voluntary sector into two categories. The first category would consist of large non-profit organisations providing services as sub-contractors or agents of public bodies and who would be fully funded by the state. The second category would be the 'authentic voluntary bodies' which would be 'free to fulfil the essences of voluntarism: vision, radical reform and social change' (p. 305). There would be no state funding for this second group. In what follows this division is not utilised, although distinctions on the basis of size and function will be fully acknowledged.

Fortunately, this chapter is not concerned with the whole range of voluntary organisations; its focus is exclusively on social welfare organisations. Even so, its scope remains uncomfortably large. The following list of the types of social welfare organisations gives some idea of the range of the voluntary sector in this area:

1. Neighbourhood organisations.
2. Self-help or mutual aid groups.
3. Organisations providing services for groups of 'clients'.
4. Pressure or advocacy groups.
5. Groups primarily concerned with medical, educational or social research.
6. 'Umbrella' or intermediary organisations concerned with the co-ordination and development of other groups.
7. Foundations.
8. International aid and development organisations.

The above categories are by no means mutually exclusive, and many groups will be hybrids. Furthermore, large organisations may be involved in a wide range of activities with specialist departments or sections. This diversity creates difficulties in attempts to devise over-arching theories as the next section will demonstrate.

Theories of the voluntary sector

Theories of the voluntary sector can be divided into five broad categories: organisational theory; theories drawn from political science and public administration; economic theories dealing with competition, markets, supply and demand; theories which seek to explain the existence of or the need for voluntary bodies; theories seeking to illuminate government/voluntary sector relationships. The first three of these are borrowed from other disciplines, and we have already addressed some of the economic and political issues. This section will therefore concentrate on the last two in the list, beginning with theories attempting to account for the existence of voluntary organisations.

Explaining the existence of the voluntary sector

Salamon and Anheier (1996) say that 'the nonprofit sector has attracted a rich outpouring of theoretical interest in recent years as scholars have sought to explain the curious persistence, and recent resurgence, of this long-neglected backwater of social and economic life' (p. 9). Many of the theories result from the work of American economists from the late 1970s onwards, although more recently the academic base of the theorising has widened. The intention is to look at six different kinds of explanations. Among the objectives of some of the theories is not simply to account for the existence of voluntary organisations, but also to suggest reasons for cross-national variations in the size and scope of the voluntary sector.

Among the earliest theories, developed by Weisbrod (1977), is what is termed either 'public goods theory' or 'market failure – government failure theory'. It rests on a general notion of demand heterogeneity and the inability or unwillingness of the market to produce sufficient quantities or variety of public goods to satisfy demand for them. Public goods are goods or services that are consumed jointly and from which it is difficult to exclude free-riders (people can benefit from the good or service whether they have paid for it or not). In these circumstances, market provision is unlikely. This is, of course, one of the classic arguments for government provision of public goods. This is where demand heterogeneity enters the picture: in culturally, ethnically or religiously diverse communities the demand for specific public goods is too great and too varied for the government to satisfactorily fill the gaps in provision left by markets. Part of the reason for this is the political necessity for government to satisfy the median voter, which leaves specialist demands unmet. In the absence of government or market provision, people turn to the voluntary sector to meet their perceived needs for a variety of public goods. It is important to note that this theory applies only to public goods and many health and welfare services (the main concern of this book) are personal or individual in nature.

James (1987) develops Weisbrod's model by adding supply-side considerations. She stresses the significance of heterogeneity and agrees with Weisbrod about the importance of unsatisfied demand for public goods, but argues that voluntary organisations will emerge only if there is also a supply of social entrepreneurs to respond to unmet demand. A recent study by Leadbetter (1997) says:

> Social entrepreneurs will be one of the most important sources of innovation. Social entrepreneurs identify under-utilised resources – people, buildings, equipment – and find ways of putting them to use to satisfy unmet social needs. They innovate new welfare services and new ways of delivering existing services.
>
> (p. 8)

What then are the incentives of social entrepreneurs? We can understand the profit motive in the commercial world and even the vote maximisation behaviour of politicians and the bureau maximisation tendencies of bureaucrats, but what drives social entrepreneurs to expend time and energy in a voluntary organisation? The rewards that have to be maximised in the case of social entrepreneurship are essentially non-monetary, unless success leads to higher salaries. James emphasises the importance of religion, and especially religious competition for members, but status, influence and power might also furnish effective incentives.

Hansmann (1980, 1987) proposes a third theory based on the assumed trustworthiness of voluntary organisations. This is particularly important in conditions of information asymmetry when the suppliers have more information than their users and when monitoring and evaluation impose heavy transaction costs. The theory applies with particular force in welfare services, the quality and effectiveness of which are notoriously difficult to measure. There may also be difficulty when the purchaser is not the consumer but someone acting on his/her behalf. Hansmann claims that in these circumstances potential customers are more prepared to trust a voluntary provider because one of the essential characteristics of a voluntary agency is that it is constrained by the requirement that profits may not be distributed to shareholders and owners. The absence of the profit motive, it is claimed, makes voluntary organisations more responsive to client needs.

A fourth attempt to explain the voluntary sector comes from Ben-Ner and Van Hoomissen (1993) who claim that voluntary organisations are governed by groups of stakeholders who control the delivery and distribution of collective or trust goods, to third parties. In self-help or mutual aid organisations the governing stakeholders may also be beneficiaries. Again, the possibility of information asymmetry is highlighted as an important factor contributing to the desirability of stakeholder control. The profit motive is absent and it is assumed that stakeholders can be trusted not to cut corners and to provide a quality service.

Salamon and Anheier (1996) claim that most of these theories were not supported by the cross-national empirical evidence generated by the Johns Hopkins international research project, although there was some heavily qualified endorsement of the heterogeneity thesis. Their chief criticism of the other approaches is their assumption that 'choices about whether to rely on market, third-sector, or state provision of key services are . . . made freely by individual consumers in an open market' (p. 15). Salamon and Anheier are the originators of the fifth theory in our review, the social origins theory. This is based on a re-working of Esping-Andersen's three worlds of welfare capitalism and the earlier work of Moore (1966) in a study of the social origins of fascism and democracy. The authors accept Esping-Andersen's three clusters of welfare regimes; liberal, corporatist and social democratic, but add a fourth category of statist. Their analysis is limited to two key dimensions: the extent of government welfare spending and the scale of the non-profit sector. They make the following observations:

- Liberal regimes are characterised by low public expenditure on social welfare and a relatively large voluntary sector.
- In corporatist regimes high government welfare spending co-exists with a large voluntary sector.
- Social democratic regimes are distinguished by high government spending and a relatively restricted voluntary sector.
- In the statist model the state is dominant, but it works in its own interest or in the interests of business and economic elites rather than in the interests of a powerful middle class or an organised

working class. Government welfare spending and voluntary activity are both relatively restricted.

The social origins theories are at a very high level of abstraction and deal in whole societies. They are also difficult to test empirically. Nevertheless, they do allow international comparison, offering tentative explanations of cross-national variations in the size and scope of the voluntary sector, and from this point of view they are extremely useful.

The final theoretical approach to understanding the voluntary sector is provided by Billis and Glennerster (1998). The authors are working towards what they call a theory of comparative advantage. The theory begins by identifying different forms of social disadvantage affecting particular groups in the population: financial disadvantage; personal disadvantage; societal disadvantage; community disadvantage. The second stage is to identify the main structural and organisational features of public, private and voluntary agencies. The final stage is to bring these two together. The suggestion is that voluntary agencies are less well-equipped than the public bodies to deal with financial disadvantage. On the other hand, voluntary organisations come into their own in dealing with personal, societal and community disadvantage. Billis and Glennerster state that their intention is to 'open up a line of enquiry which brings together the supply side characteristics of welfare agencies in the different sectors with the demand side characteristics of a number of different categories of disadvantage' (p. 94).

This brief review of theories explaining the existence of, or the need for, a voluntary sector is far from complete. The aim has been to give some indication of the richness of the theorising about voluntarism. It should be noted that many of the theories lack adequate empirical verification. Indeed, attempts to test some of the theories empirically are fraught with difficulties. By comparison theories illuminating government–voluntary sector relationships, to which we now turn, are much more amenable to empirical investigation.

Theorising government–voluntary sector relationships

Among the earliest attempts to construct theories of government–voluntary sector relationships were those devised in nineteenth century Britain as the state began to take a more prominent role in welfare. One of the main concerns of the sector at this time was with the provision of financial assistance, and this raised questions about the relationship between the Poor Law and financial aid from voluntary organisations. One attempt to devise principles to govern this relationship was known as the parallel bars theory, promoted by the Charity Organisation Society and supported in the Majority Report of the Poor Law Commission of 1909. If there are two parallel systems of poor relief, then some means has to be found to separate applicants into two groups, one to be catered for by the Poor Law and the other to be the preserve of the voluntary sector. The Charity Organisation Society initially argued that a distinction should be made between applicants for relief with some but inadequate resources (dealt with by the voluntary sector) and the absolutely destitute (dealt with by the Poor Law). This gave way to the notion that the division should be made on the grounds of desert: the undeserving poor would be directed to the Poor Law Guardians and the deserving poor would be helped by the voluntary sector. Another suggestion was that the voluntary sector should deal with those who could be helped back to independence leaving those who could not to the Poor Law.

An opposing theory, devised by the Webbs in the early years of the twentieth century, became known as the extension ladder theory, in which the state would be responsible for providing a national minimum, and that anything on top of that should be left to individuals or the voluntary sector.

MacAdam (1934) rejected both of these theories and argued that a new philanthropy had gradually emerged during the first quarter of the twentieth century, the distinguishing feature of which was a close partnership between the state and voluntary organisations. The idea of partnership was taken up by Owen (1965, p. 527) who described the voluntary sector as 'the junior partner in the welfare firm'. The role of the voluntary sector was to supplement and complement state provision, or to be the sole provider of services which the state could not or would not provide. The voluntary sector was said to have an important pioneering role in identifying new needs and developing new ways of meeting them.

The theme of partnership has been taken up by many commentators. For example, Salamon (1987) has argued strongly against those who characterise voluntary sector–government relationships in the United States as essentially competitive: collaboration is a more accurate description. Extending this notion internationally, Gidron *et al.* (1992) distinguish different models of government–voluntary sector relationships; but, although the models range from systems in which the government is the dominant partner to those in which the voluntary sector is dominant, the major change is 'in the direction of further elaborating collaborative partnerships between the third sector and the state' (p. 27). Kuhnle and Selle (1992) also stress collaboration, but distinguish between integrated dependence, in which voluntary welfare production is integrated in the overall welfare state system, and separate dependence, in which communication and contact between government and voluntary organisations is shallower and less frequent in spite of the voluntary sector's dependence on government funding. The growth of contracting in many countries has formalised collaboration with provision in the hands of voluntary organisations, but with the retention by the state of its financing and regulatory role. One of the policy dilemmas stemming from the increased dependence on government funding, and particularly the increased use of contracts, is the degree to which it poses a threat to the independence of voluntary organisations. Wolch (1990) believes the threat to be real and potentially sinister. She argues that the closer relationships between government and the voluntary sector have led to the emergence of a 'shadow state' in which voluntary agencies are increasingly dependent on government funding. Wolch claims that the shadow state phenomenon 'poses several dilemmas for voluntary organizations and for society in general'. She believes that these dilemmas 'are potentially very serious and threaten both the maintenance of independent organizational missions and the social welfare protections of individuals' (p. 215).

In her discussion of the shadow state, Wolch raises questions about the role of the voluntary sector in protecting and promoting democracy. This will be considered in the next section in the broader context of the voluntary sector's social significance.

The social significance of the voluntary sector

In the next section of this chapter the functions of voluntary organisations will be examined. The purpose of this section is to look not so much at specific functions (for example, service provision) but to consider the broader social and political roles of the voluntary sector. We will begin by looking at the contribution of the voluntary sector in creating and sustaining a democratic society, followed by a consideration of cross-national variations in the voluntary sector's importance.

Democracy, solidarity and civil society

This section will consider the claim that the voluntary sector promotes democracy by facilitating solidarity and fostering the development of civil society. Although the meaning of civil society is contested, the simplest interpretation of the term will be used here: a distinct area of social activity between individuals and the primary group of the family, on the one hand, and the state on the other. The notion of civil society has been particularly influential in Central and Eastern Europe where it is seen as essential for securing individual rights and liberties and acting as a bulwark against unwarranted extensions of state power.

A thriving voluntary sector is seen as an indispensable component of a civil society and of a democratic political system in Central and Eastern Europe. Siegal and Yancey (1992) claim that:

> The promise of the post-communist era rests largely on the potential for creating a more vibrant and deeply rooted network of organizations and institutions that mediate between the citizen and the State: the connective tissue of a democratic political culture.
>
> (p. 15)

The sentiments expressed in this quotation have strong connections with the frequently claimed capacity of the voluntary sector to promote solidarity or social integration. As evidence of this tendency note Salamon's (1992) statement that the non-profit sector in America 'is a response to the need for some mechanism through which to give expression to sentiments of solidarity' (p. 9). Anheier and Seibel (1993) writing of Germany say that 'participation in society via associational membership and volunteering has long been identified as a major ingredient of social integration' (p. 12). Voluntary bodies, it is claimed, both demonstrate and facilitate joint, co-operative action.

It is possible to argue, however, that voluntary organisations, and the civil society of which they are a part, also have the capacity to be divisive and particularistic. Solidarity *within* groups may actually work against broader constellations of solidarity. It was such considerations that led to the banning of guilds and associations in France immediately after the Revolution in 1791. Particularistic groups would, it was argued, thwart the expression of the general will of the people and were thus inimical to democracy.

Salamon (1993) questions the 'conventional wisdom' on the relationship between the non-profit sector and democracy 'which takes it as given that non-profit organizations are essential for democracy' (p. 3). He argues that non-profits may be either a prerequisite to democracy (for example in Central and Eastern Europe), an impediment to democracy (because of particularism and the inequities of pressure group politics) or they may be an irrelevance (when voluntary organisations are not involved in political activity).

Hirst (1994) provides an interesting and provocative contribution to the democracy debate in his work on associative democracy. The main themes of this work are decentralisation of the state and a challenge to its claims to sovereignty. The basic units would be self-governing voluntary associations accountable to their members. Hirst is proposing nothing less than governance through voluntary associations. He says of associationalism:

> It treats self-governing voluntary bodies not as secondary associations, but as a primary means of both democratic governance and organizing social life. A self-governing civil society thus becomes the primary feature of society. The state becomes a secondary, but vitally necessary, public power that ensures peace between associations and protects the rights of individuals. It also provides the mechanisms of public finance whereby those forms of provision that are regarded as necessary and available as of right to all members of society are administered through voluntary associations that those members elect to join in order to receive such services.
>
> (p. 26)

Such arrangements would give to communities the power to create their own moral and political frameworks and to participate in deciding what services should be provided and how they should be delivered. As the quotation indicates, the finance would come from public sources. Hirst claims that this scheme is not utopian: he sees it as a supplement to representative democracy and market economies. It is certainly utopian in that the chances of such a scheme being implemented are remote. Nevertheless, Hirst's ideas are worth further exploration, and though a fully-fledged scheme of associative democracy may be unattainable, democratic benefits may arise from moving in the general direction he suggests.

In the preceding section in the discussion of theory we had cause to refer to Wolch's (1990) work on the shadow state. Wolch is more sceptical about the contribution of voluntary organisations to democracy. She agrees that they have the capacity to encourage participation and empower users, but dangers arise when voluntary organisations are too heavily dependent on government finance and other forms of support. In these circumstances the independence of the voluntary sector may be compromised, and voluntary agencies may become little more than extensions of the state – indeed they may become agents of social control, losing in particular their important role as critics of government policy. Wolch does not believe that these undesirable developments are unavoidable, but vigilance and commitment is required if the democratic potential of a strong voluntary sector is to be realised:

> Without resorting to one-way pluralist arguments, our political eco-
> nomic analysis of voluntarism shows that voluntary action expands
> the realm of democratic participation and can influence state policy.
> The capacity of the sector to limit state powers and, in the extreme
> case, to smash the state is precious indeed and must be protected
> from the possible deformations of the shadow state.
>
> (p. 221)

There are two other issues to consider in any assessment of the relationship between the voluntary sector and democracy. The first is the extent of internal democracy in voluntary organisations. Kramer (1987) says that:

> The celebration of voluntary organizations as an important democra-
> tizing force has . . . been called into question by the composition and
> the decision-making processes of their governing bodies and the
> prevalence of minority rule . . . policy-making tends to be concen-
> trated in a small number of self-perpetuating board members –
> disproportionately self-selected white males from the corporate
> business and professional community.
>
> (p. 245)

On the other hand, as organisations become increasingly professionalised, and their work increasingly complex, there may be a
shift in power from voluntary governing bodies to paid executive

staff. Contracting, because of its complexity, may intensify this trend (Billis and Harris, 1992; Harris, 1996; Hedley and Rochester, 1992).

The second issue is concerned with the external relationships of voluntary organisations – more specifically, with their accountability. Leat (1988; 1990a; 1996) has done much to focus attention on this important question. She makes an initial distinction between political accountability (policy and priorities) and operational accountability, which is further sub-divided into fiscal accountability (the proper use of money), process accountability (the use of proper procedures) and programme accountability (the quality of their work). Leat also makes distinctions between accountability enforceable through sanctions and accountability that simply requires explanation or response. The picture becomes even more confused when the multiplicity of groups to which voluntary agencies may be considered accountable is included. Clear lines of accountability are an essential feature of democracy, and Leat considers the present lack of clarity to be a serious disadvantage:

> Despite the rhetoric of user-empowerment, and the role of voluntary organisations in democracy, we are a long way from understanding the principles, the aspirations and the practice of voluntary organisations in making themselves accountable.
>
> (Leat 1996, p. 77)

Taylor (1996) also views accountability as a major issue if voluntary organisations are to contribute fully to a democratic society. She distinguishes three facets of accountability: giving an account; holding to account; taking into account. Taylor states:

> Voluntary organisations are expected to be accountable for their role in providing welfare. But they also act as watchdogs on the state, holding it and other actors to account, and they play an important role in developing an informed and active citizenship, which not only holds to account but demands to be taken into account.
>
> (p. 58)

Taylor identifies the tensions surrounding accountability in voluntary associations. In doing so, she examines the relationships between trust and accountability, process and task, diversity and equity and the problems arising from a multiplicity of interests. She argues that if voluntary organisations are to remain at the forefront of democratic innovation, they need 'to develop more rigorous and sophisticated conceptions of accountability' (p. 57).

Cross-national variations

There are obvious difficulties in attempting to measure cross-national variations in the significance of voluntary organisations in welfare states. Part of the problem is how significance is to be defined and measured. Another difficulty is patchiness of the information, particularly in the less developed countries of the world. This is demonstrated by the international study conducted under the leadership of Salamon and Anheier: of the twelve countries studied, only seven produced sufficient data for detailed comparisons to be made. The five countries with insufficient data were Brazil, Egypt, Ghana, India and Thailand. This lack of information is likely to be a temporary phenomenon: in all five countries, and in other developing nations, academic and political interest in the voluntary sector is a relatively recent phenomenon, but is now growing quickly.

To some extent the size of the voluntary sector may be taken as an indicator of its significance in particular countries. Size on its own, however, is not a satisfactory criterion: it is possible to conceive of a small, but highly influential, voluntary sector. Nevertheless, a social and political system that fosters the growth of a large voluntary sector is one which is likely to recognise the sector's potential. Fortunately, size is not the only indicator available to researchers; there is ample evidence of the voluntary sector's role in welfare in most of the developed countries in the world and there are some statistics to indicate the importance of its contribution to national economies. For example, Table 4.1 gives an indication of the contribution of the voluntary sector to the economies of the seven countries in the Johns Hopkins study for which reliable figures were

Table 4.1 Voluntary sector – employment and expenditure

Country	Employment as % of total employment	Operating expenditure as % of GDP
France	4.2%	3.3%
Germany	3.7%	3.6%
Hungary	0.8%	1.2%
Italy	1.8%	2.0%
Japan	2.5%	3.2%
United Kingdom	4.0%	4.8%
United States	6.8%	6.3%

Source: Johns Hopkins Comparative Nonprofit Sector Project (Salamon and Anheier, 1994)

available and it also allows comparisons of the size of the sector in each of the countries to be made.

Table 4.1 uses the number of people employed in the voluntary sector as a proportion of all people in employment and operating expenditure as a proportion of GDP as reasonable indicators of economic significance. On both counts, the voluntary sector in the United States is by far the most extensive with Hungary at the other end of the scale. The contribution of the voluntary sector to the economies of Italy and Japan is relatively modest. The United Kingdom, France and Germany lie somewhere between the two extremes. However, these figures do not tell the whole story. They take no account, for example, of the enormous contribution of unpaid volunteers.

The last two decades have witnessed a rapid increase in many countries in the number of voluntary organisations. For example, Kramer *et al.* (1993, p. 112) refer to 'the unprecedented explosion of peer self-help groups and community-based organisations with advocacy and/or social service functions.' The authors claim that this is a worldwide trend related to the growth of social movements 'for greater citizen participation . . . in the formation and implementation of public policy and for greater decentralization of governmental functions.' Kramer and his colleagues found evidence of growth in three of the four countries they studied: England, Italy and Norway; in the fourth country, The Netherlands, the government had been attempting to reduce the huge number of organisations concerned with the provision of health, welfare and education services by offering special funding to organisations agreeing to merge.

Single country surveys almost invariably reveal expansion since the 1960s in the number and variety of voluntary organisations, growth being particularly marked in the 1980s. Although the general picture is one of expansion, the pace of development and the size of the voluntary sector vary from country to country. In the countries of Central and Eastern Europe voluntary organisations independent of the state virtually disappeared during the communist period. There was some development of the voluntary sector in the mid-1980s, but the most rapid development occurred after 1989. Direct suppression of voluntary organisations also occurred during the 1930s and 1940s in Japan and Germany. In both countries, however, there has been a period of 50 or 60 years for the effects of suppression to be overcome, and the German voluntary sector, in particular, is very large and very powerful.

In seeking to explain the differential development of the voluntary sector in different countries, careful attention must be paid to cultural and political influences. Hungary, France, The Netherlands, Sweden, and the United States will be used to illustrate this point. Hungary will serve as an example of one of those countries in which the voluntary sector was virtually absent for more than forty years. As Kuti (1993) explains:

> Rooted in Leninist ideology, the new communist regime considered individuals as part of a potentially hostile 'bourgeois' mass that needed to be re-educated and re-oriented as socialists. Inherent in that concept was a fear that social movements might fall outside Party control. In order to counteract this fear, foundations were liquidated, and voluntary associations were banned in the 1950s.
>
> (p. 5)

There is perhaps another point to be made: the problems that voluntary welfare associations were set up to solve would not arise or would be quickly eradicated in a socialist system.

There was some relaxation of Party control in the 1980s before the fall of the regime in 1989 and voluntary organisations began to emerge – many of them 'substitutes for political parties' (Kuti, 1993, p. 5). Since 1989 the development of voluntary organisations has been rapid. Kuti estimates that by the spring of 1992 there were about 17,000 voluntary organisations among a total population of 10 million (p. 6). This remarkable growth has been achieved in the face of several difficulties. One of these is that there had to be a steep learning curve; knowledge of how to establish, maintain and manage voluntary organisations was limited to a very few people. Furthermore, some of the leaders of voluntary organisations became more active in the new political parties or were lost to the private sector. Initially, too, the legal position was unclear, although new laws have now rectified this. Collaboration with the state was problematic, partly because of the deep suspicion of the state that followed the changes. It must be remembered that reconstruction was taking place on several fronts at once – economic, political and social.

Until the 1980s, France lagged behind most other countries in Western Europe and the United States in terms of the size and significance of its voluntary sector. The reasons are largely historical. Archambault (1993) talks about France's 'historical lag' and claims that 'the relative underdevelopment of France's non-profit sector had its roots in the 1789 French Revolution' (p. 2). The 1791 *Le Chapelier* Act banned guilds and other associations: no intermediary institutions were to be allowed to stand between the citizen and the state. This led to the centralisation of power which, until the 1980s, was one of the hallmarks of the French political system. The right of free association was not granted in France until 1901, but Seibel (1992, p. 213) argues that the Jacobin tradition in France 'is still alive, and suspicion of the associations, most of them still close to the Catholic laic movement, has never completely disappeared.' There are undoubtedly still traces of this suspicion, but the number of associations began to expand from the mid-1960s. Massive development, however, had to wait until 1982 with the implementation of a policy of decentralisation. In 1990 over 60,000 declared associations (those registered or 'declared' at the *prefecture*) came into being, and an informed guess puts the total number of such associations at between 600,000 and 700,000 (Archambault, 1993, p. 10).

The Netherlands, by contrast, has a very long history of voluntary sector provision of health, education and welfare services. Kramer *et al.* (1993, pp. 70–1) claim that 'three sociopolitical traditions played crucial roles in the development of the Dutch pattern of service delivery: egalitarianism, the absence of a powerful central state, and religious pluralism.' Within this context, two major principles guided the provision of health, education and welfare services. The first of these was subsidiarity – a principle equally important in the German system and in the European Union. The term, which has general applicability, implies that lower levels in the hierarchy take precedence over higher levels, and indeed the higher level has a responsibility to protect and help the lower level. In social policy, it means that private provision of services is to be preferred to public provision and government has an obligation to help private providers to achieve their goals. In the Dutch system this means that most services are provided by voluntary associations. The number of such associations is considerably increased by the second principle of service provision in The Netherlands; the principle of pillarisation. Kramer *et al.* (1993, p. 71) explain that pillarisation is based on the view that 'a citizen's educational, social welfare and health needs should be met by providers from the same religious background.' This meant that in each locality there were several providers of the same services to different groups in the population. In more recent years a combination of greater secularisation, government attempts to curb costs and rationalise provision by promoting mergers, has resulted in the virtual abandonment of pillarisation, but provision is still almost wholly by voluntary sector suppliers.

The case of The Netherlands illustrates the contribution of religious and ethnic heterogeneity to the development of a vigorous voluntary sector. This contrasts with Sweden in which, as Gould (1993, p. 164) indicates, 'the population, in terms of religion and ethnicity, was fairly homogeneous, and remained so until well into the latter half of the twentieth century.' The existence for some centuries in Sweden of 'a strong centralised state with sophisticated administrative machinery' (Gould, 1993, p. 164) also provides a direct contrast with The Netherlands. It is often asserted that the Swedish voluntary sector is relatively undeveloped, but this is disputed by Lundström and Wijkström (1995) who claim that concentration on service provision has led to an underestimation 'of the size and importance, as well as the independent role, of the Swedish non-profit sector' (p. 1). Lundström and Wijkström argue that there is a large voluntary sector in Sweden, but that it has 'developed less in the fields of health and social services, and more in the areas of culture, leisure, and advocacy' (p. 1).

In spite of recent setbacks, the Swedish health and welfare system is still predominantly state-dominated with a generous and extensive state welfare system which leaves little room for the development of a vigorous voluntary sector. The long uninterrupted period of social democratic government is largely responsible for this position. In 1995, however, the Social Democratic minority government announced austerity measures which included substantial cuts in welfare spending. It will be interesting to see what effects the cuts have and whether they will lead to a compensatory increase in voluntary activity.

The United States has frequently been characterised as 'a reluctant welfare state'. Wilensky and Lebeaux (1965) provided one of the earliest and most convincing explanations of this reluctance. They argued that the principal reasons for the American reluctance were to be found in the dominant cultural values of American society: individualism, an emphasis on private property rights and the free market and a distrust of government. It is interesting that Wilensky and Lebeaux also cite racial, ethnic and religious heterogeneity as contributing to the relative under-development of the American welfare state. As we have noted, heterogeneity is one of the factors affecting the size and significance of the voluntary sector.

Somewhat ironically, Wilensky and Lebeaux were writing during the era of the Great Society when new social programmes were being established, welfare expenditure was rising faster than GDP and the involvement of the federal government was increasing. For a very short time it looked as though the United States was moving towards a European style welfare state, but by the mid-1970s the welfare backlash had begun.

Although it experienced considerable growth in the 1980s, the size and scope of the American voluntary sector is by no means a new phenomenon. The attitudes and approaches described above have a long history and have ensured a prominent role for the voluntary or non-profit sector in the American welfare system. Clotfelter (1992, p. 1) makes the following claim:

> . . . the collection of institutions loosely referred to as the non-profit sector has been playing an important part in education, health and other social services from the nation's earliest days. To a degree unparalleled elsewhere, the nonprofit sector in the United States is enshrined in constitutional law, instrumental in the delivery of many essential social services, and inextricably bound up with broad social processes of change and governance.

This section of the chapter has been concerned with the social significance of the voluntary sector emphasising its role as a repository of values, and as a contributor to the maintenance and development of democracy, solidarity and civil society. We also looked at the growth of the sector which has generally added to its significance. We noted briefly the voluntary sector's varying contribution to national economies. In order to carry out these roles effectively, however, voluntary organisations need to acquire legitimacy in the communities in which they operate. Legitimacy is most likely to come from the practical value of what they do – they need to appear not only worthy but also useful. It is in this context that we now turn to the specific functions of voluntary organisations.

Roles and functions

Service provision

William Beveridge's influential book, *Voluntary Action*, was published in 1948. In this publication Beveridge made a distinction between philanthropy and mutual aid. The first was concerned with service to others – an unequal activity in which one group of people provide services for another group of people who are perceived to be in need. In mutual aid there is a much greater emphasis on reciprocity: those participating in the activities of a mutual aid or self-help organisation are both providers and recipients. These two categories will be given separate consideration, beginning with service provision.

Voluntary organisations have long been providers of services, the significance of their contribution varying from country to country. In The Netherlands, Germany and the United States, for example, the voluntary sector has always played a prominent role in service provision. Some explanation of the voluntary sector dominance in health and welfare provision in The Netherlands has already been offered. Since the 1930s, government funding of services, either directly or through social insurance, gradually increased: by the 1960s almost the entire expenditure was publicly funded. In 1974 a government consultative committee criticised the fragmentation and lack of co-ordination, resulting in unevenness of provision, duplication, gaps and an uneconomic use of resources. The government responded by what it called a 'judicious funding policy' under which government subsidies became dependent on the acceptance of rationalisation (mergers) and the provision of more detailed information. In spite of these interventions by the government, the production and delivery of health and welfare services remains in voluntary sector hands.

In Germany, the principle of subsidiarity, the result of accommodation between the Catholic Church and the state, means a substantial role for voluntary sector providers, especially in the areas of health and social services. The six free welfare associations, the main providers of social services, are heavily dependent upon public subsidies, but they have been sufficiently powerful to retain managerial independence.

The size of the voluntary sector's contribution to health and welfare services in Germany is overshadowed by the role played by the non-profit sector in the United States. It is in the area of health care that the American non-profit sector is most significant. The significance of the voluntary sector in the areas of hospital care, home health care and specialised clinics has already been noted. Their contribution to nursing homes is dwarfed by the commercial establishments. Salamon also identifies the importance of non-profits in higher education and in social services. Non-profit agencies control 74 per cent of total social service revenues.

The three countries so far discussed have a long tradition of voluntary sector health and welfare provision. In the UK the voluntary sector has played a relatively minor role in health care services, and, until recently, a supplementary or complementary role in the personal social services. Housing associations, again until recently, made a comparatively minor addition to the supply of social housing. By far the biggest field of voluntary sector involvement in the UK is education: this stems from the award of charitable status to private schools and universities.

During the last twenty years the voluntary sector has come to occupy an incomparably more prominent role in the production and delivery of welfare. As 6 (1994) says in relation to Western Europe: 'voluntary, non-profit and co-operative agencies have, in recent years, moved centre stage in the delivery of social welfare services' (p. 401). However, it is not just in Western Europe that this has happened: the change is to be observed 'in the developed countries of Western Europe, North America and Asia; in the former Soviet bloc; and in the developing countries of Africa, Asia and Latin America' (Institute for Policy Studies, 1994, p. 1). There are several possible explanations of this increase in government attention. Stoesz and Midgley (1991) see it as a direct consequence of the growing influence of the New Right:

> To the extent that welfare is beyond the means of the family and the informal sector, the radical right prefers that assistance be provided through the organized voluntary sector. The voluntary sector embodies virtues that are dear to traditionalists such as neighbour-liness, self-reliance and community solidarity.
>
> (p. 37)

The aim of the New Right is to roll back the state and cut public expenditure – especially social expenditure. This is a theme already addressed in Chapter 2.

Irrespective of New Right ambitions, there is suspicion of the state and government not only in the United States but also in the former communist countries and some of the countries that have experienced military rule in South America, Africa and elsewhere. More generally, Kramer *et al.* (1993, p. 196) see voluntary sector provision as a response to 'the decline in legitimacy ascribed to government'. The claimed advantages of the voluntary sector in promoting solidarity, supporting democracy and nurturing civil society have already been addressed.

Salamon and Anheier (1994) point to a general dissatisfaction with current methods of provision:

> Prompted by dissatisfaction with the cost and effectiveness of exclusive reliance on government to address the social welfare and developmental challenges of our time, efforts have been launched to find alternative ways to respond.
>
> (p. 1)

Although greater use of the voluntary sector in service delivery does not automatically bring about reductions in public expenditure, governments have inevitably seen this as one of its possible benefits. Governments committed to privatisation programmes and the promotion of competition through marketisation, may also see the voluntary sector as a component in their more general strategy. Illustrations of this approach can be seen in the UK under a Conservative government; in New Zealand under a Labour government during the 1980s and more recently under a conservative National Party government; and in the United States under both Republican and Democratic administrations.

A steadily growing feature of voluntary sector provision of services are purchase-of-service arrangements – the provision of services on the basis of contracts drawn up between government agencies acting as commissioners or purchasers and voluntary associations or commercial undertakings as providers. This has enormous significance for voluntary organisations – with implications for their functions, their organisational form, their independence, and their accountability. Contracting has been common in the United States for many years, and it is now well-advanced in the UK where the 1990 NHS and Community Care Act produced a purchaser/provider split and where quasi-markets have been introduced in most areas of social provision (Bartlett *et al.*, 1994; Le Grand and Bartlett, 1993).

Contracting for care has been developing since the 1970s in Italy, and more modest beginnings have been made in France, Germany, The Netherlands, Australia, New Zealand, Argentina and Brazil.

Contracts affect not only the voluntary sector but also commercial undertakings. Furthermore, they crucially influence the relationships within and between these two sectors and the ways in which both relate to the state. They are therefore a very significant element in mixed economies of welfare, and we have had cause to refer to the issue of contracting in earlier chapters. Before moving on, however, it might be as well to recall what was said in Chapter 2 about the different interpretations of contracts in different countries.

Self-help

Beveridge used the term mutual aid for what is now more frequently referred to as self-help. In some ways mutual aid is a more satisfactory term since the notion of mutuality has 'connotations of solidarity' (Davis Smith, p. 28). Beveridge said that mutual aid stemmed from:

> a sense of one's own need for security against misfortune and realising that, since one's fellows have the same need, by undertaking to help one another all may help themselves.
>
> (pp. 8–9)

Beveridge laid great stress on friendly societies and building societies, but these are very different in character from the voluntary bodies considered in this chapter, and in Britain, at least, many are shedding their mutual status. Because it is more commonly understood, the term self-help will be used in this section.

The classic treatise on self-help is that written by Samuel Smiles in Victorian England. But Smiles was writing about individuals rising from humble circumstances to achieve fame and fortune through showing initiative, enterprise, perseverance, diligence and thrift. Self-help in this sense is not our concern here. We are more concerned with self-help groups 'formed by people who have a shared problem, or concern, joining together for mutual support and the provision of services to members; most will also be concerned with pressing the case of the particular social, medical or cultural group from which members are drawn' (Johnson, 1987, p. 102).

There has been a rapid and substantial increase in the number and variety of self-help groups in recent decades. Such groups have contributed in large measure to the general expansion of the voluntary sector. Lorenz (1994a, p. 108) writes of 'new self-help initiatives manifesting themselves in stunning diversity'. Lorenz was here talking of health issues in a European context, but the same comment could be made worldwide and extended to every area of provision. Within Europe, the greatest expansion has occurred in Germany: Nowak (1988) estimated that in Western Germany in the mid-1980s there were as many as 40,000 self-help groups (including co-operatives) covering mental and physical health, homelessness and housing issues, youth, unemployment, women's issues, older people and peace groups. Richardson (1984, p. 2) describes similar developments in Britain:

> Self-help groups have burgeoned in recent years, taking on not only common and familiar problems but also those of a much rarer nature. There are groups for people with all sorts of handicaps . . . for people with all sorts of diseases . . . for people who face . . . widowhood, a stillbirth, infertility or bringing up a family on their own.

Evers (1990, p. 12) shows how the development of self-help organisations has been a Europe-wide movement. He writes of:

> small-scale forms of social self-organization which have been a product of the social and cultural movements which crosscut the societal landscape at the end of the 60s in West-European countries and are actually showing up in the post-communist European countries: associations, organizations for mutual help which strongly depend on a local or regional setting and community.

Wollert and Barron (1983, p. 105) estimate that in the early 1980s there were well over half-a-million self-help groups in the United States. They describe the emergence of these groups as 'a robust social phenomenon.'

An indication of the rapid development of self-help initiatives is the growth of self-help clearing houses which act as information and resource centres and as facilitators. In 1983 the World Health Organisation published the results of a workshop on self-help and health. It recommended the establishment of local and national support systems and issued guidance about how this might be best achieved. The clearing house idea began in the United States, where clearing houses are now widespread and firmly established. Germany has a national clearing house and 120 spread throughout the country. Belgium, the UK and The Netherlands also have self-help clearing houses, and several are being established in the countries of Central and Eastern Europe. A clearing house should provide a forum for the exchange of ideas and information and should be able to advise those wishing to establish self-help groups how to proceed. Another clearing house task is the maintenance of a directory. Even when directories exist, however, it is difficult to be precise about the number of groups in any one country, because many groups are small and local and the picture is constantly changing as some groups disappear and new ones emerge.

There are four possible explanations for this quite remarkable upsurge of self-help initiatives: 1. government encouragement; 2. dissatisfaction with current provision and the desire for more participatory services; 3. the emphasis on consumerism; 4. the search for identity and the struggle against oppression. We will look at each of these.

1. Government encouragement
Governments frequently have an ambivalent attitude towards self-help. They applaud the principle of self-reliance, but they are often less enthusiastic about self-help *organisations*, particularly when such organisations are militant. Governments also view self-help as a means of cutting public expenditure, and reducing the role of the state. Self-help clearly fits in with prevalent attitudes to welfare in the United States, and Presidents Reagan, Bush and Clinton have all endorsed it. In the UK, Mrs Thatcher's contention that the welfare state creates dependency and the government's promotion of 'active citizenship' had implications for self-help. In Germany, Chancellor Kohl took a similar line to Mrs Thatcher and attempted to halt the continued growth of the welfare state through a group of policies given the title of *Wendepolitik*. A central feature of the policy was to be a 'new subsidiarity' which, among other things, would encourage a much greater emphasis on self-help.

2. Dissatisfaction
Dissatisfaction with present forms of provision is said to have given added impetus to the movement towards self-help. The evidence about dissatisfaction is not entirely unequivocal. In Britain and

elsewhere New Right and government denigration of public services has created a climate in which private is said to be superior to public provision (Deakin and Wright, 1990). However, there have also been criticisms from the anti-state libertarian left and from middle left governments in Australia and New Zealand, for example.

In relation to Germany, Freeman and Clasen (1994) are firmly of the view that shortcomings in current arrangements have contributed to the rapid development of self-help:

> To an extent, the growth of self-help reflects a multi-faceted dissatisfaction with the German welfare system. What is in principle a system of pluralist decentralisation, organised through many local agencies and insurance funds, comes to be in practice one of corporatist centralisation, in which arrangements are in fact negotiated between representatives of enormous associations of organisations. Furthermore, the formulation of policy tends to be determined . . . by the interests of employees rather than those of users or beneficiaries.
>
> (p. 13)

Although he does not relate criticisms of the welfare system specifically to self-help, but to grassroots pressure, Walker (1993) says of Britain:

> More and more users of the social services have been complaining about their bureaucratic organization, complexity and lack of responsiveness to felt needs. In fact there is a long series of research studies pointing to the divergence between the perceptions of need held by users and professional providers in the social services.
>
> (p. 74)

These quotations, which could easily relate to other countries, offer some clues as to the precise nature of the criticisms of present provision and the benefits anticipated from their replacement by self-help. The dissatisfaction focuses on the dominance of bureaucrats and professionals and on the highly centralised nature of the administration of services.

The arguments relating to bureaucracy are the familiar ones of remoteness, inflexibility and unresponsiveness to needs. Rules, regulations and formal procedures are possibly appropriate in the case of standard cash benefits, but they become less so when dealing with more individual and more personal needs. Because some needs are not being adequately met, and because people feel powerless when faced with a large bureaucracy, clients and potential clients become disenchanted with statutory services and turn to self-help as a viable alternative.

By its very nature self-help is participatory, although the degree to which members wish to be involved will vary, some being continuously active, some taking part from time to time and some whose membership entails little more than the payment of a subscription. Because of its participatory nature, self-help, it is claimed, can be a means of giving people more control over their lives by reducing their dependence on both statutory help and professional workers.

Relationships between health and welfare professionals and their clients, between providers and recipients, are unequal. They are unilateral in that the client has nothing to offer in exchange for the service which therefore takes the form of a gift (Titmuss, 1970). Clients are forced to accept professionals' definition of problems and needs which may not accord with their own interpretations. It should be noted that these problems are not restricted to statutory agencies; they might just as easily arise when services are received from large voluntary providers who employ professional staff. By contrast, in self-help organisations the distinction between providers and recipients is blurred or non-existent, and it is members who control both the organisation and the definition of problems and needs.

Not only do such organisations have the potential for reducing stigma by reducing dependence, but they may very well produce a more accurate and acceptable identification of need. For example, people who have themselves experienced a disability, or those who have cared for someone with a particular disability, are likely to know much more than doctors or social workers about its impact and management. In a self-help organisation the combined knowledge of the membership is potentially at the disposal of all those who need to avail themselves of it.

Relationships with professionals have been a matter of some discussion within the self-help movement. In mental health, for example, Judi Chamberlin, probably the most influential figure in the United States and worldwide, has written about the survivors' movement which started in the early 1970s in the United States and Italy and in the late 1970s in Britain and other European countries. Chamberlin is on the more radical wing of the survivors' movement, which she refers to as the mental patients' liberation movement. In her first and still her most influential book (1977) she identified three models of providing alternative services:

- The partnership model where professionals and non-professionals work together in service provision.
- The supportive model which abandons the distinction between the helper and the helped and in which professionals provide external support.
- The separatist model in which patients provide support for one another and run the service completely excluding all non-patients and professionals.

Chamberlin supports the separatist model because she believes that the other models do not allow for full self-definition or self-determination and they hinder consciousness-raising. She also claims that groups that do not adopt the separatist model soon move from liberation to reform.

Adams (1990) identifies three levels of social work involvement in self-help organisations:

- Integral self-help in which the social work agency funds the initiative and provides direct professional leadership, but in which the goal is client involvement and self-help is encouraged.
- Facilitated self-help in which 'professionals provide some support and a degree of indirect leadership' (p. 35).
- Autonomous self-help which is 'initiated, organized, resourced and run entirely independently of professionals' (p. 36).

It will be observed that Adams is prepared to see a role for professionals within a general philosophy of self-help. This is in marked contrast to Chamberlin's anti-professional separatist view.

3. Consumerism
In most advanced industrial countries, there is considerable interest in consumerism in public services. It is closely related to participation which was so popular a prescription in the late 1960s and early 1970s. Like participation, consumerism is supported by people with widely divergent political standpoints. Consumerism is said to have two main aims: the extension of choice and empowerment.

Beresford (1988) identifies three models for 'hearing the voice of the consumer'. The first he calls the market research model which is 'essentially concerned with information and intelligence gathering'. (p. 37). The second model is the consumerist approach – an extension of the market research model. Of this model Beresford says:

> Its recent emergence has coincided with the expansion of commercial social services provision. Service users or clients are now conceived of as consumers, and issues are reframed in terms of market preferences, consumer rights and product developments, echoing the language and conceptions of the market economy from which they have been borrowed.
>
> (p. 38)

The third model is the democratic approach in which 'the concern is with enabling the involvement of consumers so that they may have a greater say in and control over the services that are provided' (p. 38).

Consumerism then is not simply concerned with market research, nor simply with consultative procedures. In both of these the consumer is relatively passive, and the term consumerism, in its fullest sense, implies the more active involvement of consumers or users. A fully developed form of consumerism would involve users in the identification of need and with the expression of views about what resources and services are required to adequately meet needs. Users would also be involved in decisions concerning both policy and practice and possibly in the management of services or facilities. They would be given the opportunity to evaluate performance through the appraisal of such matters as the speed and method of delivery, the quantity of services provided and their quality. There would also be adequate machinery for the hearing of complaints and for the redress of grievance.

One of the objectives of mixed economies of welfare is the extension of choice. Baldock (1991, p. 3) identifies the demand for greater service variety:

> Research has shown that one of the chief ways that the dependent and their carers believe that their welfare could be enhanced is if there was a much greater variety of services available for them to choose from. They would particularly like more choice of types of domiciliary and respite care between the extremes of full-time family care and full-time institutional care. They may not be particularly concerned which organisations actually supply these services, simply that they should exist.

The debate about participation and user-involvement has been a debate about empowerment and citizenship. Empowerment is currently a very fashionable term in social policy discourse; it is concerned with both attitudes and strategies. The most important attitude is a respect for all service-users and the recognition by professionals and bureaucrats of the ability of people to contribute to service delivery and, more importantly, policy formulation. In this context empowerment is about the self-image of both professionals and users and about the image they have of each other. Professionals have to be prepared to give up some of their power and accept a different definition of their roles. This may imply the need for developing new skills. The most widely favoured strategy is self-help.

4. Identity and oppression

Goffman (1968) described stigma as 'spoiled identity'. The main groups used as illustrations by Goffman were mentally ill people, physically disabled people and ex-prisoners. One of the functions of self-help groups is to overcome stigma. The notion of stigma is closely connected with discrimination and oppression which affect not only the groups highlighted by Goffman, but also women, ethnic minorities and older people. Knight (1993) says that:

> the pursuit of identity is an important aspect of voluntary action. It almost always means group action both to combat external forces that impair identity and to bolster internal forces that promote identity. Thus, the group will tend to use methods of mutual aid.
>
> (p. 94)

The interaction between social movements and self-help initiatives is interesting. Some of the most innovative self-help schemes have sprung from the civil rights, women's, peace and green movements. The women's movement is probably the most widespread of these; the peace movement is also widely spread, but may have lost some momentum in recent years; the civil rights movement is strongest in the United States, though it is not restricted to that country; the environment is of worldwide concern, but as a political force the green movement has been particularly strong in Germany.

Lorenz (1994b) makes a very direct connection between social movements and the rise of self-help groups in Germany:

> Their rise in Germany during the 1970s and 1980s was closely associated with the emergence of new social movements. With their

critique of established bureaucratic and neo-corporatist structures and their challenges to positions of power, including those of the professions, social movements have become a considerable force in Germany as in other societies. Spearheaded by the women's, ecology and peace movements, local initiatives and self-help groups began to question the authority of the state and to speak and act on behalf of all sections of society.

(pp. 163–4)

Women's groups have been particularly innovative in self-help, but often the way matters are handled, the structure and the relationships within the organisation, are as important as the type of activities. Such groups are frequently based on less hierarchical more co-operative forms of organisation than some of the more traditional associations. Among the self-help services organised are well-women clinics, pre-school playgroups and kindergartens, the provision of refuges (shelters in America) for women subjected to domestic violence, the provision of support for victims of rape, theatre groups, specific groups for older women and for black women. Self-help may be combined with consciousness-raising and action designed to secure and extend rights. In a paper on community action in the United States, Miller *et al.* (1995) state:

> Organizing around race/ethnicity and gender has become a major focus, often as part of broader social movements using extra-institutional channels to challenge attitudes or institutions. Organizing around identity seeks to break conventional ways of 'conducting business' by reframing issues along new principles of justice or equality.

(p. 115)

Some of the issues raised by combining social movement, self-help and political action will be considered when we look at the pressure group activities of voluntary organisations. Before leaving the topic of self-help, however, some of its possible dangers and drawbacks need to be identified.

The first is the danger of tokenism. Professionals and bureaucrats may talk about self-help and empowerment, but take few practical steps to facilitate the process. The control of resources of all kinds may remain in the same hands. For example, a prime requirement for self-help is the free flow of information in a form which users can assimilate and utilize. The control of information is an immense power which is largely in the hands of professionals and bureaucrats.

This is a particularly sensitive area in mental health services (Brandon, 1991). Frequently professionals will seek to justify the withholding of information on the grounds that disclosure would be harmful to the patient/client. In some circumstances this may be a perfectly sound reason, but it may also be based on false assumptions about the recipient's capacity for understanding and coping with the information.

Information is just one of the resources needed if self-help is to lead to empowerment. Financial support is also needed. Beresford (1991) emphasises the importance of funding when he writes of 'an essential new agenda for politicians and service providers who want to do more than just talk about involvement'. He describes this new agenda in the following terms:

> First they must offer greater support to service users and carers and their organisations so they develop their own voices. Second they must commit themselves to a changed value system that values the contribution of service users and carers. Policy makers, researchers, consultants and academics may all have their own claims on resources to enhance people's participation in community care. But it's vital that the bulk of funding and support goes to people at the hard end – to carers and service users themselves – if their participation is to be a reality.
>
> (p. 12)

If resources are not forthcoming, the suspicion must be that governments see self-help as a means of reducing public expenditure and curtailing the role of the state. Mayo (1994) maintains that self-help groups are not 'attempting to supplant professional services, but rather to make professional services more responsive and appropriate, whilst offering complementary self-help' (p. 140). Self-help, therefore, need not necessarily imply a reduction in formal provision. Paradoxically, tokenism subverts the principles of self-help and may lead to greater control by the state.

Lack of support is connected to another possible problem: exploitation. This is clearly stated by Finch (1984) in an interesting study of pre-school playgroups. She argues that the promotion of self-help playgroups is essentially deceitful for three reasons:

> First, encouraging the women to run their own pre-school facilities rather than seek an extension of statutory resources is deceitful because it promotes a form of provision which such women cannot

supply for themselves. Second, the idea of self-help obscures the fact that what is being sought are facilities on the cheap, incorporating the unpaid labour of mothers themselves. . . . Third, as a form of pre-school provision, playgroups make no contribution whatsoever to the needs of parents in paid work, since they both assume and encourage full-time mothering.

(pp. 17–18)

Part of the thrust of Finch's argument is that setting up and operating a self-help group is largely a middle-class activity. This is a view confirmed by Lawrence (1983) who says of self-help groups that 'the skills, time and energy required to organise such groups may result in their being either more successful and sustained in middle class areas or dominated by an unrepresentative section of their membership' (p. 16). Similarly, Svetlik (1991) says that the experience of self-help groups in Berlin seems to show that, 'more often than not, self-help groups are middle-class' (p. 12). Not only is there a middle-class bias in self-help but also a white bias. Although a high proportion of the black or ethnic minority groups are indeed based on the principles of self-help, there is evidence to suggest (Johnson, 1991) that they are poorly funded, and that they often experience difficulties in securing access to policy-making and funding agencies.

The social class and racial biases in self-help raises questions about the overall impact of the self-help movement on equality. Radical support for self-help stems from its potential as a participatory alternative to state services. It is claimed that self-help gives working-class and disadvantaged people more control over their lives and enables them to articulate demands for a greater share of resources. In so far as these demands are met, self-help may lead to a reduction in inequality. For this to be realised, however, requires a greater degree of equality within the self-help sector itself. Even so, changes in service delivery are unlikely to have more than a marginal effect on inequality. While self-help groups may give a voice to consumers, and to some extent challenge professional dominance, no great disturbance of power relationships is involved.

Community development

Community development, in some of its manifestations, has strong connections with self-help, but it is a much broader term which is used to cover a wide range of different agencies and strategies. In industrial countries, it includes everything between very small neighbourhood projects, possibly focusing on housing, social facilities, vandalism and crime, and very large urban regeneration programmes with huge resources and collaboration between government, private industry and the local community. In developing countries, it includes everything between small grass roots self-help groups and co-operatives and major projects financed in part by international agencies or by foreign agencies working within the country. Fortunately, we do not have to survey the whole of this field: our task is to identify the role of the voluntary sector in community development initiatives.

The beginnings of community development can be traced back to the settlement movement in Britain and the United States. The first university settlement, Toynbee Hall, was founded by Canon Barnett in Whitechapel in 1884. The main aim of settlement houses was to bridge the gap between the well-educated and affluent and the poor. Another root of community development can be found in the 'Third world under the Colonial Service where the problems facing the administration were immense and the resources slim' (Knight, 1993, p. 50).

One of the most widely known names in the more recent history of community development is Saul Alinsky whose main work was in inter-war Chicago. Alinsky's method was to form coalitions of existing community organisations, and to focus their combined attention on easily identifiable and winnable issues. The tactics were overtly political and confrontational, and early success was thought to be an important incentive for continued campaigning. Churches were often the core groups in Alinsky's coalitions, and this has continued in the successor organisations in the Industrial Areas Foundation.

The American War on Poverty in the 1960s, which was meant to involve 'maximum feasible participation', gave a renewed boost to community development in the United States. The civil rights movement played a prominent part, although some sections within the movement were suspicious of government motives and feared co-option. The Community Development Project (CDP) in the late 1960s in Britain was said to be modelled on the American War on Poverty, but Mayo (1994) says that the British projects lacked the emphasis on economic development that was such a prominent feature of the American Poverty Programme. She says of the latter:

In the USA jobs and training issues have been clearly on the agenda for community development.... The Poverty Programme, which was provided with federal financial backing in 1965, had a major focus on economic issues.

(p. 70)

The relationship in community development between economic and social development is of great significance. The CDP's failure to address economic issues limited its ability to bring about lasting social change. But a balance has to be found: if economic objectives become completely dominant, the poor are unlikely to benefit and community involvement is likely to become peripheral. Job creation, job retention and retraining have to be concentrated in the poorer areas of cities. Massive programmes to re-vitalise prime sites (such as waterfronts in Baltimore, Boston, Genoa, Liverpool, London) do little to benefit either poor people or poor areas and community involvement is minimal. Such schemes are a far cry from those based in small neighbourhoods which address the needs of economically disadvantaged residents.

In the 1980s market-led approaches to development predominated in both the United States and Britain: the emphasis was on property development, and financial and property companies, backed by central government in Britain and by federal state and local government in the United States, were making the strategic investment decisions. Claims were made that commercial confidentiality had to be protected. Towards the end of the decade, however, community involvement and empowerment were in vogue, and those responsible for development projects felt bound to listen to demands for greater participation.

In Britain, for example, the Urban Development Corporations, after criticism from the Audit Commission and other sources, began to acknowledge the desirability of greater community participation. However, although some tentative moves were made, the rhetoric exceeded the achievement. The Urban Development Corporations have now been wound down. According to 'exit strategies' they are supposed to leave local communities in a position to sustain the economic improvements. More recent initiatives by the British government have given greater recognition to the place of community participation in development. The City Challenge and the Single Regeneration Budget (an amalgamation of twenty different programmes) are intended to involve the principle of partnership.

As Atkinson and Cope (1997) say:

> The key notion developed in both City Challenge and SRB is that of local partnership between local government, the private sector, voluntary bodies, local communities and where applicable other government agencies such as training and enterprise councils and English Partnerships.
>
> (p. 41)

The authors note, however, that 'problems are beginning to emerge in securing community participation'. Voluntary agencies appear to be only very marginally engaged. The voluntary sector has some representation on training and enterprise councils, but the role of voluntary agencies as providers of training, particularly for disadvantaged groups, has declined substantially (Finn, 1994).

It would be mistaken to give the impression that no progress has been made and that future prospects are entirely gloomy, but the successes, while demonstrating what can be achieved, are outweighed by the failures. One example which seems to gain general approval is Chicago under Mayor Washington (1983–87), programmes which were continued under Sawyer after Washington's death. Wiewel and Gills (1995) argue that the success in Chicago would not have been possible had the neighbourhood movement been less well-developed. This in no way detracts from the Washington–Sawyer achievement:

> The enduring elements of the legacy of the Washington–Sawyer era ... are that it demonstrated that a progressive coalition can be built which pushes forward the material, democratic and communal–egalitarian interests of most of the city's residents; it also demonstrated that significant changes can take place in the political culture of governance, embracing broad citizen participation. This era represented an unique attempt at fusing expertise with social activism in decision-making and implementation on the basis of shared values about fairness, equity and openness.
>
> (p. 132)

There are similar success stories in other countries. Mayo, for example, cites Harlow in Britain, but there are many small grass-roots developments which receive little publicity. Some of these, in a variety of locations, are described by Knight (1993). It is worth noting that the third European Poverty Programme, launched in 1989, placed much more emphasis on partnership and participation than its predecessors. Voluntary organisations were to be included in partnerships, and this has been a feature of other European Union initiatives since that date. The European Union has also set in train a number of employment and training initiatives which have encouraged developments in all member states.

Employment and training initiatives are only one aspect of community development. Environmental and social improvements of all kinds may be involved: play space, leisure facilities, reclamation of waste land, community transport, meeting places, community shops, credit unions, neighbourhood councils, information and advice centres, carers groups, mothers and toddlers groups, measures to combat crime, vandalism and substance abuse. Some of the groups may be based on gender and/or ethnicity. These activities and groups may exist singly or in any combination, although it is most unlikely that a neighbourhood will be able to sustain the full range. Examples of neighbourhood organisations in a variety of countries may be found in Evers and Svetlik (1993).

Housing is a major concern of many neighbourhood organisations, and indeed housing problems may have been the spur to many community groups which subsequently widened their activities beyond housing. The voluntary sector may be involved in two ways: housing associations or co-operatives may build, refurbish and manage properties; tenants' groups may be involved in various aspects of the management of housing estates and they may campaign on a wide range of housing issues. Many countries have a voluntary or non-profit housing sector with particular responsibilities for social housing. In Britain, for example, most social housing is provided and managed by voluntary sector housing associations. The position is similar in Germany and The Netherlands, but in Japan and the United States the voluntary sector is little involved in social housing. In a book analysing the American non-profit sector (Salamon, 1992) housing is barely mentioned, and then in relation only to government expenditure. In developing countries where housing problems are acute voluntary organisations do sometimes engage in housing provision, but there are also self-build housing schemes supported in some instances by the World Bank. Mayo (1994) reports on two relatively successful schemes in Zambia and Nicaragua.

Tenants' groups have proliferated everywhere. Their functions, powers and influence vary considerably even within a single country. The main growth of such groups occurred in the 1970s in, for example, Britain, France, Germany, The Netherlands and the USA. Willmott (1989) estimated that in Britain in the late 1980s there were 2,000 tenants' organisations. In spite of this large number of organisations, the Nolan Committee still felt compelled to recommend in May 1996 that housing associations should pay particular attention to securing genuine tenant involvement (Edwards, 1996). In relation to the United States, Atlas and Dreier (1983) claimed that tenants' groups 'existed in every city and many suburbs' (pp. 166–7). Tenants' groups differ in size: they may cover a single block of flats or large areas with many units of accommodation. Atlas and Dreier also identified citywide and statewide tenants' groups and in both Britain (in 1977) and the United States (in 1980) national organisations have been formed. In 1991 a Tenants' Resources and Information Service was established in Britain. At the other extreme, tenants' associations in the former GDR covered only ten to twelve households, although their activities were co-ordinated by neighbourhood committees each of which was responsible for between fifty and eighty tenants' associations (Chamberlayne, 1990). The groups were chiefly engaged in repairs and maintenance. In most of the countries of Western Europe and in North America tenants' groups might begin with issues concerning repairs and maintenance, but would anticipate going beyond this to address a wider range of concerns. In 1983 Richardson wrote of tenant participation schemes:

> Some operate as *de facto* complaint forums, in which tenants raise specific problems concerning housing maintenance and other local management issues. Others involve regular discussion of broader issues, such as estate modernisation plans or proposed changes in administrative procedures. Some explicitly preclude consideration of any financial issues, such as rents, but others enable these matters to be discussed along with any other issues tenants wish to raise.
>
> (1983, p. 36)

This was written some years ago, and wide though Richardson's list is, it needs updating with some of the more recent developments. Among the most radical schemes are those involving tenant self-management through co-operatives. Mayo (1994) describes a tenant management co-operative in Camden, and there are some well-known examples in Glasgow. The Netherlands also has tenant management co-operatives. Emms (1990) reports an interesting German example of tenant involvement on the Woltmannweg estate to the south of Berlin. This was a new development to replace a run-down, insanitary estate built in the 1950s as 'temporary' accommodation for homeless refugees and people from clearance areas. Tenants 'were directly involved in the design of the buildings and layout . . . the landscaping, ecological and environmental principles, the range of social facilities . . . shops and commercial facilities, public transport needs, and provision for children and older people who together form over a third of the population' (p. 183). Emms adds, however, that 'Woltmannweg is a rare and possibly unique example in Germany of intensive co-operation between the tenants and the various providing agencies'.

Housing initiatives are also a feature of both rural and urban programmes in developing countries, but although the concerns of developing and developed countries might be similar, the problems facing community development programmes in the Third World are of a quite different order. Community development in developing countries also introduces some additional considerations, one of which is the presence of international or foreign voluntary organisations and their relationship with indigenous agencies. Anheier (1987), in a study of development in Africa, says:

> . . . international NPOs [non-profit organisations] preempt some of the potential areas for indigenous NPO activity. African countries act as hosts for American and European NPOs, and it is the interaction between international and indigenous NPOs that seems to set agendas for the growth and direction of the latter.
>
> (p. 419)

This comment could equally well apply to other parts of the world such as Central and South America. In spite of these problems, however, indigenous agencies are gaining in strength and confidence in most of the developing countries.

Voluntary organisations have substantially expanded their role in international development over the last thirty years. Smith (1993), using OECD and other sources, states that between 1970 and 1988 the transfer of funds from European, Canadian and US non-governmental agencies to developing countries increased from $2.7 billion to $5.2 billion in real terms. In 1980 the number of North Atlantic voluntary agencies involved in foreign aid stood at 1,600: by 1989 this figure had risen to 2,500. Smith also notes that there has been a movement 'away from an exclusive emphasis on relief to include a long-term focus on structural change', tackling the causes of poverty rather than alleviating its symptoms (p. 327). The large financial institutions such as the World Bank and the International Monetary Fund are increasingly channelling funding through voluntary agencies rather than governments, in the belief that this will achieve greater community, grassroots participation and more effectively reach poor people.

Smith (1993) notes that governments in the developed countries have traditionally provided a major part of the resources of voluntary agencies (Smith refers to NGOs) engaged in foreign aid. However, government subsidies have now levelled off, and in some countries, notably the United States and Britain, there have been attempts to reduce dependence on government funding. Even more serious is the growing trend 'for legislatures and foreign aid ministries to offer additional monies to NGOs ... but for specific purposes or regions of the world not of NGO choosing' (p. 330). Government funding comes to reflect 'foreign policy priorities of home governments ... or specific issues of domestic public concern'. In the United States there have been suggestions that the benefits accruing to the American economy should be the main determinant of the scale and direction of expenditure on foreign aid – including grants to voluntary agencies. Smith sees this as a major change, but national self-interest has always been a feature, and possibly the dominant feature, in foreign aid. This makes it all the more important to fully engage indigenous voluntary agencies and local communities in determining their own priorities. A participatory approach, coupled with training programmes, will also help to ensure sustainability – a crucial requirement in all community development whether in the Third World or in advanced industrial countries.

Lack of sustainability was one of the failings of the CDP in Britain and of the War on Poverty programmes in the United States. To some extent this resulted from unrealistic assumptions about what might be achieved. Knight (1993, p. 51) says that the British CDP and similar schemes had over-optimistic aims: 'just as Third World community development was expected to usher in democracy, First World community development was expected to cure poverty – a false hope in both cases.' Some of those involved in these programmes questioned the degree to which voluntary neighbourhood projects could be seen as offering solutions to the problems of deprived areas. Davidoff and Gould, writing of the American poverty programmes, say that all of them shared a common 'underlying strategy based on a false assumption – the assumption that because the problems of race and poverty are found in the ghettos the solution to these problems must also be found there . . .'. Benington (1974) the Director of the Coventry CDP, makes a similar comment about the British anti-poverty programmes:

> Because their causes do not operate at the local level alone, many of these problems are not susceptible to solution at the local level alone. Self-help and community action may help to gain marginal improvements and some compensatory provision. But the crucial determinants of the residents' quality of life remain unaltered.
>
> (p. 275)

Knight (1993) claims that a combination of over-optimistic aims, an initial under-estimation of the system's capacity to resist change and a belief that local action was almost totally ineffective, led to 'the demise of the free-standing community project'. Deakin (1994, p. 67) describes the 'disillusioning effects of the CDP experience, with its bleakly negative message about the irrelevance of local action', but notes that by the end of the 1970s the local perspective began to be re-established.

Knight (1993) and Taylor (1995) both point to the decline in the number of community workers in the UK and Lorenz (1994a) records a decline in The Netherlands from over 3,000 in the 1970s to about 700 in 1990. Lorenz also quotes evidence which suggests that community work in The Netherlands is less concerned than formerly with politically contentious issues such as unemployment, poverty and inequality. It was a similar story in those countries selected as crisis areas in the EU Combat Poverty Programme: Greece, Ireland, Southern Italy, Portugal and Spain. Meekosha and Mowbray (1995) demonstrate that the same process has occurred in Australia where community workers are now less likely to be viewed as radicals fighting for rights and combating oppression. This is a gloomy picture, but there are also more hopeful signs. We have already identified some of these and pointed to examples of successful community involvement. There is a renewed interest in participation and empowerment, and it is in this area that community workers and community groups may rediscover greater radicalism. Helping voluntary agencies to express the needs and views of the groups they represent, and ensuring that this process does not exclude sections of the more disadvantaged members of society, is an important aspect of community development work. This raises issues relating to advocacy and campaigning, and it is to these that we now turn.

Advocacy and campaigning

It should be clear from the discussion of self-help and community development that voluntary agencies frequently engage in pressure or interest group activities. Self-help groups, for example, may be concerned to protect or promote the interests of their members or of the group from which their members are drawn. Neighbourhood groups may press for resources or services to improve the local environment. Service-providing groups may take action in support of their client group. Yet other groups are concerned almost solely with advocacy and campaigning either on behalf of particular social groups (e.g. people with learning disabilities, homeless people, refugees) or to promote a particular cause (e.g. penal reform, pro- or anti-abortion, temperance). It would be misleading to interpret these distinctions too inflexibly. In many respects the groups have similar aims and adopt similar tactics.

For some groups advocacy is their sole or main purpose, attempting to change public attitudes and campaigning for better provision of services. In Britain the Child Poverty Action Group (CPAG), Shelter, the Low Pay Unit and the Unemployment Unit are good examples of groups in this category. All four groups carry out careful research into the issues falling within their sphere of interest. The results are used to challenge official statistics and government interpretations of needs and problems. They comment upon proposed policy changes and keep a watching brief on new legislation. There are similar groups in other countries. An interesting example in the United States is the Center on Budget and Policy Priorities based in Washington, DC which describes itself as 'a non-profit, tax-exempt organization that studies government spending and the programs and public policy issues that have an impact on low-income Americans'. The Center's output, since its establishment in 1984, is impressive: for example, between 1984 and 1995 it published analyses of over twenty tax plans. The tax series is one of three, the other two being (i) hunger and welfare, nutrition and health and (ii) labour issues, unemployment insurance and minimum wage. In

1994 it published several documents on the Clinton health care plans.

The Gray Panthers, in Germany and the United States, are also concerned with pressure rather than service provision. Within a general platform of opposition to ageism, the organisation campaigns on a wide range of issues. In the United States it is particularly powerful. Founded in 1970 by six friends, it now has 40,000 members in thirty-two states. Another influential campaigning body for older people in the United States is the American Association of Retired Persons. There are similar pensioners' groups in most countries.

Some voluntary associations combine advocacy with either self-help or service provision. Many neighbourhood organisations fall into this category, but so do some of the more traditional service-providing agencies. Many of the groups for disabled people combine both functions. The exact balance between service provision and advocacy will vary from one organisation to another: in some instances advocacy will be a major concern while in others it will be peripheral to their main activities and employed only intermittently. A study of voluntary organisations for disabled people in England, Italy, The Netherlands and Norway (Kramer *et al.*, 1993) demonstrates these variations. An interesting but unexplained discrepancy between The Netherlands and the other three was that in the former combining service provision and advocacy was uncommon. It is worth noting that the combination of advocacy and service provision in a single agency is at odds with the Knight's proposal for a split between the two which was referred to earlier.

Kuti (1996) writes of the prevalence of organisations combining advocacy and service provision in Hungary. She explains that such organisations believe that 'practical achievements are more convincing than petitions, demonstrations and theoretical arguments' (p. 139). One of their purposes in beginning to provide services is to alleviate specific problems or fill gaps in provision 'but they also have in mind that making needs explicit is a possible method of advocacy' (p. 139). Kuti calls this 'everyday advocacy'. She distinguishes two other approaches: 'responsive', in which agencies comment upon government policies and proposals, and 'creative', in which voluntary agencies take the initiative and put forward their own policy proposals. Although Kuti is of the opinion that voluntary organisations will eventually become 'a significant force in shaping government policy in Hungary', she is well aware of the constraints arising from lack of knowledge and current experience, ineffective communication within the voluntary sector and some reluctance to co-operate. She also says that 'the service-oriented, multipurpose character of most of the Hungarian voluntary organizations is becoming an obstacle to professional advocacy work in some cases' (p. 140). This is a concern being expressed in Britain as contracting spreads. The fear is that contracts may be granted only for direct service provision and that the time and energy put into negotiating and managing contracts may diminish advocacy.

There are a few voluntary organisations which deliberately eschew advocacy. The best example of such an organisation is Alcoholics Anonymous which 'is not allied with any sect, denomination, politics, organisation, institution; does not wish to engage in any controversy; neither endorses nor opposes any causes' (National Council for Voluntary Organisations, 1984, p. 4). A similar stance is taken by organisations, such as Gamblers Anonymous and Recidivists Anonymous, which have modelled themselves on Alcoholics Anonymous. These organisations have shunned advocacy as an act of deliberate policy, but there are many, particularly local, groups who feel uneasy about advocacy and avoid political controversy. Sometimes the tension between service provision and advocacy may cause dissension in voluntary agencies. There were some members of Gray Panthers in the United Sates who were alienated by the radical politics and militant tactics of their founding member, Maggie Kuhn who died in 1995. Local branches of medical research organisations are often engaged exclusively in fund-raising and would not usually be regarded as interest groups.

Despite these exceptions, however, advocacy constitutes one of the main distinguishing characteristics of voluntary agencies. In the United States, the Filer Commission (Filer, 1975) said that 'the monitoring and influencing of government may be emerging as one of the single most important and effective functions of the private nonprofit sector', (p. 45). The Wolfenden Committee (Wolfenden, 1978) noted that voluntary organisations 'are well placed to act as independent critics and pressure groups' (p. 27). Kramer (1981) goes even further when he claims that the advocacy role 'comes close to being a unique organisational competence of the voluntary agency' (p. 231). Much more recently, the Report of the Commission on the Future of the Voluntary Sector (1996) unambiguously states the importance of these roles:

... the need to carry out other functions usually associated with the sector – campaigning and advocacy – has not diminished. Quite the contrary, in fact. For example, the experience of recession across the European Union has exposed the persistence of racism and prejudice against minorities of all kinds, who have been disproportionately affected by loss of jobs and shortages in the housing market. Other forms of campaigning have also taken on new significance. For example, there is greater awareness of the problems of environmental pollution, which does not respect national boundaries.

(p. 37)

Petracca (1992) claims that the period from the late 1960s has witnessed an 'advocacy explosion'. Petracca's analysis relates principally to the United States, but he cites evidence of a similarly dramatic increase in other countries, including the UK, France and Canada. A relatively recent phenomenon has been a very substantial increase in the number of what Petracca calls citizen or welfare groups.

In exerting pressure on government, either directly or through influencing public opinion, the groups are attempting to secure more favourable treatment for those they represent. They are therefore participating in the process of policy formulation in a variety of ways:

1. By identifying, quantifying and publicising 'problems'.
2. By trying to force issues on to the political agenda and to keep them there.
3. By pressing for or opposing legislative change.
4. By commenting upon government policies and suggesting alternatives.
5. By encouraging statutory agencies to more fully implement policies and thus improve provision, and resisting attempts to reduce provision.
6. By securing a larger share of resources or resisting cuts in expenditure.

Groups may also place emphasis on welfare rights, trying to ensure that potential claimants know their entitlements and how to go about obtaining them. Welfare rights campaigners will be concerned not only with the level of provision, but also with eligibility criteria and procedures. It should be noted that groups not only press for changes they perceive to be beneficial to those they claim to represent, but will oppose changes perceived to be harmful. They may oppose changes on ideological, moral or religious grounds. The Charity Organisation Society in nineteenth century Britain provides a historical example of ideological opposition to extending the state system of cash benefits. More recent examples from the political right would include the American Enterprise Institute, the Hoover Institution and the Heritage Foundation in the United States and the Institute of Economic Affairs, the Adam Smith Institute and the Centre for Policy Studies in Britain. All of these overtly political organisations argue for a reduction in the role of the state in welfare.

While interest groups work on several fronts simultaneously, they attempt to concentrate their efforts on those parts of the political system where pressure is most likely to bring about the desired results. This varies from one country to another depending upon the nature of the political system. In countries with a federal rather than a unitary constitution, the United States, Canada, Switzerland, India, Germany and Australia, for example, the groups are obliged to divide their attention between the federal and state governments. The precise nature of the division will depend upon the division of power between the central and state governments – especially the power to legislate and to decide policy.

In the United States, while not ignoring local, state and federal bureaucracies, groups concentrate their main efforts on Congress and state legislatures because this is where their influence on legislation is most effective. In Britain, by contrast, Parliament has little chance to seriously amend legislation. Although groups are fully aware of the value of the House of Commons as a forum for the airing of issues, their main concern is to influence government departments because it is in these that policies are formulated and legislative proposals are drafted. A similar focus on bureaucracies is common in many European countries. The methods used to influence a representative assembly are entirely inappropriate in dealing with a bureaucracy. Consequently, in the United States the lobby is the most common strategy, while in Britain and many other European countries direct and private negotiations with government officials is more usual. The more public nature of the lobby also encourages much greater use of the mass media in the United States.

Advocacy has the potential to bring voluntary organisations into direct conflict with government. In the United States lobbying is expressly sanctioned by law, but there has been much heated discussion about the right of voluntary bodies in receipt of federal funds to use them to finance lobbying. Several countries impose constraints on the 'political activities' of voluntary organisations. This is a complex legal and regulatory area and the constraints vary considerably from one country to another. Fortunately, Randon and 6 (1994) have conducted some preliminary research into the constraints placed upon public policy campaigning in twenty-four countries. The countries fell into two groups: those which organise the legal status of voluntary bodies around the concept of a charity and those that do not. It is only in the former that constraints are imposed: in non-charity law countries there were no legal impediments to policy campaigning and advocacy. The charity law countries studied were Australia, Canada, England and Wales, India, Ireland, Northern Ireland, Scotland and the United States. All of these countries had some form of legal restrictions on campaigning. In Canada and the United States, for example, limits were placed on the proportion of an organisation's expenditure which could be spent on campaigning. England and Wales is unique in having a Charity Commission; in other countries the law is applied by the tax authorities. It must be stressed that this account deals only with the law, and a great deal depends on how the law is applied. Certainly, there seems to be as much and as vigorous campaigning in the eight countries mentioned above as there is in non-charity law countries such as Belgium, Denmark, France, Germany, Italy, The Netherlands and Nigeria. The absence of legal impediments to campaigning is no guarantee that a repressive government will allow criticism of its activities. Similarly, the existence of apparently restrictive law does not necessarily lead to reduced emphasis on advocacy: much more depends upon the ways in which the laws are interpreted. For example, England is a charity law country, but advocacy remains a key activity of voluntary organisations. The Commission on the Future of the Voluntary Sector (1996) unequivocally endorses the rights of voluntary organisations to campaign:

> In a plural society it is impossible, and probably undesirable, that government and voluntary organisations should always see eye-to-eye on ends or on means. Voluntary organisations can and should provide information, stimulate debate and provoke dissent, whether or not these activities are welcome to those in power. In doing this voluntary organisations are playing their proper role in a democratic society. . . . Government should recognise this, and should

acknowledge its own obligation to support and promote a healthy voluntary sector as a major player in the democratic process.

(p. 49)

In the United States, lobbying is intense. It is heavily concentrated in Washington which, according to Petracca (1992, p. 14) has increasingly 'become a headquarters for national non-profit associations'. Advocacy is big business in the United States. The large organisations employ highly paid legal and public relations teams, and there are richly rewarded companies selling their advocacy and campaigning skills to any organisation willing to pay the very substantial fees. This poses equity issues. The rich business interests predominate and the voice of welfare organisations, and still more the voice of the consumer, may be shouted down. An illustration of this, is the fate of the Clinton health reform proposals which were defeated by a combination of business, insurance and professional interests.

But inequalities also arise even where the business interest is more muted. The power to influence is not equally distributed among different sections of the population. A newspaper report by Walker (1996), for example, claimed that in the United States the 'children of poor families look like footing some of the bill for America's highly vocal elderly population, as politicians shy from tackling soaring Medicare and Medicaid budgets'. Benefits for elderly people are buttressed by middle class support, 'while cuts and savings target the poor who are less adept at lobbying the political system'. Furthermore, as Kendall and Knapp (1996) argue, while voluntary organisations have played a pivotal role 'in changing ideologies, values, responsibilities and policies . . . they have also been reactive vessels for the perpetuation of existing ideologies, attitudes and patterns of privilege and power, and they have acted as mechanisms for social control, not always of the benign variety' (p. 1).

It is clear that some voluntary advocacy groups are more acceptable to governments than others. The more radical, non-traditional groups find it more difficult to raise funds, and their access to the policy-making process is more limited. Governments look much more favourably upon voluntary agencies which provide direct services for approved groups. This preference may lead government agencies to divert voluntary organisations from advocacy to service provision – a trend that may be reinforced by the move to contracting.

Conclusion

There can be no doubting that the voluntary sector now occupies a more substantial role in the provision of welfare in all welfare states than it did in the 1960s and 1970s. There are still wide variations, with Sweden at one end of the spectrum with a relatively small voluntary sector in welfare, and the United States, Germany and The Netherlands at the other. Even in the United States, which has always had an extensive voluntary sector, there was further expansion between 1977 and 1989 when expenditure by the voluntary sector in real terms increased by 79 per cent (Salamon, 1992).

In all welfare states there is substantial dependence on government funding, although the proportion of resources from this source varies from 68.2 per cent in Germany and almost 60 per cent in France, down to 29.2 per cent in the United States. In Central and Eastern Europe revenues coming from government are lower: in Hungary, for example, they amount to 22.9 per cent of the total.[3]

One of the main issues facing voluntary organisations in many countries is the degree to which acceptance of government funding threatens their independence. This danger is perceived to be greater when funding is in the form of contracts rather than grants. Contracts constitute a form of regulation, specifying how much of a service is to be provided, for which clients and at what cost. Quality standards will be laid down and even procedures and processes may be prescribed. Contracts do, however, vary in their specificity and monitoring contract compliance is expensive and time-consuming. More generally, Kramer *et al.* (1993) argue that:

> For government, the costs of more systematic supervision and control are often too great fiscally and politically, hence the typical lack of governmental incentive and capacity to assure adequate accountability from its private public-service providers.
>
> (p. 195)

Nevertheless, a number of studies identify independence as an issue in several countries. The report of the Johns Hopkins University twelve-country project states:

> Few issues are as crucial to the future of the non-profit sector . . . as determining how to fashion cooperation with the state in a way that

protects the non-profit sector from surrendering its basic autonomy and thus allows it to function as a true partner with the state and not simply as an 'agent' or 'vendor'.

(Salamon and Anheier, 1994, pp. 103–4)

The need for vigilance to maintain the independence of the voluntary sector is a theme running through two British studies (Knight, 1993; Commission on the Future of the Voluntary Sector, 1996) and a study looking at the lessons to be learned from the American experience (Richardson, 1993). The Japanese voluntary sector provides an example of a system almost totally lacking in independence with the social welfare corporations restricted to carrying out the work assigned to them by central and local government. Salamon and Anheier (1994, p. 82) say that 'no concept of an independent, private, voluntary sector existing apart from, and to some extent in opposition to, the state exists in Japan'.

The policy dilemma for voluntary organisations is how they are to co-operate with government and at the same time retain their independence. They have to decide whether the acceptance of state funding in any way compromises their freedom to criticise government agencies. An associated dilemma is whether an enhanced role in service provision interferes with their roles in advocacy and community development.

Participation in quasi-markets poses another set of dilemmas for voluntary organisations. They may be forced to compete one with another and with commercial operators. There may be a reduced willingness to share information among voluntary organisations as more of the information becomes commercially sensitive. A balance has to be struck between co-operation and competition. If competition predominates, then voluntary organisations can easily take on the characteristics of commercial enterprises, and what is valuable in being 'voluntary' may be lost.

Government policy determines the social policy context in which the voluntary sector operates, but the capacity to influence that policy varies cross-nationally. We have just seen that no such opportunity arises in Japan. In corporatist Germany, by contrast, the peak voluntary organisations are consulted about any major legislative changes and there are permanent arrangements, involving representatives of the trade unions, employers, insurance associations and government, for discussion of economic and social policy.

Particular examples of the impact of government policy include reduced government support for publicly provided services in Britain and the United States in the 1980s. Both Reagan and Thatcher sought to reduce public expenditure and shift responsibility for meeting need to non-state providers, including the voluntary sector: their successors have not significantly changed this approach. The notion, once common in Britain, of the voluntary sector complementing and supplementing state provision is being replaced by a policy of substitution. It may very well be that complementing and supplementing state provision accurately described the role of the voluntary sector in Britain, but it understated the sector's role in Germany, The Netherlands and the United States and overstated it in France and Italy (before the 1980s) and Sweden.

The example of The Netherlands seems to indicate that the voluntary sector has the capacity to substitute for the state in service provision. However, the role of the voluntary sector in The Netherlands derives from a particular set of cultural and historical circumstances. Furthermore, the system is currently experiencing some strain with the government using its dominance in funding to foster greater integration and amalgamations. Kramer *et al.* (1993, p. 83) claim that the 'relations between the service organizations and the government are becoming ever more ambivalent' and that 'the growing influence and intervention of government have provoked complaints and fears'.

In the United States, the voluntary sector is already prominent in certain aspects of health care and in the personal social services, but in many other countries, the voluntary sector may be in no position to substitute for the state in health, social security and educational provision. Substitution is more feasible in the personal social services, and substitution in this sphere has already taken place in the United States and is in the process of doing so in Britain. France and Italy are some way behind in this respect, and the reborn voluntary sector in Central and Eastern Europe is still too weak to serve as the major provider of a range of adequate services.

Voluntary organisations, however, are not simply providers of services. They are also repositories of values. Voluntarism gives opportunities for service to others; it offers a practical means of expressing a sense of civic pride and duty. The voluntary sector, itself diverse, contributes to social diversity and constitutes an essential ingredient in a civil society and a democratic polity. The Report of the Commission on the Future of the Voluntary Sector (1996) states:

> The value base of voluntary organisations is one of their defining characteristics. It is an essential part of the answer to the question 'if not for profit then for what'? Within this value base are several clear strands that include caring, user involvement and, in its widest sense, equal opportunities. These stem from a concern with issues of fairness and equity.
>
> (p. 113)

While there is no doubting the voluntary sector's concern with equity and fairness, there are circumstances, paradoxically, in which increased use of voluntary organisations may lead to greater inequity. This arises because of the unevenness of voluntary provision. Urban areas are better served than rural ones and affluent areas are better served than deprived areas. This raises doubts about the sector's ability to achieve equity. Leat (1990b) argues:

> The voluntary sector does not have the capacity adequately to administer and regulate provision in such a way as to ensure equity and wide coverage. The sector has difficulty in coping with equity not least because voluntary initiatives do not flourish most easily in areas of high need.
>
> (p. 282)

Leat's analysis relates to Britain, but Sosin (1986) found a similar discrepancy between levels of need and voluntary action in the United States. If this is the case in Britain and the United States, with relatively well-developed voluntary sectors, it is likely to apply with equal or greater force to many other countries. Nor are the inequities related only to territorial areas and social class. There is also uneven distribution among client groups. Children, physically disabled and elderly people tend to be well-served by voluntary organisations, whereas mentally ill people, alcohol and drug abusers, single homeless people, certain ethnic minorities, gay men and lesbian women, and lone parents are poorly served.

This general tendency among voluntary organisations to distribute resources in such a way as to benefit certain sub-groups in the population is usually referred to as particularism or clientelism. In some respects this may be thought of as a strength of the voluntary sector, but as Salamon (1987, p. 112) says it 'also has its drawbacks as the basis for organizing a community's response to human needs'. The major drawback is the greater inequity resulting from it. In some welfare states, public services also exhibit strong elements of clientelism. In Italy, for example, there is 'a long-standing tradition of rewarding various constituencies with social policies that benefit only them' (Kramer *et al.* 1993, p. 52). Lorenz (1994a) describes a similar situation in Greece where newly created participatory structures have been expropriated by the political parties. In welfare states already clientelist, an augmented role for the voluntary sector may lead to increased particularism. In relation to one such country Kramer *et al.* (1993, p. 195) say: 'Because Italy's welfare state . . . is already notoriously particularistic, extensive delegation of service delivery to voluntary agencies could erode even more rapidly its nominal universality'.

As long as voluntary organisations were limited to complementing and supplementing statutory provision, a consideration of the sector's strengths and weaknesses was of only marginal relevance to the overall analysis and evaluation of welfare states. Now that voluntary organisations have moved centre stage, an assessment of their advantages and deficiencies becomes increasingly more relevant. The aim of this chapter was to look at the growing body of available evidence about the role of the voluntary sector in a wide variety of welfare states. A realistic appraisal, however, is possible only if the sector is considered as a component in mixed economies of welfare, and the chapter has therefore paid some attention to the voluntary sector's relationships with markets and the state. The next chapter examines the informal sector. There are few studies that examine voluntary sector/informal sector relationships, but a useful framework for analysing voluntary-informal relationships was suggested by the Wolfenden Report (Wolfenden, 1978). The Report identified three roles for voluntary organisations in relation to the informal sector: (i) replacement where family or neighbourhood arrangements do not exist or have broken down or cannot cope; (ii) relieving the pressure on families by providing respite care in the form of day centres or short-term residential care; (iii) reinforcing informal caring arrangements by providing various forms of psychological and practical support. This provides some clear points of connection between this chapter and the one that follows.

Notes

1. 6 (1995) disagrees with this requirement because it becomes very difficult to handle non-profit co-operatives.
2. Note here the impact of the single market in the European Union.
3. The source of these figures is Salamon and Anheier (1994).

CHAPTER 5

THE INFORMAL SECTOR AND SOCIAL WELFARE

Introduction

What is normally understood by the informal sector in social welfare is the provision of social and health care by relatives, friends and neighbours. It is extremely difficult to measure the extent and importance of such care because much of it is unrecorded, both carers and the recipients of care regarding their actions as 'natural' and unremarkable. Even if the number and range of contacts could be accurately recorded, there would still be problems. For example, it would be difficult to decide upon an appropriate unit of measurement which takes into account not only the frequency and duration of contacts but also their intensity and the subjective meaning attached to them by the participants.

There was a heightening of interest in informal care during the 1980s and the 1990s. Most of this work was concerned with care by families; much less attention was paid to the role of friends and neighbours. The increased volume of studies concerned with families was particularly marked in Europe, with many people and institutions contributing to the growing body of work. Among the institutions taking an active interest were the Social Policy Research Unit at the University of York, the Joseph Rowntree Foundation, also located in York, the Family Policy Studies Centre in London and the European Centre for Social Welfare Policy and Research in Vienna. The European Commission was also actively engaged in promoting work on families through the European Observatory on National Family Policies, and 1994 was the International Year of the Family. Most of the studies were comparative, and we will have cause to refer to them as the chapter progresses.

Lewis (1989) says that during the 1950s studies of the family were dominated by functionalists such as Talcott Parsons. The 1960s and the early 1970s saw few innovative studies, but there was a revival of interest beginning in the mid-1970s and gathering pace in the 1980s. Lewis claims that feminist theorists have been chiefly responsible for the new prominence being given to studies of the family:

> In large measure it was feminist analysis that brought the study of the family back to life. Particularly crucial have been the distinction between sex (the biological) from gender (the social) and the conceptualization of women's labour as wives and mothers as unpaid work.
> (1989, p. 132)

There is a great deal of truth in this observation, but other factors have also been at work. Among these may be mentioned: policies which emphasise care in the community; the desire to reduce expenditure and shift costs from the state to families; the pressure from the political and religious right for a return to 'traditional family values', coupled with a concern, not restricted to the New Right, that the family is in decline. Family decline is seen as both a symptom and a cause of social and moral instability and disintegration. This is a debate we will return to later in the chapter.

Although difficulties of measurement and incomplete evidence make the precise quantification of the informal sector problematic, there can be little doubt that in all welfare states its contribution is considerable. In the case of elderly and disabled people not living in institutions (and most are not in residential care) the informal system is almost certainly more important by a considerable margin than either the statutory, voluntary or commercial sectors. Child care is overwhelmingly provided by parents, and where these are not available, by other relatives.

An international perspective, focusing specifically on family care for frail elderly people, is provided by the OECD (1994):

> As elderly people become more frail and in need of care, it is usually the network of family members which responds first, and which is responsible for the greatest proportion of care for elderly people. . . . Attempts to estimate the value of family care, using even modest rates for bought-in care, suggest that it exceeds by a ratio of at least 3

or 4 to 1 the value of formal services, even in countries with highly-developed social services.

(1994, p. 41)

Evidence in support of this statement will be the main focus of this chapter, but first, a conceptual and theoretical framework must be established. To this end, the next section considers three issues: community care; theories of the family; and politics and the family.

Theoretical and conceptual framework

Community care

Neither of the two words in the term community care is unproblematic, and the first task is to consider some of the alternative meanings ascribed to each of them. We can begin looking for the meaning of community by referring to the work of two nineteenth century German social theorists: Tönnies and Durkheim. For Tönnies (1887), the change to an industrial society had malign effects on community relationships. He distinguished between *gemeinschaft* (community) and *gesellschaft* (associations); industrialisation involved a movement in the ordering of social relationships from the former to the latter. Thus pre-industrial society was characterised by strong ties of kinship, friendship, neighbourliness, community and tradition, whereas industrial society was based on more impersonal, associational patterns of relationships. Durkheim (1893) took a different approach to the impact of industrialisation on community relationships, arguing that the change from pre-industrial to industrial society was accompanied by a shift from mechanical to organic solidarity. Mechanical solidarity was characterised by tradition, known rules and shared tasks. Organic solidarity was characterised by differentiation and the division of labour, with the family giving ground to the workplace and relationships being governed by the roles people played. Tönnies considered the possibility of recreating the more traditional, informal and personal relationships in modern society. Similarly, present-day communitarians lament the lost ideals of community on which American and other societies used to be based, but believe that a return to community styles of living is both desirable and achievable. Whether such an ideal state ever existed is open to question. At the very least, as Abrams (1977; 1980) argued more than twenty years ago, such small, tightly-knit communities as existed in the past were based on isolation and shared adversity – there may have been a sense of community in the nineteenth century urban slums, but any loss of community consequent upon urban regeneration and improvement seems a small price to pay.

One of the problems of defining community is the unrealistic and romantic interpretations of the term. Nowhere is this more apparent than in the fashionable doctrine of communitarianism which Amitai Etzioni (1995) has been promoting with an almost religious zeal since 1990. He has won the support of Clinton and other political leaders in the United States, Prime Minister Blair in the UK and Chancellor Kohl in Germany, but his influence spreads well beyond these three countries.

The emphasis in communitarianism is on duties and responsibilities rather than rights; indeed it calls for a moratorium on any new rights and some existing rights may have to be foregone so that people can focus on service. American society, it is argued went astray in the 1960s encouraging selfishness, greed and materialism, and too great a dependence on the state. The cure is a return to traditional family values, reversing the 'parenting deficit'. Greater attention would be paid to service to others and civic duties. Divorce would be made more difficult, and moral education would be introduced into the school curriculum. Crime would be dealt with by a mixture of peer pressure (including public humiliation), random alcohol and drug testing, community policing and crime watch schemes. Communitarianism is at its strongest in exposing the shortcomings of stark individualism. Bell (1993) for example, sees communitarianism as presenting a challenge to liberal individualism, and he criticises western governments for failing to recognise the importance of both local democracy and community.

Many of these ideas have been taken up by the Labour Party in the UK under the leadership of Blair. In fashioning the new Labour Party, Blair constantly emphasised the importance of community which he claimed was the true basis of socialism. In this philosophy, responsibilities are given at least equal weight with rights and social class is not even mentioned. Socialism defined in terms of duties is the main theme of a work by Selbourne (1994) who argues that the notion of civic duty should be given more prominence in theories of socialism. Young (1994) says that Selbourne's work should 'become a significant text for the socialism-of-community that Blair is seeking to define'. The idea of community as a principal element in socialism has a much longer history than new Labour. It has close connections with the fraternity associated with the French Revolution, and the term was used by Owen and Morris in the nineteenth century. Also in the nineteenth century, the notion of solidarity and fraternity informed the nascent labour movement.

Mayo (1994, p. 48) says that 'the concept of "community" is notorious for its shiftiness'. She argues that the difficulties of definition are compounded by disputes about alternative sociological approaches and competing political orientations:

> It is not just that the term community has been used ambiguously; it has been contested, fought over, and appropriated for different uses and interests to justify different politics, policies and practices.
>
> (1994, p. 48)

Among the most obvious ways of defining community is with reference to sets of relationships. These relationships may be based on geography, with people interacting with others who live in close proximity to them. Such interactions most commonly take place in relatively restricted areas or neighbourhoods. However, people have different sets of relationships which may be based on work or occupational group, religion, ethnic origin, political affiliation, leisure pursuits, or even shared adversity. This formulation ignores the quality of the relationships. Feelings of belonging, sharing a common identity, solidarity and comradeship are what most people have in mind when they talk of community.

We can begin to understand why some commentators express doubts about the usefulness of the term. Mayo (1994, p. 48) for example, says that 'there is a case to answer as to whether "community" should actually continue to be used at all'. To avoid some of the difficulties and restrictions arising from the use of the term community, Bulmer (1987) suggests that the focus should be on primary groups and networks. He distinguishes between primary group relationships or personal relationships and institutionalised or socially structured relationships. Personal relationships are characterised by informal ties, principally between friends, neighbours and kin. Such ties, Bulmer argues, are 'established on the basis of affect, tradition or propinquity (in the case of neighbours)' (p. 38). These personal relationships are compared with formal institutional relationships based upon 'roles, offices, formal rules and patterns of expectation' (p. 38). This analysis has particular relevance for the study of informal care which is the concern of this chapter. Bulmer argues that:

> A major benefit of shifting the emphasis from the study of 'community' to the study of the primary group – whether made up of neighbours, friends or kin – is that it gets away from the metaphysical problem of community.
>
> (1987, p. 39)

Bulmer also uses the term 'social network' as a means of avoiding the more ambiguous 'community'. As a way of encapsulating informal care in the community, social networks is a useful concept because it does not have the territorial limitations of some of the definitions of community. It also allows for the consideration of a wide range of informal relationships, suggesting complex, possibly interlocking, patterns of interaction which can nevertheless be mapped and evaluated. Bulmer summarises the advantages of network analysis in the following way:

> Personal relationships are at the heart of informal care, but they are also a mainstay of local social relationships. The value of the term network lies in avoiding the reification involved in talking about 'community', yet enabling one to talk about a wider set of informal relationships than just the family or the extended kin group. The set of relationships has broadened to include friends, neighbours and work associates.
>
> (p. 109)

Unfortunately, the use of the term 'network', without qualification, shares some of the problems of the term 'community'. The problem is one of scale. Networks can cover a small local area or a whole city or a whole country or may stretch to larger political groupings or even the whole world. The use of the word 'local' may help, but 'local' is capable of varying interpretations. In looking at informal care we are concerned with personal relationships and what might be termed 'informal networks'. Another term that is in common use is 'helping networks'. For example, the following passage, taken from a book by four American writers, emphasises the significance of 'helping networks':

> We have chosen to use the term 'helping networks' to describe a wide
> range of informal helping activities . . . we believe that emphasizing
> informal helping within the context of a network of relationships has
> distinct conceptual advantages to more traditional ways of viewing
> social relationships. The concept of a network in its most general
> form draws our attention to the *structure* of relationships among a set
> of actors as well as the specific *exchanges* which take place among
> them and the *roles* they play with each other.
>
> (Froland *et al.*, 1981, p. 19)

The idea of helping networks brings us closer to what is usually
implied by informal care. However, the term 'care' is itself ambiguous, and some clarification is required. A useful, and now quite
common, distinction is made between 'caring about' someone and
'caring for' someone. Although this distinction is now well-known, its
origins are relatively recent. Parker (1980; 1981) was among the first
to make explicit the difference between the two uses of the term
caring, and Ungerson (1983, p. 31) warns of the dangers of making
'the all too easy, but mistaken, elision between caring *about* someone
and caring *for* that person'. Caring *about* someone refers to feelings
of affection and attachment. Caring *for* someone means attending to
their everyday needs – making people's lives more comfortable.
Graham (1983) makes a similar distinction between caring as labour
and caring as love. She talks of 'a labour of love' and contends that
much of the analysis in both Psychology and Social Policy fails to take
account of the ways in which these two aspects of caring are closely
interwoven. She also argues that caring is about both activity
(labour) and identity. Caring is integral to the way in which women
construct their identities. Finch (1993) uses the phrase 'emotional
labour' and sums up her own and Graham's argument:

> Caring is bound up with the construction of women's social identities
> in a way which is simply not true for men. Labour and love are
> intertwined in a way which is specified for women, and which makes
> the experience of being a female carer different from being a male
> carer, even if a man and a woman are performing the same physical
> tasks.
>
> (1993, p.16)

This is not the end of the terminological tangle. The motivations
for caring for a family member will vary from person to person. It can
not be assumed that care, even within families, is automatically an

expression of affection and nothing else. People may help others out of a sense of duty or obligation. Children caring for elderly parents may see it as a repayment for the care which they received when they were younger. Again, the repayment may be seen either as an expression of gratitude or as a more general obligation to repay debts. The importance of duty or obligation in propelling people (particularly women) into caring relationships is demonstrated in work by Lewis and Meredith (1988) and Ungerson (1987). A very influential book by Finch (1989) is called *Family Obligations and Social Change*. In the conclusion to the book, after reviewing the evidence on the practical aspects of caring, Finch states:

> The other dimension to family support is what I have called throughout the 'sense of obligation'. This is the 'ought' dimension, reflected in political debate by the belief that people *should* be prepared to assist their relatives, even if this does not always happen in practice. For many people this sense of obligation is the key defining characteristic of family ties, especially between close kin. You feel 'duty-bound' to help your family, and this gives kin support an inescapable quality.
>
> (1989, pp. 240–1)

However, duty and affection are as inextricably intertwined as are love and labour. The relative strengths of the two elements can not be determined empirically with any degree of confidence.

Another issue that has come to the fore since the mid-1980s is a questioning of the sharp distinction that is frequently drawn between formal and informal care. Ungerson (1990) explains why the split has been perpetuated among British scholars:

> Perhaps because the word 'caring' has slipped into the British vernacular to refer largely to the *informal* caring which – by definition – only exists within the private domain, it is noticeable that the British feminist literature on caring has tended implicitly to accept the conceptual division between public and private and stress the private context of caring.
>
> (1990, p. 10)

Ungerson expresses doubts about the utility of such a conceptual split, and notes that Scandinavian scholars 'appear to have shaped not only a vocabulary, but also a mode of analysis which crosses the public/private conceptual division and allows them to analyse aspects of the two domains together' (p. 13). The distinction between formal and informal care becomes increasingly blurred as payments for care grow in significance. This is an important topic, but since it is tied in with social security provision for those receiving and providing care, consideration of it will be delayed until a later section of the chapter when policies designed to promote informal care are examined.

The concepts of care and caring, which at first glance seem so simple, become increasingly complex the moment one scratches the surface. The greater subtlety of the debate surrounding the notion of care is due almost entirely to nearly two decades of feminist scholarship.

Having separated and unpacked the terms 'community' and 'care', it is now time to re-unite them and to look at community care which is now the preferred policy option in just about every welfare state. When community care began to grow in popularity during the 1950s, it was defined as care *in* the community as opposed to care in institutions. The explanation of this shift in emphasis from institutions towards the community as the location for care is multi-faceted. The reasons may be divided into two broad categories: those relating to the alleged harmful effects of institutional life and those relating to the positive advantages of remaining in the community.

Prominent among the factors contributing to the declining popularity of institutional care was research in the late 1950s and the 1960s demonstrating the harmful consequences of living in what were referred to as total institutions: the break with familiar surroundings and relationships, the humiliating admission procedures, the submission to rigid regimes, the loss of the ability to determine one's own routine and activities add up to what Goffman (1961) calls 'the mortification of self'. Total institutions, often physically and socially isolated, were defined by Goffman in the following way:

> A total institution may be defined as a place of residence and work where a large number of like-situated individuals, cut off from the wider society for an appreciable period of time, together lead an enclosed, formally administered round of life. Prisons serve as a clear example, providing we appreciate that what is prison-like about prisons is found in institutions whose members have broken no laws.
>
> (1961, p. 1)

Other prime examples of total institutions include enclosed religious orders and military barracks. In the field of social and health care are mental hospitals, homes and hospitals for the chronic sick, residential establishments for older people and children and boarding schools. Much of Goffman's work was concerned with mental hospitals, and it was in mental health that the process of large-scale de-institutionalisation first began. Goffman was not the only influence on these developments. The anti-psychiatry movement, led by Laing (1959; 1961) and Szasz (1961), also flourished in the early 1960s. Both Laing and Szasz were psychiatrists, but they claimed that there was no such thing as mental illness, and that psychiatrists were agents of an oppressive society. The most blatant expression of this oppression was to be observed in the psychiatric hospitals. The earliest response to these ideas came in Italy in about 1963, although *psichiatria democratica* did not reach its fullest expression until 1978 when a new law was passed which brought about the wholesale closure of hospitals. The plan was to replace these with non-oppressive community facilities, and where these facilities were made available (as in Trieste, for example) the lives of patients were greatly improved (Basaglia, 1980; Ramon, 1985). The reforms were more successful in Northern and Central Italy than they were in the South. But there were large areas throughout the country where no extra community facilities were made available, and mental patients were turned out of the hospitals to wander the streets. Such people became known as the *abbondonati* – the abandoned ones.

No other country went as far or as fast as Italy, but changes did occur in most European countries and in the United States in the late 1960s. Although there were differences in approach, the general trend was away from institutional care with a greater emphasis on community care. Care in the community came to be based in many countries on multi-disciplinary teams. In the United States the plan, never fully realised, was to establish a nationwide network of one-stop mental health centres. Thus, the institutional population in mental health declined from the late 1960s onwards. Mental health services have been singled out for more detailed treatment because the changes have been more marked (and more controversial) in this area than in any others. Mental health also demonstrates better than any other service the ways in which the development of community care was partly a response to the shortcomings of institutional care. There can be no question, though, that these socio-psychological studies were given added weight by economic considerations and the assumption that community care would be less costly. Cost considerations were particularly relevant in the 1950s and 1960s because of the poor state of repair of many of the mental hospitals. Hughes and Lovell (1986, p. 161), for example, claim that one of the reasons for the de-institutionalisation programme in American mental health services was that 'the existing physical plant of the public asylum system – a legacy of the nineteenth century – was rapidly approaching a state of total decrepitude that made their renovation or replacement mandatory'. The same legacy was apparent throughout Western Europe, although a partial exception has to be made of the Scandinavian countries.

As already indicated, the argument for community care did not rest solely on the negative aspects of institutions; there were also more positive arguments stressing the benefits of care in community settings. At the same time as total institutions were being vilified, a number of studies emphasised the importance of community relationships. Indicative of the interest in community was the foundation in 1954 of the Institute of Community Studies. Much of the work emanating from the Institute was concerned with the durability and the continuing role of the extended family. Examples of such studies include: *The Family Life of Old People* (Townsend, 1957); *Family and Kinship in East London* (Young and Willmott, 1957); *Family and Class in a London Suburb* (Willmott and Young, 1960).

In the 1960s community care in Britain was generally interpreted to mean care by statutory personnel working within the community. This is clear from the community care report issued by the Ministry of Health in 1963. The fact that this report was issued by the Ministry of Health has some significance in that community care was usually assumed to concern only health and personal social services: the importance of housing and social security for community care was not always appreciated.

A shift in meaning of community care began to emerge in the 1970s; a shift from care *in* the community to care *by* the community: a distinction first made by Bayley (1972). It is difficult to overstate the significance of this change of meaning. Care *by* the community is care by family, friends and neighbours. This was most clearly stated in a White Paper on the care of elderly people in Britain:

> Whatever level of public expenditure proves practicable, and however it is distributed the primary sources of support and care are informal and voluntary. These spring from the personal ties of kinship, friendship and neighbourhood. They are irreplaceable. It is the role of public authorities to sustain and, where necessary, to

develop – but never to replace – such support and care. Care *in* the community must increasingly mean care *by* the community.

(Department of Health and Social Security, 1981, p. 3)

Community care became popular with governments because it seemed to offer the opportunity to cut public expenditure and reduce the role of the state. The Commission of the European Community in its Report on Social Development in 1981 stated:

> Throughout the Community, the tendency has for some years been to reduce the number of people in residential institutions, caring for them instead in their own homes or families with the assistance of out-patient services and day-care centres. Some governments are now in favour of speeding up movement in this direction both on humanitarian grounds and with a view to economising resources.
>
> (Commission of the European Communities, 1982, p. 119)

In the following year, the Commission claimed, 'the policy of community care was promoted with increasing vigour by governments anxious to transfer the cost of such care away from their budgets' (Commission of the European Communities, 1983, p. 127). The economic imperatives leading to community care could hardly be more plainly stated. It should be noted that the costs were transferred to informal carers.

By the beginning of the 1980s, then, community care was firmly established as the preferred policy option. The balance of evidence suggests that, given the option, most older disabled and chronically sick people prefer to remain in the community rather than enter an institution. Nevertheless, the demand for residential care, particularly among the elderly population, remains high. The older, frailer and more dependent people become, the more they (or their relatives) are likely to contemplate residential care. Residential institutions differ in the degree to which they exhibit the characteristics of total institutions identified by Goffman. Smaller institutions, near to or in major centres of population, are very different from the large and isolated psychiatric hospitals. Hospital treatment itself has undergone changes with the integration of mental health services into the general hospital system and the introduction of therapeutic communities. The stark choice between institutional life and community care was being modified by different forms of sheltered accommodation and by the acceptance of the practice of spending short periods in an institution interspersed with longer periods in the community.

The definition favoured by governments was care *by* the community. Criticisms of this new formulation, and of the romantic vision of community care were already being voiced in the late 1970s. Abrams (1977), for example, did an effective demolition job on the romantic views of community care. Abrams defined community care as 'provision of help, support and protection to others by lay members of societies acting in everyday domestic and occupational settings' (p. 125). Community care is thus distinguished by its agents (lay people) and the setting in which it occurs (open). Abrams rejects spontaneity as an important distinguishing characteristic of community care:

> I would like deliberately and specifically to avoid any suggestion that spontaneity is a defining feature of community care . . . there is no evidence . . . that would suggest that spontaneity is in any way an important source of the type of sustained altruistic practice which community care embodies.
>
> (1977, p. 128)

Abrams's general view is that community care in modern industrial societies is 'typically volatile, spasmodic and unreliable' (p. 130), but that if we are looking for a firmer basis for community care, then we must look to reciprocity. Romantic notions of selfless caring relationships in a community setting must be discarded: 'The relevant finding seems clearly to be that effective community care is almost invariably tied to perceptions of long- or short-term reciprocal advantage' (p. 132).

More prosaically, the financial advantages claimed for community care may be illusory, in that a full range of community services will not necessarily cost less than institutional care. If community care means leaving people with inadequate care, or if it means privatising the finance and provision of care by transferring responsibility to families, then the only gains will be reduced public expenditure. In other words, what may be achieved is not a reduction in total costs but a redistribution of responsibility for meeting them.

Higgins (1989) goes further than most in entirely rejecting the use of the term community care which she describes as 'an unnecessary and complicating element in social policy analysis and can be abandoned without any real loss to meaning or understanding' (p. 15). Higgins argues that the distinction between institutions and community is not at all helpful:

The real distinction is actually between the institution and home, and
services are normally available either in the institution or *from* home
(in the case of day care) or *at* home (in the case of domiciliary care).
. . . Adding in the concept of community implies care by anonymous
others and conceals the great volume of care which is carried out by
kin (especially female kin) in the home.

(1989, p. 15)

Higgins refers, in the above quotation, to the predominance of
women as providers of care in the home, and it has already been
noted how feminist writers throughout the 1980s and into the 1990s
have criticised the gendered nature of community care. The in-
equitable distribution of caring work is closely related to care within
families, and a fuller treatment of this important aspect of
community care is to be found in a later section of the chapter. The
discussion will be informed by some of the theoretical work concerning families.

Theories of the family

One problem in trying to construct theories in this area is the variety
of family types that any theory must encompass. It is misleading to
talk of the family as though all families were much the same: an
assumption, perhaps, that the typical family consists of two married
adults with dependent children. As Campling (1985, p. ix) says,
'Historical and contemporary evidence shows that the only real
defining characteristic of families is their variability'. A basic
distinction is between nuclear families of two generations (one or
two adults with children) and extended families including grand
parents, aunts, uncles, cousins and more distant relatives. This
distinction, however, barely makes a beginning in exposing the
diversity. If, for example, we look at couples or partnerships then we
find considerable variation:

- Married couples with children.
- Unmarried couples with children.
- Married couples without children.
- Unmarried couples without children.
- Retired couples.
- Gay/lesbian couples with children.
- Gay/lesbian couples without children.

In addition, there are lone mothers and fathers, and if households as well as families are considered, then people living alone without children have to be included. Adult couples may live with one of the two sets of parents and older people may live with their adult children. There may be rural and urban variations and families will be affected by the social and cultural environment in which they are placed: for example, tribal and caste systems will have a substantial impact. It should be noted, too, that this catalogue concentrates on the structural aspect of families, taking no account of diversity of relationships within families.

There is a continuing debate about the extent of change that has occurred in family structures and relationships. Part of this debate concerns the claim that the extended family has disappeared to be replaced by the nuclear family. On the one hand, Laslett (1980) disputes the claim that the nuclear family is the result of urbanisation and industrialisation arguing that this particular family form has been common since the Middle Ages. On the other hand, as we shall see when we examine family care, the extended family is not dead. This is certainly true of Japan and other East Asian countries and of Southern Europe, but it also lingers on in Western advanced industrial societies.

Another debate about family change is concerned with relationships within families, and a move from an instrumental role of the family to a more affective one (Shorter, 1975). According to this approach, family units have become closer and more private. As a consequence, relationships within the family are more equal. This view is disputed by Delphy and Leonard (1992) who claim that patriarchy is still the dominant characteristic of family relationships with power in the hands of husbands and fathers. Thus the family is essentially oppressive and women are the oppressed. Dalley (1988) sums up the radical feminist perspective:

> Feminists are mostly agreed in linking women's subordination today to the structure of the nuclear family and the ideology which underpins it, and identify the development of these and their hegemonic nature to the rise of capitalism.
>
> (p. 36)

A midway position is taken by Fox Harding (1996) who argues that the patriarchal nature of marriage has declined giving women greater freedom and more choices of lifestyle. Nevertheless, although patriarchy has been weakened, it has not disappeared. She seems to support Walby's (1990) view that private patriarchy within house-holds has been partially replaced by public patriarchy based on institutions outside of the family and marriage. Fox Harding (1996, p. 105) believes that in recent decades the family has undergone fundamental change, 'but that the importance of close relationships continues in a modified patriarchal framework'. The weakening of patriarchy has made families and marriage more fragile.

It is important to realise that most of the theorising about families is concerned with white people living in Western industrial societies. Cultural and religious factors are of prime importance in deter-mining family structures and roles: examples might be Confucianism in East Asia and Catholicism in Latin America and Southern Europe. Equally, tribal systems in Africa and the caste system in India have an impact upon families. Developing countries may adopt different family patterns from those common in the developed nations. Furthermore, there are likely to be regional, class and ethnic variations within countries. Thus social provision and support for families should ideally recognise cultural differences. This raises a number of political considerations and it is to politics and the family that we now turn.

Politics and the family

Jones and Millar (1996, p. 4) say that 'the ways in which governments do, or should, intervene to alter existing family patterns, or behav-iour within families, is central to political debate in Britain'. It is also a matter for debate in many other countries around the world, and as will be seen in the discussion of social policy and the family later in this chapter, there are several different models of state–family relationships.

In this section we will be dealing largely with the ideological elements in the debate, beginning with the views of conservatives because they have always been supporters of the family, frequently bemoaning its decline, which they see as the cause of declining stand-ards of discipline among the young and, more broadly, of declining moral and religious standards throughout society. The family, when properly functioning, is seen as an effective means of socialisation and social control: it is a source of stability in the married partners, and it provides a stable background for the rearing of children who develop into well-adjusted adults. According to Berger (1993) in an Institute of Economic Affairs publication, the conventional two-parent family, what she calls the 'bourgeois family', is the source of economic prosperity in Western industrialised countries. She writes: 'This type of family . . . is particularly suited for producing self-reliant, morally accountable and entrepreneurial individuals who become the carriers of political responsibility and economic prosperity' (p. 24). She argues from this that 'the fate of the bourgeois family and the fate of our type of society are inexorably intertwined (pp. 24–5). This is a view not too dissimilar to that expressed by conservative political leaders in Britain, the United States and elsewhere.

Since the family is such an important influence, it follows that many social problems will be seen as stemming from inadequate and unstable families. In the Foreword to a book by Morgan (1995) entitled *Farewell to the Family?*, the Director of the Institute of Economic Affairs Health and Welfare Unit, David Green, writes:

> Patricia Morgan shows how, step by step, the traditional family of man, wife and children is being replaced by the mother–child–state unit. She warns that this development is doubly harmful. First, the children of broken families tend to suffer: they under-perform at school, grow physically less well, experience more illness, and are more likely to turn to crime and drugs. And second, young men who ought to be assuming the responsibilities of fatherhood, adopt instead an unattached and predatory lifestyle which often brings them into conflict with the police.
>
> (1995, p. iv)

Morgan puts the blame for the decline of the traditional family firmly on the shoulders of militant feminists, and the access they have had to decision makers. She claims that 'while leaders of lone-parent organisations have been recruited to the kitchen cabinets of Ministers with responsibility for "women's issues", these have contained nobody with a brief for the conventional family'. The advisors listened to by ministers have urged the 'more speedy and complete plunder' of the traditional family (p. 25). This argument is the complete reversal of the more usual one which emphasises the politically dominant voice of the radical right in matters relating to the family and sexual behaviour. The best example of this influence is its dominant position within the Republican Party in the United

States. Writing about the United States, Stoesz and Midgley (1991) refer to the Institute for Cultural Conservatism which published a manifesto in 1987 in which it argued for the revitalisation of the family to enable it to fulfil its traditional welfare role. The Institute wished to see the restoration of the role of the conventional nuclear family with the mother remaining at home. Attempts would be made to bolster parental authority. Divorce, abortion and pre-marital and extra-marital sex were to be strongly discouraged. There would be action to ensure the economic sufficiency of stable nuclear families.

There has always been strong support for the family from religion. This has been particularly obvious in Catholic countries such as Ireland, Italy, Poland, Portugal, Spain and the countries of Central and South America. The Catholic Church's strictures on divorce, contraception and abortion have been given wide coverage, and the debate need not be summarised here. The Catholic Church is also responsible for the emergence of the principle of subsidiarity, and for its current significance in Germany and The Netherlands. Subsidiarity was intended to be a defence against the power of the central state, but the Catholic Church was also concerned to stress the importance of family. Spicker (1991) explains the relevance of the principle of subsidiarity for the role of the family:

> Subsidiarity is justified as an expression of the responsibilities that people have for each other's welfare. These depend on the closeness of their relationship. Because the closest relationships mainly exist within families, it is the family that bears the primary responsibility for social support. The role of others who are more remote is correspondingly reduced.
>
> (p. 4)

Equally interesting, is evangelical Christianity in the United States and its crusade for a return to traditional values. Peele (1984, p. 71) argues that 'the emphasis on family or social issues which characterized the New Right in the 1970s was in part a response to the perceived permissiveness of an earlier decade'. According to the New Right it is the welfare state and social-democratic philosophy which have led to what it perceives as a decline in the family and the consequent erosion of decent moral and religious standards. An alliance of the political and the religious right would reverse the trend by restoring the family to a centrally important place in American society. In Britain and continental Europe fundamentalist religion is not such a prominent political force as it is in the United States. There are evangelical groups, but their political significance is negligible. In Britain the Church of England, described by Sydney Smith as 'the Tory Party at Prayer', probably has more influence within the Conservative Party than has evangelical Christianity.

There is, however, a possible paradox in the New Right's approach to the family stemming from the alliance within it of two not entirely consistent ideologies: economic liberalism and conservative authoritarianism. The economic liberals advocate a minimum state in economic matters, but this view spills over into the social sphere: conservative authoritarians, on the other hand, are concerned with the re-establishment of political authority and are not averse to regulating families. The first group might argue that the best way to strengthen the family is to keep government out and leave families to make their own decisions. However, the religious right and other strands of conservatism in American politics are more closely aligned with conservative authoritarianism. It is fairly obvious, for example, that the proposals of the Institute for Cultural Conservatism require government intervention in families at a number of levels. Mishra (1989), however, sees nothing that is particularly unusual, or even paradoxical, in the alliance between these two strands of New Right thought: 'The combination of laissez-faire in economic matters with conservatism and authoritarianism in social issues is scarcely a novel departure in the history of conservatism, especially as it has evolved in the United States' (p. 174). Lister (1996, p. 19) identifies similar contradictions in the Conservative Family Campaign in Britain: 'The family crusade was not without its dilemmas and contradictions for the Conservative Party. As Margaret Thatcher recognised in her memoirs, there is a difficulty of squaring an ideological commitment to reducing the influence of the state with intervention in the "private" sphere of the family'. Lister also refers to a rather more subtle contradiction exposed by Gray (1994) in which he says that a decade and a half of neo-liberal policies had subjected the family to 'all the stresses of unchannelled economic change, leaving it fractured and resourceless in communities themselves rendered fragile and impotent by a form of public policy in which social life is reduced to a series of market exchanges'.

But it is not only conservatives who celebrate the family. In the 1997 election campaign in Britain Blair portrayed the new Labour Party as the party of the family. Clinton made similar claims in the

1996 Presidential campaign. In France and Germany, protection of the family transcends party politics: in both, the family is referred to in the Constitution, and this is reflected in ministerial appointments. In France, the *Haut Conseil de la Population et de la Famille* and the *Institut de l'Enfance et de la Famille* enjoy high prestige and merit Presidential patronage (Hantrais, 1994).

Havas (1995) writes of the family as ideology. She claims that as the nuclear family developed, it reflected 'the middle class ideal rather than a reality for all classes, since the model has always been limited by class' (p. 6). The increasingly privatised nuclear family became the model by which all families were judged. Havas describes the effects of this privatisation:

> The family as ideology denies that what happens in the wider society affects all our children and gives the illusion that we can somehow isolate ourselves. It makes the 'burden' of child-rearing a private one and it denies the notion that any child's disadvantage ultimately affects other children and the wider society.
>
> (1995, p. 7)

The family is represented as a haven from the pressures of the outside world, providing a loving and stable environment for the rearing of children and opportunities for the personal growth and fulfilment of the parents. Even at its best, the family will find it difficult always to meet this ideal, and at its worst, it falls woefully short. The privacy of families may facilitate the physical and sexual abuse of women and children.

Conservatives identify marriage and motherhood as the basis of the family. In Britain, the Institute of Economic Affairs sees the decline of marriage and the decline of the family as parallel and closely connected processes. This has led to opposition to divorce reform (Whelan, 1995). David (1986, p. 139) claims that the New Right is trying to promote a model of the private family through 'social policies which increasingly celebrate motherhood as a crucial social activity for all women'. In the traditional view of the family mothers are expected not to work. Mothering for women is seen as 'natural': since it is only women who can bear children, it is only women who can be expected to nurture them. It is a fact of biology as is a man's 'natural instinct' to provide for his wife and children. Fitzgerald (1983, p. 50) describes this socio-biological perspective as 'biological essentialism', which is 'implicit' in neo-liberalism.

In many ways the New Right is looking back with nostalgia to a largely mythical golden age of the family; this was certainly true of Mrs Thatcher's desire for a return to Victorian values, and it is equally true of much of the contemporary material stemming from the Institute of Economic Affairs and the Adam Smith Institute in Britain and the Christian Coalition and the Institute for Cultural Conservatism in the United States. It is less stridently expressed in Christian Democratic and other conservative parties in Europe. It would be a mistake, however, to dismiss this view as no more than nostalgia. The restoration of the family to a pre-eminent position in society is part of a much broader plan to privatise welfare provision. The neo-liberal vision of the minimum state implies a drastic reduction in the welfare role of the state and a transfer of functions and responsibilities to other institutions. It is assumed that families are both willing and able to take on a heavier caring role than they accept at present. The evidence suggests that this assumption may be unfounded, as the next section illustrates.

Family care

Empirical studies have demonstrated how important the family is as a source of care in all welfare states. The care of handicapped and sick people by nuclear family members and the system of reciprocal support between elderly people and their adult children are especially significant. Three studies, each roughly ten years apart, allow comparisons over time. The first of these was by Abrams (1977) who claimed that care which is identified as community care frequently proves, on closer examination, not to be based on community in the territorial sense at all, but on kinship, race or religion, kinship being especially significant. The second study was by Willmott (1986) who also stressed the importance of kinship networks. A more recent study by McGlone, Park and Roberts (1996) confirmed the findings of the two earlier studies:

> . . . the family, far from being in decline, seems to be in enduringly good shape. True, fewer people live with kin nowadays, and people are seeing slightly less of their family than they were a decade ago, perhaps on account of the changing demands of work. Nonetheless,

the family remains a key (perhaps *the* key) social network and the primary source of informal care and support for many.
(1996, p. 66)

Other studies by Finch (1989), Glendinning (1992) and Parker (1990; 1993) reinforce the dominance of families in the informal system of care. All of these studies relate specifically to Britain, but the same picture is repeated wherever one looks. This is amply demonstrated by the material emerging from the European Observatory on National Family Policies (Ditch *et al.,* 1996a, 1996b). Since this is a European Union initiative, it covers only the member states. This is also true of Millar and Warman (1996) although they also include Norway and there are also individual studies of Norway (Wærness, 1990; Leira, 1993). Studies of Central and East European countries are to be found in Evers and Svetlik (1993) which also covers Canada, Israel and most of Western Europe. Information on Japan is to be found in Gould (1993) and Okazaki *et al.* (1990).

An early study by Abrams (1977, p. 133) maintained that 'kinship remains the strongest basis of attachment and the most reliable basis of care that we have'. A more recent study by Millar and Warman (1996) sums up the evidence from a variety of studies which 'show that in all the EU countries the family is overwhelmingly the main source of non-spouse care for older people, with adult children as the most frequently mentioned carers' (p. 33). The same statement would apply to most other countries, and certainly to the rest of Europe, Australia, Canada, Japan, New Zealand, the United States and the countries of Central and South America. It is interesting to note that even in countries with highly developed welfare states, such as Sweden, 'the bulk of elderly care is provided by families' Johansson, 1993, p. 103). Gould (1993, p. 200) predicts in relation to Sweden that 'informal care will be relied on more in the future to take care of elderly people'. Although most research into informal care has focused on older people, families provide most of the care for other groups in the population: disabled and chronically sick people, for example. Children form the most numerous group of people cared for within families. Although this chapter will necessarily reflect the research bias towards the care of older people, other groups will be considered and the reciprocal nature of much caring work will also receive some attention.

So far, this discussion of family care has not gone much beyond broad generalisations. In order to add more substance, three central questions will be addressed: (i) who are the chief recipients of care? (ii) who are the carers? (iii) what services are provided?

We have already identified the people who may receive informal care: older people (especially frail people); physically disabled people; people with learning disabilities; those suffering from chronic physical or mental illness. The vast majority of dependent children are cared for in families, but separate considerations arise in their case which may make the use of the term informal care inappropriate. Nevertheless, there are important issues about who has the main responsibility for the care of children in the home and the relationship between employment and the availability of pre-school facilities.

Among the elderly population, about two thirds of those being cared for are women. The reason for this is very obvious: most frail older people are in the 85+ age bracket and, given women's greater life expectancy, they easily outnumber men among the older age ranges. In 1991, in the United Kingdom for example, there were three women aged 85+ to every man. The exact proportions of women among those being cared for will depend upon the demographic characteristics of the country being studied, but since older women outnumber older men in all advanced industrial countries, there are unlikely to be huge variations.

Much recent research attention has been directed towards the characteristics of carers, and particularly to the division of caring work between men and women. The weight of the evidence suggests that women are seen as 'natural' carers and that, conveniently for men, there is an expectation that women will take on the prime responsibility not only for child care but also for elderly and other dependent relatives. A very influential and much-quoted article by Finch and Groves (1980) talks of a 'double equation': community care = family care = care by women:

> The cultural designation of women as carers in the family setting is reflected in the available evidence about what happens in practice: in terms of primary responsibility, wives care for husbands, mothers for handicapped children and daughters for their elderly parents or disabled siblings. Care is also provided by female neighbours and volunteers.
>
> (1980, p. 499)

Some more recent work tells a similar story. For example, Baldwin and Twigg (1991, p. 120), although recognising that care by men has been under-estimated, conclude that 'the general understanding of caring as a predominantly female activity remains'. Wærness (1990, p. 114), summarising work in Norway, states that 'studies of inter-generational care in the family show that it is first and foremost daughters who do the care-giving work'. McGlone and Cronin (1994) and Ungerson (1995) looked at caring in a European context and found a gender bias in the countries studied.

However, according to Parker (1993, p. 6), many of the studies concluding that women did most of the caring took insufficient account of the 'increasing evidence that the marriage relationship is the prime location of care, certainly for older people'. This partly helps to explain the results of the British General Household Survey (GHS) of 1990. The GHS found that 17 per cent of women (3.9 million) had caring responsibilities as compared with 13 per cent of men (2.9 million). Although these figures represent an increase in the discrepancy as compared with the 1985 survey (15 per cent women and 12 per cent men) they suggest that the differences are not so striking as had been supposed. In cases where one spouse is caring for another, the carer is just as likely to be a man as a woman. Who provides care for elderly parents depends upon distance from the potential carers. A recent study by McGlone, Park and Roberts (1996) indicated that about 30 per cent of adult children and their parents lived within a journey time of less than fifteen minutes, and that 74 per cent of parents lived within one hour's journey of an adult child. Qureshi and Simons (1987) found that sons and daughters were not expected to care if they lived more than two hours away. Thus, if a daughter lived more than two hours' journey from her parents and a son lived in close proximity to the parents, then the son would be expected to help rather than the daughter; if a son lived with his parents, then he rather than a daughter would be the main carer. The importance of shared residence is confirmed by Levin *et al.* (1989) who say that shared residence overrides gender in decisions about who should care. These cases apart, there is a hierarchy of preferences, expectations or obligations in which spouses take precedence, followed by daughters, daughters-in-law, sons, other relatives and non-relatives.

However, more detailed analysis of time spent in caring work and of the services performed, begins to re-assert the dominance of women in caring. The 1990 GHS revealed that in Britain 21 per cent of male carers, as compared with 24 per cent of female carers, spent twenty or more hours a week in a caring capacity. Those doing twenty or more hours of caring a week either lived with the person being cared for or very close by. At the other end of the scale, 38 per cent of male and 30 per cent of female carers spent less than five hours a week engaged in caring work. The kind of work done also varies with the gender of the carer. Parker and Lawton (1994) make a distinction between what they call the 'heavy end' of caring and informal helping. Heavy end caring, consisting of *personal* care such as washing, dressing, toileting, feeding and general attention to bodily needs and comforts, was predominantly done by women; men were more likely to be involved in informal helping – gardening, jobs around the house and driving. This distinction, however, does not apply to spousal care.

Most of the above data relates to care for elderly relatives. If other groups are considered, the dominance of women as carers is confirmed. Parker (1990) makes the following comment in the second edition of a book first published in 1985:

> By contrast with the evidence about care of elderly people, recent research has done little to challenge the analysis presented in the first edition of this book about the care of children with disabilities. As in the great majority of families with children, the bulk of caring for a disabled child is done by his or her mother with little help from other family members.
>
> (p. 47)

The most common age for both men and women to be engaged in caring work is 45–64: the GHS survey of 1990 reported that 27 per cent of women and 20 per cent of men in this age range were carers. It is, of course, people between the ages 50 and 64 who have parents in the 70+ age bracket. The daughters and sons of people aged 85+ are themselves going to be approaching pensionable age in most countries.

In the course of looking at the cared for and their carers, there has necessarily been some reference to the kind of services that are provided, but this now needs to be treated more systematically. We will begin by looking at a useful early categorisation which Willmott (1986) adapted from work conducted two years earlier by Seyd *et al.* (1984). The first four in the following list are adaptations of the categorisation used in the earlier study; the fifth is a category added by Willmott:

1. Personal care, which includes washing, bathing, dressing, feeding and toileting – this corresponds to Parker's (1981) notion of 'tending'.
2. Domestic care – cooking, cleaning and laundering.
3. Auxiliary care – mainly less onerous tasks such as odd-jobbing, gardening, transport and baby-sitting.
4. Social support – visiting and companionship.
5. Surveillance – keeping an eye on vulnerable people.

Although there are several excellent studies of informal support in specific caring situations, probably the fullest *general* account of the range of help available within families is provided by Finch (1989). She divides help into various groups: (i) economic support; (ii) accommodation; (iii) personal care; (iv) practical support and child care; (v) emotional and moral support. Each of these categories is further sub-divided. Finch also looks at help between different members of families, including siblings, children and grandparents and other relatives. She also emphasises that help may be given reciprocally and at different stages in the life cycle: by parents to adult children (financial assistance and accommodation, for example) and by adult children to frail elderly parents.

Reciprocity implies some form of exchange, but the exchange may not resemble the kind of exchanges which take place in the local supermarket; they are somewhat closer to a bartering system, and closer still to long-term credit. In some relationships, there may be almost instant and continuous reciprocity, so that people are simultaneously givers and receivers. Thus an elderly parent may perform child-minding services for their adult daughters and sons, and daughters and sons may help their parents with jobs around the house or gardening. Reciprocity may not involve simply two parties. For example, one son or daughter may provide most of the daily care for an elderly parent because they live closer to hand than siblings, but the sister/brother who lives further away may have their nephews and nieces to stay with them while their parents take a holiday. No doubt readers can think of even more complex permutations. Reciprocity may be very long term, and reference has already been made to the possibility of sons and daughters providing care for elderly parents as a form of repayment for the care they themselves received as children. This analysis has important implications for those who are dependent upon others with little hope of reciprocating.

Although family care is important everywhere, it is not equally important in all countries. Its significance will depend on a complex set of variables: cultural expectations and practices; the availability of residential facilities; the effectiveness of policies for supporting families and carers (including social security provision); working practices and the structure of the labour market; housing policies. Although some of these variables will be briefly considered in later sections of the chapter, it would take up too much space to cover all of them.

Ditch *et al.* (1996a) in a study of families in the European Union point to marked differences between northern and southern Europe. In Greece, Italy (especially in the South), Spain and Portugal, residential care is undeveloped, and the authors claim that the lack of development 'may have its roots both in traditional values and in the less well developed public sector' (p. 118). Ditch and his co-authors refer to work by Finch and Mason (1993) which indicates that in the UK caring obligations are negotiated both within the family and over time. They contrast this with southern European countries:

> By contrast, traditional expectations appear to remain very strong in the southern European countries such as Greece, Italy, Portugal and Spain, where there appears to be little negotiation, and caring responsibilities tend to be regarded as an inevitable part of family relationships, rooted in the private sphere and independent of state purview.
>
> (1996a, p. 113)

As a consequence of these factors, 90 per cent of the care of elderly people in Spain is provided by families, and in Italy 80 per cent of severely disabled elderly people receive help from relatives. In Greece, less than 1 per cent of the elderly population are in residential accommodation. Traditional values in East Asian countries, especially Japan, also make for strong emphasis on the family as a source of care. Goodman and Peng (1996, p. 207) say: 'At the simplest level, we might argue that Japan is characterized by . . . a system of family welfare that appears to negate much of the need for state welfare . . .'. This may be something of an over-statement, but it is in marked contrast to a statement in Ditch *et al.* (1996b, p. 76) about Denmark: 'It is not common for adult children to be the prime carers of the elderly nor is this likely to change in the near future'.

It is clear that where alternatives are not readily available, as we saw in southern Europe, there is no choice: it is family care or nothing. In northern Europe, North America, Australia and New Zealand, one of the main arguments advanced for developing informal care is that it is the preferred option of recipients who have no wish to become dependent upon the impersonal professional care of the state. This assumption is based on very little research evidence.

State services may sometimes create dependency, but the danger of community care is of creating new, and possibly less acceptable, forms of dependency. This is certainly true when unsupported kin are expected to provide the necessary care. Dependency on kin may be even harder to come to terms with than is dependency on public services. The wish not to be a 'burden' on relatives is very common among older and disabled people. Craig and Glendinning (1993), having commented upon the social construction of dependency, and the rejection of the label 'dependent' by disabled people, continue:

> It is important to note that these views are not just the sole prerogative of the more politically active members of the disability movement. There are strong similarities here with the expressed wishes of older people for 'intimacy at a distance' – for relationships which do not make them feel unduly dependent on and indebted to their relatives.
>
> (p. 177)

Phillipson (1988) also challenges the orthodox view that elderly people turn to formal agencies for help only when informal support is absent or inadequate. He summarises American research which indicates that elderly people are turning away from informal care based on kinship towards formal professional support. He writes:

> This is not to say that people will not give the support (as we know they do and invariably at great sacrifice); but it does suggest that care by the community is seen as a less attractive option than care from professionals, but with the support and involvement of the family.
>
> (1988, p. 8)

Qureshi (1990, p. 68) also argues that 'taking account of the views of elderly people and their families, it is clear that the assumption of a general preference for informal care is too simple a view'. In the main, frail older people, who may themselves have been carers at an earlier stage in their lives, are not unaware of the pressures placed on family members when they take on caring roles. It is to these pressures that we now turn.

The impact of caring

It is difficult to convey the impact of caring upon the carers themselves or upon their families. Statistics cannot give any idea of the unremitting drudgery which caring often entails. An incontinent, frail elderly person will have to be toileted, washed, dressed, fed and put to bed; clothing and bedding will have to be changed and washed frequently. Care is almost constant throughout the day and frequently at night. The interrupted sleep and hard physical work lead to tiredness and possibly ill-health. Charlesworth, Wilkin and Durie (1984, p. 7) say that 22 per cent of the carers in their study felt that health problems 'had either been caused or worsened by caring for the elderly person'. Slightly more women than men reported a deterioration. Nor is it only physical health which is affected: the largest single category of problems identified by carers was depression and anxiety attributable to the stresses of caring over a long period of time. There is a big discrepancy between these earlier results and those of a study published in 1992 which reported health problems attributed to caring in 65 per cent of the carers in the survey. It is difficult to find a wholly convincing explanation for these divergent findings. The more recent survey was conducted among members of the Carers National Association (CNA), and it is possible that people join the Association only after several years of caring; we know that the longer the period involved, the more serious the effects upon health are likely to be. It is also possible that members of the Association are caring for more heavily dependent people, but this is no more than speculation. Even more speculative is the suggestion that in the eight years between the two surveys, the problems of carers have received greater prominence and this may have made it easier to admit to health and other difficulties associated with caring. However, the divergence is huge, and it cannot be explained satisfactorily.

The tenor of the two reports, however, is similar. The sheer physical labour involved can be damaging; 28 per cent of the CNA respondents, for example, mentioned back problems. It should be noted, however, that many carers are in late middle age when health may deteriorate. Parker (1990) claims that a *causal* link between 'caring and physical ill-health is, as yet, unproven' (p. 93). Since Parker arrived at this conclusion, however, we have had the CNA study which, while it does not *prove* a link, at least gives a strong indication of a relationship between caring and physical ill-health. Parker does, however, state that 'there is clear evidence of the toll imposed on the mental well-being of carers' (p. 93).

There are several factors contributing to mental ill-health among carers. One such factor is the unremitting nature of some of the work and the social isolation that often accompanies heavy caring responsibilities. The CNA survey reported that 20 per cent of carers never had a break. Even when regular breaks were taken, the majority (62 per cent) were for half a day or less. The majority (59 per cent) of occasional breaks were also short-lived – less than a week. These findings confirm those of the Charlesworth *et al.* study (1984) which found that 44 per cent of both male and female carers reported restrictions on their leisure time, 'although men appeared to resist more strongly encroachment on their leisure activities' (p. 18). Further evidence comes from Chetwynd's (1985) study of the factors leading to stress among mothers of children with learning disabilities: the absence of breaks and the restriction of the mothers' social life were major contributors to stress.

In addition, there may be increased tension in the home. Children and husbands may resent the presence of, for example, a frail elderly relative, particularly if the elderly person appears to monopolise the time of the mother/wife. Arguments may develop, and the woman may find herself in the middle attempting to keep the peace. In a study by Nissel and Bonnerjea (1982), family members complained of a loss of privacy, and both husbands and wives reported a deterioration in marital relationships. Some parents thought that children's school performance had suffered – yet another source of worry. Clearly, problems of this nature are more likely when the person being cared for lives with the carer's family, but time spent away from the family home looking after a relative may also give rise to tensions.

A more subtle danger is that the affection for the person being cared for may be stretched to its limits, and this may lead to feelings of guilt. What was once a cause of satisfaction, may become a resented duty. This may be most likely when the behaviour of the person being cared for changes – a physically frail elderly person may, for example, develop behavioural symptoms of mental distress. This is naturally a cause for anxiety, but it also makes caring more difficult, particularly if there are problems of rational communication.

Reduced financial circumstances may present an additional problem for carers. Levels of deprivation/affluence among carers depend on individual circumstances, but from a social policy point of view, the major influences are social security arrangements, labour market policies, the availability and cost of child-care facilities, fiscal policies and the legal enforcement of maintenance payments. We will look at some of these issues in a later section. Our concern here is with the financial problems faced by carers. There are several ways in which carers may be disadvantaged. The most serious restriction is on the type of employment that can be undertaken. It has to be close to the carer's home and the hours of work will have to make allowance for caring responsibilities; this may involve working part-time. This makes it extremely difficult to find work, so that carers are more likely to be unemployed. If they do find work, it is often low-paid with little job security and no prospects of advancement. Even those in reasonably paid occupations may have to forego promotion, if it would involve longer or less predictable hours. Work by Baldwin (1985), Joshi (1987; 1991), Glendinning (1989), Parker (1990), Noden and Laczco (1993); the Nuffield Provincial Hospitals Trust (1993); and the Caring Costs Alliance (1996) provide evidence of reduced work opportunities and lower pay. Lower pay can be measured by comparing a group of carers with a control group, but it is much more difficult to quantify loss of training and promotion opportunities, and the part that they play in reducing carers' incomes. The losses involved in moving from full-time work to part-time or from part-time work to not working at all can be calculated, as can (with a little more difficulty) loss of pension entitlements, but it is not possible to measure in monetary terms the lower levels of job security.

There is another side to the financial equation: expenditure. There are extra costs associated with caring for a frail elderly person or a disabled child. Pioneering work in this area done by Baldwin (1977; 1981; 1985) and work carried out by Smyth and Robus (1989) produced similar patterns of extra expenditure in the case of disabled children. Among the items identified were purchases of special equipment; house adaptations; food; clothing; bedding; transport; laundry; heating. Putting together reduced employment opportunities and additional expenditure means that extra expenses have to be met out of a reduced budget.

The problems associated with family care most seriously disadvantage women. We have established that women are more involved than men at the heavy end of caring. Women also take on the major role in child care and may also do more than their fair share of household chores. If all of these roles are combined, the stress is incalculable. As will be seen in the next section, it is usually women who give up paid work entirely or move from full-time to part-time work when caring responsibilities increase, and it is women who have to cope with the day-to-day problem of managing a reduced family budget.

Social change and family care

This section will consider a range of social changes as they affect family care. Among the changes to be examined will be worldwide increase in the elderly population; changing patterns of partnership and family forms; labour market changes.

Ageing populations

Every industrial country has experienced an increase in the proportion of elderly people in its population. In many cases this is a long-term change beginning in the early years of this century, but the increase has been more marked in the last forty years. All forecasts predict that the trend will continue until well into the next century. There is much talk of an alarmist kind: in earlier chapters reference was made to the European Commission's (1995) fears of a 'demographic time-bomb', and an item in *The Guardian* newspaper commenting on a World Bank report in 1994 had the headline *'Ageing population threatens global crisis'*. The OECD and the IMF have expressed similar concerns. As one would anticipate from the source of the comments, the main worry is an economic one. How are the pensions for the increased numbers to be paid for and what long-term effects will an ageing population have on productivity and therefore living standards? There are numerous calculations of what is called the dependency ratio: a full dependency ratio has to take account of all non-employed people, which includes older people, young people in full-time education, unemployed people and those prevented from working by severe physical and mental disabilities.

This sum is then divided by the number of economically active people. More frequently the ratio is arrived at by adding together those between the ages of 0 and 14 and those who are aged 65+ and then dividing this sum by the number aged between 15 and 64. If the purpose is to highlight the 'problem' of elderly people, then figures are produced which indicate the number of working-age people for every person of 65+ in the population: Table 5.1 is an example of such calculations taken from an OECD Report (1994). All of the countries in Table 5.1 are moving in the same direction, but at different speeds. Japan merits special mention with a very rapid decline between 1960 and 1980 and a steady decline thereafter. Turkey also stands out, but for the opposite reason: by the year 2000, Turkey will still have at least twice the number of working-age people for every elderly person.

The figures in Table 5.1 are important indirectly for informal care. If the predictions are accurate, there is going to be increasing pressure on pensions and other age-related expenditure; this is certainly governments' main concern. This in turn may mean more pressure on family budgets, more charging and more means-testing.

Perhaps more significant for informal care is that growing proportions of elderly people mean more people requiring care. OECD figures suggest that the proportions of older people in all OECD countries have been increasing since at least 1950 and that the increase will go on until the middle of the next century. The OECD (1994) forecasts a doubling of the population over 65 between 1950 and 2050 'from an OECD average of less than 10 per cent to an

Table 5.1   Working-age population per elderly person in selected OECD countries

Country	1960	1980	1990	2000	2020	2040
Australia	7.2 (1961)	6.6 (1981)	6.0 (1991)	5.5 (2001)	3.7 (2021)	2.9 (2041)
Austria	5.4	4.2	4.5	4.3	3.3	2.1
Denmark	6.0	4.5	4.3	4.4	3.3	–
Finland	8.5	5.6	5.0	4.6	2.9	2.7
Japan	11.2	7.4	5.8	4.0	2.4	2.1
New Zealand	9.0 (1961)	6.4 (1981)	5.8 (1991)	5.6 (2001)	4.1 (2021)	2.7 (2041)
Norway	5.7	4.3	4.0	4.3	3.6	2.8
Spain	7.6	5.6	5.0	4.2	3.7	2.1
Sweden	5.5	3.9	3.6	3.7	3.0	–
Turkey	15.1	11.3	13.8	11.3	11.0 (2005)	–
United Kingdom	5.5	4.3	4.2	4.1	3.5	2.8
United States	6.5	5.9	5.3	5.4	3.6	2.7

Source: OECD (1994)

average of more than 20 per cent' (p. 37). The European Commission claims that by the early years of next century those over 65 will overtake the number of children for the first time. This is not all, however. The OECD states:

> Within this major shift in population balance, a second demographic change is beginning. . . . A secondary ageing process, sometimes termed the ageing of the aged, is under way in OECD countries and will lead to a substantial increase in numbers of people aged 80 or over. This increase in numbers ranges from up to 50 per cent in Western and Central European countries to over 200 per cent in Australia and Canada.
>
> (p. 37)

Table 5.2 shows the increase in two age groups, 65–79 and 80+, as a proportion of the population. Although the proportions of those aged 80+ seem small they have been increasing at a faster rate than those aged between 65 and 79. By the year 2000 the proportion of the population aged 80+ in most countries will have increased by between two and three times since 1960. In the same period, Japan will have experienced a fivefold increase. It is in the 80+ group that the heaviest care needs are likely to be found, so that as the proportion of this group increases so does the demand for care.

Earlier in this chapter, the physical distance between the homes of an older person and his/her adult children, was identified as an important determinant of the caring relationship, of who cared and of the intensity of the care. Shared residence was particularly significant. The frequency with which elderly people live with their children varies enormously from country to country. An illustration of this diversity may be provided by comparing Japan with Sweden, Denmark, The Netherlands and Norway. In Japan it has long been customary for older people to live with their children or grandchildren. In spite of a decline in the proportion of those aged 65+ living in two generation or three generation households, the proportion in Japan remains incomparably higher than in the countries of Western Europe or North America. In 1960, 87.4 per cent of people aged 65+ lived with their children or grandchildren, but by 1985 the proportion had declined to 65.5 per cent. There has been a further reduction since 1985, but the proportion remains well above 50 per cent. This compares with 5 per cent or less in Sweden and Denmark, 8 per cent in The Netherlands and 11 per cent in Norway.

Table 5.2   People aged 65–79 and 80+ as percentage of total population – selected OECD countries

Country	1960/61	1980/81	1990/91	2000/01	2020/21
Australia					
65–79	7.27	8.07	8.98	9.30	13.78
80+	1.24	1.74	2.18	2.99	4.12
Austria					
65–79	10.44	12.74	11.43	–	–
80+	1.77	2.68	3.69	–	–
Belgium					
65–79	10.28	11.53	11.35	13.43	15.28
80+	1.94	2.69	3.47	3.65	5.55
Canada					
65–79	6.38	7.85	9.11	10.19	15.38
80+	1.25	1.85	2.37	3.53	5.06
Denmark					
65–79	9.01	11.57	11.92	11.10	15.23
80+	1.63	2.78	3.67	4.10	4.29
Finland					
65–79	6.45	10.25	10.59	11.42	17.18
80+	0.93	1.81	2.88	3.34	4.35
Japan					
65–79	5.00	7.71	9.66	13.34	18.09
80+	0.72	1.39	2.39	3.60	7.10
New Zealand					
65–79	4.95	8.26	8.94	8.78	12.18
80+	1.51	1.70	2.29	2.79	3.73
Norway					
65–79	9.15	11.85	12.74	–	–
80+	1.98	2.96	3.76	–	–
Portugal					
65–79	–	9.74	10.34	11.18	14.58
80+	–	1.71	2.73	3.09	6.13
Spain					
65–79	7.01	9.32	10.67	12.70	14.13
80+	1.41	1.94	2.87	3.43	4.46
Sweden					
65–79	10.03	13.21	13.46	11.91	15.32
80+	1.94	3.17	4.30	5.01	4.83
United Kingdom					
65–79	9.80	12.26	11.98	11.51	13.48
80+	1.92	2.70	3.67	4.08	4.55
United States					
65–79	7.84	8.99	9.71	9.51	13.57
80+	1.40	2.28	2.79	3.49	4.11

Source: OECD (1994)

In Western Europe, Italy comes closest to the Japanese figure with 39 per cent, followed by Spain at 37 per cent, Poland at 29 per cent and Austria at 25 per cent. Germany, Switzerland, the United Kingdom and the United States are within two percentage points of one another, varying from 14 to 16 per cent. France is somewhat higher with about 20 per cent of older people living with their children. These figures, taken from an OECD report (1994), suggest similarly wide variations in the proportions of elderly people living alone. As would be anticipated, Japan has the smallest proportion of older people (12 per cent) living in single person households. This compares with 53 per cent in Denmark, 40 per cent in Germany, Sweden and the United Kingdom and just over 30 per cent in France and the United States.

To understand the full significance of the demographic changes we need to know what is happening to the supply of potential carers. The next two sub-sections look at various aspects of this issue.

Changing patterns of partnership and family forms

I have borrowed the useful terms partnership and partnering from Millar and Warman (1996): the terms are useful because they include both formally married partners and cohabiting or unmarried partners. Millar and Warman also divide the European Union countries (plus Norway) into three groups. The first group includes the four Scandinavian countries and the UK, characterised by lower marriage rates, higher rates of cohabitation, higher numbers of extramarital births and higher rates of divorce. Care must be taken in interpreting the grouping of countries in this way. For example, Denmark (after an increase in 1994) now has the highest marriage rates in the European Union, followed by Portugal and the United Kingdom. It is possible to widen the analysis to cover countries outside Europe. Simply on the basis of divorce rates, we could add to the group containing the UK and Scandinavia: Australia, Canada, Estonia, Israel, Latvia, Lithuania, New Zealand and the United States. Among industrial countries, the United States has the highest divorce rates in the world. Within the European Union, the UK has the highest rates, although rates actually fell in 1993 and 1994. Millar and Warman's second group are the diametric opposite to the countries just identified. Greece, Ireland, Italy, Portugal and Spain

Table 5.3   Divorce rates[1] in selected countries: 1992 (latest year)

Australia	2.6[2]
Austria	2.1
Belgium	2.2
Canada	2.9[3]
Denmark	2.5
Finland	2.5
France	1.9[2]
Germany	1.9
Italy	0.4
Japan	1.4
Luxembourg	1.9
Netherlands	2.0
New Zealand	2.6
Norway	2.4[2]
Poland	0.8
Portugal	1.3
Spain	0.7
Sweden	2.6
United Kingdom	4.3
United States	4.8

Sources: Millar and Warman (1996) and UN Demographic Yearbook, 1992
Notes
[1]   Number of divorces per 1000 of population
[2]   1991
[3]   1990

have high rates of marriage, low rates of divorce, cohabitation and extramarital births. Again taking divorce as the measure, we could add Japan, Poland and many of the countries in the Middle East, the Far East and (with a number of exceptions) Central and South America. Millar and Warman's third group consist of Austria, Belgium, France, Germany, Luxembourg and The Netherlands, all of which on most measures fall between the two extremes. There is one measure, extramarital births, that does not conform to the pattern. All but Austria and France in this group have lower rates of extramarital births than Portugal and Ireland.

Divorce (and possible remarriage) has important implications for caring for two main reasons. First, divorce and any subsequent re-marriage or cohabitation considerably complicate kinship networks, and we still know far too little about the impact of this on caring. Do obligations to other family members survive divorce? Does subsequent remarriage cancel out former obligations and substitute new ones? Second, divorce contributes substantially to the growth in the number of lone-parent families.

The proportion of couples cohabiting varies considerably. Sweden has the largest proportion in this category – 48.1 per cent. The proportions in the other Scandinavian countries are all around 23 per cent. We need to know more about the precise relationship between cohabitation and caring. There is no obvious reason for supposing that stable, cohabiting relationships are any less likely to result in caring obligations than are relationships based on marriage, but research in this area is needed.

The evidence that most non-spouse informal care for older people is provided by adult children is incontrovertible, and this implies that smaller family size is bound to reduce the pool of potential carers. Lone parenthood itself means smaller family size. It also means that looking after children unaided, housework, possibly working outside the home, leaves little time for carrying out caring work.

Table 5.4 shows lone-parent families as a proportion of all families with children. The data in the table confirm Millar and Warman's claim (1996, p. 21) that 'the growth in the number of lone-parent families has been one of the most striking trends in many countries over the past 20 or so years'. The vast majority of lone parents are women: in the European Union 83.3 per cent of lone-parent families

Table 5.4 Lone parent families as a percentage of all families

Australia (1994)	18
Austria (1993)	15
Belgium (1992)	11
Denmark (1994)	19
Finland (1993)	16
France (1990)	12
Germany (1992)	19
Greece (1990/91)	11
Ireland (1993)	11
Italy (1992)	6
Japan (1990)	5
Luxembourg (1992)	7
The Netherlands (1992)	16
New Zealand (1992)	25
Norway (1993)	21
Portugal (1991)	13
Spain (Madrid) (1991)	7
Sweden (1990)	18
United Kingdom (1992)	21
USA (1991)	29

Source: Bradshaw *et al.* (1996)

were headed by women (Ditch *et al.*, 1996a, p. 34). Lone mothers may be single (never married), separated/divorced or widows. Bradshaw *et al.* (1996) identify the proportions of lone mothers in each of these categories in twenty countries. Japan has the lowest proportion of single mothers (5 per cent) which compares with 49 per cent in Austria, 46 per cent in Sweden, 42 per cent in Norway, 38 per cent in the United Kingdom and New Zealand and 37 per cent in the US. Separated and divorced women, taken together, are the largest single category of lone mothers with the exception of Ireland, Portugal and Spain where more than half of lone mothers are widows. In Ireland, where divorce became legal only in February 1997, 61 per cent of lone mothers were widows.

Family size is a direct function of the total period fertility rate: the number of children born to women during their child-bearing lives. The number of children needed to replace the population is an average of 2.1 per woman. Table 5.5 shows how fertility rates have been falling steadily since 1970 in EU countries. The rates for non-EU countries have been added to the original table, even though they are non-historical, in order to extend the comparison of the current

Table 5.5   Total period fertility rates in selected countries

Country	1970	1980	1990	1993
Belgium	2.25	1.69	1.61	1.59
Denmark	1.95	1.55	1.67	1.75
France	2.48	1.95	1.80	1.65
Germany	2.02	1.45	1.50	1.28
Greece	2.34	2.23	1.43	1.34
Ireland	3.87	3.23	2.17	1.93
Italy	2.43	1.69	1.29	1.22
Luxembourg	1.97	1.50	1.62	1.70
The Netherlands	2.57	1.60	1.62	1.57
Portugal	2.76	2.19	1.48 (1989)	1.52
Spain	2.84	2.22	1.30	1.26
United Kingdom	2.45	1.89	1.84	1.75
Australia				1.85 (1991)
Austria				1.50 (1991)
Canada				1.83 (1990)
Finland				1.78 (1992)
Japan				1.53 (1991)
New Zealand				2.12 (1989)
Sweden				2.12 (1991)
USA				2.02 (1989)

Sources: Ditch *et al.* (1996a) and UN Demographic Yearbook, 1992

position beyond the EU. Commenting on the EU figures, Ditch *et al.* (1996a) state:

> Every country in the EU had a fertility rate in 1993 below replace-
> ment level. . . . Although in southern EU countries fertility levels
> began to fall in the late 1970s (about a decade after the northern
> countries), they have rapidly caught up and indeed, overtaken the
> northern countries. For example Spain and Italy now have the lowest
> rates in Europe and indeed the industrial world.
>
> (pp. 28–9)

It will be seen from Table 5.5 that of the countries not included in the historical comparisons, Australia, Austria, Canada, Finland, Japan and the United States have fertility rates below population replacement rates. Sweden and New Zealand are marginally above that level. China and Israel (not in table) have fertility rates of 2.38 and 2.91 respectively. Clearly, declining fertility has important economic implications, but our concern here is with its impact on family size and a reduction in the pool of potential carers.

Labour market changes

Traditionally in all countries women have been the main non-spouse carers. The picture may have been modified in recent years, but it has not been transformed. Women's increased participation in the labour market is therefore likely to have an effect on time available for caring.

An OECD (1984) study of women's employment refers to 'the dramatic global development of female participation in the labour market over the last 30 years' (p. 10). Taking all twenty-one member countries together, the number of economically active women increased by 74 per cent between 1950 and 1980. During the same period the number of economically active men increased by 25 per cent. Only Japan showed virtually no increase in female partici-pation.

The study demonstrated that participation rates varied with age: the highest participation rates usually occurred between the ages of 20 and 24 and between 40 and 44, while rates declined between the ages of 25 and 34. There were exceptions to this, however. In Sweden and the United States, for example, female participation rates remained the same over the whole of the age range of 20 to 54. In Belgium, by contrast, there was a steady decline in female participation after the age of 29.

The extent of participation also varied very substantially from one country to another. This variation is confirmed by a more recent OECD (1994) study covering all twenty-one member states. The study produces figures showing average participation rates from 1980 (the end year of the previous study) until 1990 or 1991.[1] The percentage change over the same period is also calculated. The average participation rates show a variation from 75.88 per cent in Sweden to 29.11 per cent in Spain. Denmark, Finland and Norway all have rates in excess of 65 per cent, and at the other end of the scale there are four countries with less than 40 per cent: Ireland (33.05%), Italy (34.23%), Greece (36.31%) and Luxembourg (39.33%). The rate given for the United Kingdom is 55.84 per cent and 59.65 per cent for the United States. While these figures are useful for purposes of comparison, they seriously understate levels of participation. Women in work are measured against all women between the ages of 15 and 64. Many women will still be in full-time education at 15, and the retirement age for women was in many countries below 64 in the period covered by these statistics. In Britain, for example, the school-leaving age was 16 and the retirement age for women was 60 during this period. In 1996, comparing working women against all women aged between 16 and 59 gave a proportion of economically active women of 71 per cent. The discrepancy is not entirely due to the different basis of the calculation, however. The period 1981–1991 included two periods of recession.

There were some differences among countries in the proportions of women working part-time. Between 1980 and 1990/91 there were more women working part-time than full-time in both Norway and The Netherlands, substantially more in the latter in which the whole of the 15.4 per cent increase in female participation was accounted for by part-time employment. Portugal's experience was exactly the opposite in that the whole of the 17.51 increase in the ten-year period was accounted for by full-time employment. Spain, Greece, Ireland and Italy all had part-time rates of under 5 per cent and Luxembourg had a rate of only 6.23 per cent. It is significant that these five countries are those with low overall rates of female participation, and it could be the lack of opportunities for part-time work which restricts women's entry into the labour market. In the United States the proportion in full-time work is almost three times that in part-time work. In the United Kingdom the disparity is much smaller: a calculation for 1996 shows that 45 per cent of all employed women are in part-time jobs.

The much greater propensity of women to be in part-time employment may be associated with caring work. The European Commission (1995) says:

> If the working patterns of women are examined, it is evident that in most Member States, women with children are much more likely not to work or to work part-time than those without. Although there are no comparable figures for those who care for adults it may well be that the pattern is similar since the constraints on working full-time are much the same.
>
> (p. 141)

An interesting study as part of the European Observatory on National Family Policies (Bradshaw *et al.,* 1996) examines the employment of lone-parent families. This is a crucial topic, since lone parents are greatly over-represented among the poorer members of the community in most countries. The value of the study is increased by its coverage of twenty countries. Variations among countries are considerable. Simply taking one indicator – the percentage of lone mothers in paid work – the study reveals that 87 per cent of lone mothers in Japan are in paid employment as compared with Ireland's 23 per cent. France, with 82 per cent in paid employment, comes second to Japan; Belgium, Denmark, Spain, Italy, Sweden and Luxembourg all exceed 65 per cent. In Australia, Germany, Ireland, The Netherlands, New Zealand and the United Kingdom less than 50 per cent of lone mothers are in paid work. Finland (65 per cent), Norway (61 per cent) and the United States (60 per cent) are in the middle rank of countries in terms of the employment of lone mothers. The percentage of those employed who are in full-time work is generally high, varying from 59 per cent (Sweden) to 94 per cent (Finland), with The Netherlands and the UK as two major exceptions (40 per cent and 41 per cent respectively).

The reasons for these variations are a complex mixture of demographic factors (age, marital status, number and ages of children and the level of education of the mothers); labour market characteristics; and the facilities (e.g. pre-school nurseries or other forms of day care) and support (e.g. child benefits, paid parental leave) available to lone parents. These are social policy issues, and it is to social policy in relation to the family that we now turn.

Social policy and the family

The nature of family policy

Family policy has to be considered within the context of a more general discussion of family–state relationships.[2] It would be too extensive a task to discuss all of the possible models of these relationships, but a simple and very useful model is suggested by Fox Harding (1996). The model requires the establishment of two extreme positions as ideal types. At one extreme is the authoritarian model which 'is extremely *dirigiste* in its approach to family life, with the clear intention of enforcing certain preferred behaviour patterns and family forms and prohibiting others' (p. 179). At the other extreme is the *laissez-faire* model, in which 'the state seeks to exercise *no* influence over what families do or should be like; the position of government and the other institutions of the state is libertarian, in that family life is regarded as an area of complete individual freedom and choice' (p. 183). It must be stressed that these two extreme positions are not intended to describe specific states: they act as parameters for analysis. Fox Harding makes this point herself: 'In the real world such models are unlikely to be found in a pure form. In most cases an intermediate position is occupied by the state in relation to families, with some (but not draconian or totally limiting) control over how families operate' (p. 186). The elaboration of the model therefore requires these intermediate stages to be further clarified. Fox Harding explains:

> Five possible intermediate models are posited, ranging from the relatively more authoritarian to the relatively more *laissez-faire*. It is difficult to place these precisely on a continuum of control, but in general terms the sequence . . . represents a shading from a clear attempt to control families, at least in particular areas, to a more reactive stance which responds to family patterns and changes but does not attempt to explicitly influence, let alone direct, them.
>
> (p. 186)

There are several problems associated with any discussion of family policy. One problem is that many countries do not have any clearly identifiable policy which may be termed family policy. Kamerman and Kahn (1978), in a study of government policy towards families, divide the fourteen countries covered into three categories:

1. Those with an 'explicit, comprehensive family policy' (e.g. France, Norway and Sweden).
2. Those with an 'explicit but more narrowly focused family policy' (e.g. Austria, Denmark, Finland and Germany).
3. Those 'without any explicit family policy and where the notion of such a policy is rejected' (e.g. Canada, Britain and the United States).

Although this categorisation is two decades old, it still has relevance as an analytical framework – the details may of course need modifying. Work by Zimmerman (1988; 1992) distinguishes between explicit/manifest and implicit/latent family policy: the former is characterised as 'policy choices into which family considerations are deliberately structured' while implicit or latent family policy refers to 'policy choices into which family considerations are not deliberately structured but affect families nonetheless' (1988, p. 176).

Another problem relates to ideologies surrounding the family and to the disparity between rhetoric and action. Political ideologies in relation to the family have already been considered in an earlier section of the chapter, but it may be worth reiterating that strongly expressed sentiments in support of the family may not be matched by positive action and resources. There may be strong resistance to state intervention in what is seen as an essentially private institution. The clearest expression of this is reluctant intervention in the area of domestic violence.

A third problem is that family structures are so varied and policies may affect different families in different ways. Policies may be universal in scope or they may positively discriminate in favour of particular kinds of family (e.g. lone-parent families, poor families). A further source of variation is that the objectives of family policy may change. Family policy in Sweden, for example, was originally concerned to encourage population growth, but it has long since been seen as an important element in the movement towards equal opportunities and citizenship rights.

Millar and Warman (1996) distinguish clear differences of emphasis in family policy in the member states of the European Union (plus Norway). Three groups of countries can be identified:

1. The Scandinavian countries in which 'the emphasis is on individual entitlements and citizenship rights available to all' and where 'those in need are most likely to expect and receive state, rather than family, provision and there are rarely any legal requirements for family to provide support' (p. 46).
2. The countries in the remainder of northern Europe (Belgium, France, Germany, Ireland, Luxembourg, The Netherlands and the UK) where the emphasis is on the obligations of the nuclear family and where 'individualisation is relatively undeveloped: benefits and taxes almost always recognise these family obligations and services are intended mainly to support family care' (p. 46).
3. The countries of southern Europe (Greece, Italy, Portugal and Spain) where the emphasis is on the extended family as a system of mutual support. 'Although there are clear obligations within the nuclear family, . . . these obligations are embedded within a much wider set of familial obligations which brings in grandparents, siblings, uncles and aunts' (p. 47).

Millar and Warman are careful to point out that their categories overlap, giving the examples of Ireland and The Netherlands, both of which are included in the group of countries emphasising the nuclear family. Ireland shares some of the characteristics of the countries of southern Europe in the significance accorded to the extended family, and The Netherlands 'combines a focus on the nuclear family with a concern for individual rights' (p. 46).

Millar and Warman's categorisation is applied to Western Europe, but it could be extended to include countries outside Europe. Thus Australia, Canada, New Zealand and the United States are firmly in the 'nuclear family category' while Japan falls some way between this group and the extended family group. Extended families are of some significance in some of the African countries and some of those in Central and South America. The categorisation has been described in some detail, because it offers a partial explanation of some of the policy differences to which we now turn. There is, however, a problem of deciding what policies to include. The distinction between explicit and implicit policies is of some help, but the difficulty with the notion of implicit policies is that there are very few social policies which do not have consequences for families. The range of material makes selection essential. Four areas will be briefly considered: support for children and families, paying for care, labour market policies and family impact statements.

Support for children and parents

All social security systems were originally based on the assumption that women were economically dependent upon men. Although this aspect of income maintenance is now changing, progress has been slow and far from complete. In the main, the effect of the changes has been to enable either partner to claim for the other, or for benefits to be paid on an entirely individual basis.

Child benefits or family allowances and maternity benefits are available, almost everywhere, and most commonly on a universal basis. In a study of child support in fifteen countries by Bradshaw *et al.* (1993) the following statement appeared:

> . . . among the countries included in this study, non means-tested systems of family allowances are still the most important part of the child benefit system – most countries have them, even in some of the countries that do not their income related systems are paid so far up the income distribution system as to be almost universal. In cash terms non income related family allowances still provide the largest proportion of the child benefit package that most families, in most countries, receive.
>
> (p. 264)

Nevertheless, The European Commission (1995, p. 78), in a review of social protection schemes, says that family or child allowances 'are the only broad function to have experienced a reduction in expenditure relative to GDP since 1980'. This was partly due to a reduction in the number of eligible children. However, there were reductions in the expenditure per head as a percentage of GDP in Belgium, Germany, Greece, Spain and The Netherlands. These figures relate to the period from 1980 up to 1993; in 1995 both Austria and The Netherlands imposed further cuts in family allowances. Maternity benefits are widespread in Western Europe, and an

EU directive on maternity leave promulgated in 1992 came into effect in 1994. This guarantees a minimum of fourteen weeks maternity leave.

It would be tedious to recount all the family benefits which vary enormously in type, amount and eligibility criteria. In addition to family allowance some countries have supplementary schemes, many of which are means-tested. There are often special benefits for lone parents and in respect of disabled children. In Sweden, there is a special allowance for parents adopting a child who is a foreign national. Some other benefits are available less widely. For example, child-raising allowances are paid in Austria, France and Germany. Home care allowances are available to parents caring for children under two or three at home in Finland, France and Luxembourg, and in the last two countries lump-sum grants are paid (subject to means tests) at the beginning of the school year. It will have been noted that France has been mentioned under every head: France has pursued pro-natalist policies for many years, and Hantrais (1994, p. 150) says that 'France has been identified as the industrialised nation with the most generous benefit and tax relief system for families, particularly large families'. Bradshaw *et al.* (1993) construct tables ranking the countries according to the generosity of provision for children and families. Whether calculations are made before or after housing costs, France, Luxembourg, Norway and Belgium head the list. Denmark, Germany, The Netherlands and the UK are in the middle of the lists. Finland and Sweden, who also have generous schemes, were not included in the analysis. The United States is bottom of the list after housing costs and fourth from the bottom before housing costs. This is a disturbing result: the children of the richest country in the world are in receipt of the lowest benefits.

The United States is virtually alone in providing no general system of child benefits or family allowances, and it shares with Australia the distinction of having no maternity benefits. The nearest approach in the United States is the Aid to Families with Dependent Children (AFDC), a means-tested scheme administered by the states, although financed partly by the federal government. The benefits are aimed at poor, lone-parent families or families in which one of the parents is disabled or, in about half the states, when a parent is unemployed. In some states, since the early 1980s, workfare schemes have been introduced. Under the schemes AFDC claimants are expected to work as a condition of receiving the benefit. It was to be anticipated that President Reagan would reduce eligibility for AFDC, but the election of Clinton on a platform of 'ending welfare as we know it' has led to some of the most drastic modifications to AFDC (see Chapter 2).

In Central and Eastern Europe, the overthrow of communist regimes has not always led to the improvements that were anticipated. Poverty has increased and this has particularly serious consequences for children. A UNICEF report published in April 1997 painted a bleak picture, indicating that the number of children living in poverty has more than doubled to 2.5 million since 1989 (see Traynor, 1997). It will take much more than reform of child support payments to overcome problems of this magnitude.

Payments for informal care

The issue of paying for informal care has been widely debated in the 1990s. It is an enormously complex issue, and only a brief overview can be attempted here. However, references to the most significant publications will help the reader who wishes to know more about the topic. The discussion will be restricted to informal care which is overwhelmingly provided by kin. I shall not be dealing with the very closely related topic of payments to volunteers.

Payments for informal care may serve several quite distinct purposes:

1. They may be a means of legitimating a reduction in the role of the state, and the transfer of responsibility, and some of the costs, to close kin. They may be seen as a politically acceptable way of achieving the privatisation of welfare.
2. Payments may also legitimate policies of community, as opposed to institutional, care.
3. They may be viewed as a symbol of the importance of informal care, recognising the value of the work being done.
4. They may be used to compensate carers, at least in part, for loss of earnings and any extra costs they may incur.
5. Payments may be used as a way of empowering care recipients and/or carers.
6. They may be aimed at encouraging carers, especially women to leave the labour market and return to the home.

Payments may take several forms: (i) cash benefits to the carers; (ii) cash benefits to the recipients of care; (iii) indirect payments in the form of tax allowances. Some indication of the variety of approaches in sixteen countries throughout Europe and North America can be found in Evers *et al.* (1994). The systems employed in the Scandinavian countries are the most radical. In Finland, Denmark, Norway and Sweden informal carers, including family members may be employed by municipalities as home helpers (Johansson and Sundström, 1994; Lingsom, 1994; Sipilä and Anttonen, 1994; Swane, 1994). In Finland, Home Care Allowances (HCA) are paid to the informal carers of disabled or elderly people (Glendinning and McLaughlin, 1993; Sipilä and Anttonen, 1994).

On the surface, the HCA may appear similar to the British Invalid Care Allowance (ICA). There are, however, some very important differences. One difference relates to the administrative structure: the ICA is part of the centralised social security system, whereas the HCA is municipally operated and there is no institutional connection with social security. More importantly, ICA is paid only to people who are not employed and who are of working age; neither of these restrictions apply to HCA, which means that a potential carer can take on waged work outside the home and use the HCA to purchase substitute care.

Both Britain and Finland also provide a range of disability benefits. In Britain we have the Attendance Allowance, the Disability Living Allowance, the Disability Working Allowance and the Severe Disablement Allowance. There is no intention in the payment of these benefits that they should be used to purchase care or to reimburse informal carers. There appears to be contradictory evidence about the degree to which the benefits in Britain are treated as a means of reimbursing carers. The ICA almost certainly is, but there is some disagreement about the Attendance Allowance. Horton and Berthoud (1990), in a study of Attendance Allowances, concluded that the benefit was used to finance general household expenses, but Ungerson (1995) refers to evidence from an empirical study of stroke patients and their carers which she conducted with Baldock that 'many households containing a disabled person understand the Attendance Allowance to be a benefit which is to be used to purchase hands-on care and to pay directly a hands-on carer' (p. 35).

This is of some significance when comparisons are made with other countries. In France, Italy and Austria there is a specific recognition that disability benefits will be used to purchase care or reimburse informal carers. Germany is planning to move in the same direction. France, Austria and Italy pay relatively generous benefits which are deemed to be sufficient to cover the costs of a carer. This method of paying for informal care has the support of the disability movements in many countries: the argument is that care recipients are given greater autonomy if they are given the purchasing power.

There are, however, several difficulties. For example, benefits are paid on the basis of financial need; they are not tied in with specific types or amounts of care. Furthermore, if systems of payment are mainly driven by cost-containment considerations, they are unlikely to be generous, and market rates of wages/reimbursement will not be possible. This will lead to a reliance on family members and there is a possibility of exploitation, with conditions of work that would not be tolerated in employment outside of the home. This implies that support of carers remains essential. Various forms of respite care are certainly necessary. Short-stay residential care, day centres and night hospitals are obviously invaluable in affording carers some respite from the daily grind of looking after frail elderly or disabled people. Some areas have experimented with 'granny-fostering'.,

The burden can also be lightened by provision of domiciliary services such as practical help in the home, meals-on-wheels, health visitors, home nursing and social work support. Such services may be provided directly by statutory agencies or they may be provided under contract by commercial or voluntary sector suppliers. Suitable housing with appropriate adaptations and the supply of aids would contribute to the reduction of stress.

Labour market policies

The belief that the proper place for women is in the home is less openly expressed than it once was. However, the debate is far from over, and even when the belief is not openly expressed, it may have a formative influence in certain areas of social policy. The strictures are now more likely to be reserved for women with children or other caring responsibilities. Right-wing parties everywhere, even in Scandinavia, believe that the state should not encourage women with children to enter the labour market; indeed many would recommend active discouragement or incentives to stay at home. An interesting feature of this debate is the assumption that women have the major responsibility for child care. The provision of a place in a crèche or nursery is to allow a *woman* to work.

I do not intend to address labour market policies in general. In the context of this chapter, the main concern is on the attempts in national policies to reconcile work and family life. Most attention will be directed to measures designed to help mothers to enter the labour market, remain in work and to return to work after the birth of a child. Two broad areas will be considered: the provision of child care facilities and flexible labour markets. Gornick *et al.* (1997) state that there is ample evidence to 'support the theoretically driven prediction that having more attractive child care options increases maternal employment' (p. 48). They say that there is less evidence on the relationship between parental leave and maternal employment, but they conclude that the most reasonable assessment is that maternal participation in the labour market increases with parental leave. Two other elements dealt with by Gornick *et al.* – school hours and cash transfers – will not be covered here.

In looking at parental leave, it is important to recognise that seemingly generous provision for extensive leave may be made infinitely less attractive by the fact that all or a substantial part of it is unpaid. Thus in France one of the two parents (can alternate) can take unlimited leave during the first three years of a child's life, but there is no provision for earnings replacement for the first child; for the second and subsequent children parents can receive the allowance for caring for a child at home. Similarly, parental leave in Greece, Portugal and Spain is unpaid. The most generous country in terms of parental leave is Sweden. Twelve months at 90 per cent of salary is available, to be divided between the parents more or less as they choose. Some restriction of choice about the division of the leave was introduced in 1994. It was found that the whole period was being taken by mothers, and in 1994 a 'Daddy Month' was introduced. This requires fathers to take at least one of the twelve months. Failing that, the total leave is reduced to eleven months. Germany also has reasonably generous arrangements in terms of time, but the rates of replacement of earnings are lower than in Sweden. In Germany there is provision for six months leave paid at a flat-rate, followed by eighteen months of income-related benefit. In Italy, there is six months' parental leave commencing after twenty-two weeks of paid maternity leave, but the pay during parental leave amounts to only 30 per cent of earnings. In 1995 Denmark extended the period of parental leave to six months, but the rate of replacement has been reduced from 80 per cent of unemployment benefit to 70 per cent, with a further reduction in 1997 to 60 per cent. The Gornick *et al.* study revealed variations in the extent of paid maternity leave from six weeks in the United States to fifty-two weeks in Sweden (this is more correctly called parental leave). Wage replacement during maternity leave varied from 46 per cent in the UK to 100 per cent in Germany, Luxembourg, The Netherlands and Norway. The percentage of employed women who were covered varied from 10 per cent in Australia, 25 per cent in the United States, 60 per cent in the UK and 100 per cent in the remaining eleven countries. Within the EU, paternal leave is provided in Belgium, Denmark, France, and Spain, but it is only two days in Spain, three days in Belgium and France and ten days in Denmark. Summing up their findings on parental leave, Gornick *et al.* say:

> . . . all but three of the countries made near-universal provisions for job protection and wage replacement in the months following the birth of a child. . . . The United States and Australia were the most prominent exceptions. The United States had no national law providing job protection at the time of childbirth; in Australia, federal law guaranteed up to twelve months of job protection but provided no wage replacement. The United Kingdom also fell short relative to other countries, primarily because eligibility restrictions (e.g. on minimum earnings and job tenure) were such that only approximately 60 per cent of employed women had access to both job protection and wage replacement.
>
> (1997, p. 55)

Child-care facilities in twenty countries are enumerated by Bradshaw *et al.* (1996). They make the conventional distinction between places for children under the age of three and those for children between the age of three and school age. Provision for the older age group is much more substantial than it is for the younger children. In five countries enrolment in child-care facilities for children aged three and over exceeded 90 per cent. The countries concerned were Belgium, France, Germany (the New Länder), Italy and The Netherlands. In the enrolment of younger children, the New Länder in Germany were well ahead of the other countries with 57 per cent; Japan came second with 49 per cent, followed a long way behind by France with 33 per cent and Sweden with 32 per cent.

Family-impact analysis

Governments find it convenient to talk about the importance of the family and the need to support it. Their support is frequently limited, however, to what they regard as the conventional nuclear family of a married couple with children in which the husband/father is the main earner. Scandinavian governments are less selective, recognising both the variety of family forms and the need to assist women to participate in the labour market. Elsewhere in the industrialised world, statements about the centrality of the family in national life are not always matched by appropriate action. As an indication of their good intentions, some countries appoint ministers for the family whose responsibility is to devise a coherent family policy and to protect the interests of families when policies likely to affect them are being discussed.

Family-impact analysis has been suggested as a means of focusing attention on the family. The aim is to evaluate policies terms of their possible impact on families of different kinds, and a family-impact statement might accompany all new legislation. Existing policies and policies in the process of implementation would be similarly evaluated and monitored. Most policies have a family dimension: social security, health services, services for elderly and disabled people, education, child care, housing, fiscal, transport and employment policies are obvious candidates for systematic family-impact evaluation. At the very least, conflicting aims and effects might be exposed. Fox Harding argues that:

> A family perspective on policy should have four premises: that the family-policy relationship is two-way; that family should be taken into account across virtually the whole range of public policy; that increasing family diversity should be recognised and respected; and that all types of family (broadly defined) should be taken into account. The latter points suggest an attempt at a value-neutral approach.
>
> (1996, p. 209)

Family-impact analysis recognises the overwhelming importance of kinship ties in informal caring. For the same reason, this chapter has also emphasised the crucial part played by families in community care. By implication, as the next section demonstrates, friends and neighbours play a secondary, though not insignificant, role. In contrast to the academic and political attention paid to families, the work on friends and neighbours as sources of care is much less extensive.

Friends and neighbours

Friends have two important characteristics which distinguish them from kin and neighbours. Friends are distinguished from neighbours by their wide dispersal, and from kin by lack of diversity in terms of age, stage of the life cycle and social class.

Friendship depends on a degree of equality between participants; it is a reciprocal relationship. A one-sided caring relationship is not likely to lead to or to sustain friendship. As Allan (1985) observes, friends must be capable of contributing 'equivalent financial and emotional resources to the relationship'. Allan's conclusion, shared by other workers in this field, is that:

> While part of friendship is caring about each other to a greater or lesser degree, caring for one another is not an element inherent in the routine organization of friendship . . . the majority of routine friendships are not particularly well suited for providing the sort of caring community care entails, notwithstanding the friendship ideals that might make one think they would be (1985, p. 137).

Willmott (1986) reaches the same conclusion. He says that people have more social contacts with friends than with kin, but that 'in terms of help the bias is the other way . . . at the critical stages, such as old age, infirmity and when babies are born, relatives outnumber friends as sources of support in the ratio of ten to one' (1986, p. 47).

There are class, gender and age differences in friendship. Middle-class people have more friends than working-class people and men have more friends than do women. Middle-class people tend to have a higher proportion than working-class people of non-local friends. The same is true of men as compared to women. Young people have more friends than older people. Friends and neighbours may of course correspond, but close proximity can also inhibit friendship because of possible invasions of privacy.

Kinship is based on blood ties, friendship on affective relationships, and neighbourliness is based on proximity. Bulmer (1987) suggests that these ties are complementary, rather than substitutes, with different kinds of relationships performing different functions:

> Kin ties are typically long-term ties, whether or not there is regular face-to-face contact with relatives. Ties with neighbours are face-to-face contacts and often time-urgent. . . . Ties with friends have an affective basis reinforced by common interests or experience, and may or may not involve frequent face to face contacts. Given these different functions, it is not surprising that as sources of care, kin, friends and neighbours tend to meet different types of need, rather than substitute for one another, though some substitution, particularly in providing psychological support and domestic care, does take place.
>
> (1987, p. 78)

We suggested earlier that personal and domestic care were overwhelmingly provided by kin, and that the services provided by both neighbours and friends are straightforward tasks implying strictly limited involvement: baby-sitting, looking after children during their mothers' temporary absence, taking in deliveries, looking after keys, shopping, sharing in transporting children to and from school, borrowing and lending. It would be a mistake to diminish the importance of such tasks, but it is quite plain that they do not even begin to form an adequate basis for the development of community care policies.

While this conclusion remains true, more recent evidence from O'Connor (1992) and McGlone *et al.* (1996) suggests that friends may be more important than they were found to be ten years previously. O'Connor found that friendships among women were very often a source of practical and other help, sometimes over a long period. Typically, such help came from friends of long-standing. McGlone *et al.* asked respondents to a *British Social Attitudes* survey to whom they would first turn if they needed different kinds of help. Friends were particularly significant in helping with marital problems or depression. The proportion of respondents who would turn to friends in the event of marital problems was 27 per cent, and for depression the overall figure was 21 per cent. This last figure, however, is given further analysis: for married people the spouse was the main source of help, but for divorced/separated people the proportion naming friends rose to 44 per cent and for single people to 40 per cent.

Conclusion

The evidence that the informal sector provides more care than the statutory, voluntary or commercial sectors is incontrovertible. That families overwhelmingly predominate in the informal system of care is equally certain. It is beyond doubt, too, that within families women are the main carers.

The lives of carers are frequently restricted, with few contacts outside the home and with little help from voluntary or statutory services. Parker (1990), in a review of research on informal care, comments:

> The evidence we are able to glean from various sources suggests that available services are likely to have little overall effect for informal carers. Firstly, few dependent people who have informal carers appear to receive services and, when they do, such services are usually crisis-orientated rather than a part of long-term support. Secondly, the criteria by which services are allocated are often irrational (not allocated in relation to need) and discriminatory (not provided where female carers are available).
>
> (p. 125)

The assumption made by conservative governments in different parts of the world that the informal system of care can compensate for a reduction in statutory services has to be seriously questioned on the basis of the evidence. In the case of families, the assumption is probably erroneous; in the case of friends and neighbours it is probably over optimistic. This is not to deny the significance of the informal sector, but rather to doubt its capacity for absorbing *extra* work. In fact, social and demographic changes may be reducing the family's capacity to care, while at the same time the number of people requiring care is increasing. Policies which take little or no account of these changes, and many appear not to, can only be unrealistic and thus fail to meet their objectives.

When the costs of community care are calculated the social costs, in terms of physical, psychological and financial strain on families, and especially on women, have to be considered, even though it may be difficult to place a money value on them. The exploitative potential of family care has constantly to be borne in mind. It makes little sense to talk about equality of opportunity for women in employment if the sexual division of labour persists in the home. The principal objective of social policy in relation to the informal sector should not be to pressurise people into taking on extra responsibility, but to provide them with a realistic choice. In cases where people *choose* to care for frail elderly or disabled relatives, they should be given every possible support. The support they know to be available will be one of the considerations when people make their choice. Those who choose not to provide direct care should feel confident that acceptable alternative services exist. If the mixed economy of welfare has any merit at all then it must be concerned to extend choice not restrict it.

Notes

1. 1988 in the cases of Luxembourg and Greece and 1989 in the case of Germany.
2. Readers may care to refer back to Chapter 2.

CHAPTER 6

CONCLUSION

Mixed economies of welfare are the new orthodoxy: they are the accepted explanation of the present and the vision of the future throughout the world. The universal hegemony of mixed economies of welfare has been aided since 1989/90 by the collapse of the regimes in Central and Eastern Europe and the states of former Soviet Union. Even avowedly communist countries, such as the People's Republic of China, are embracing markets and competition in the economic system and the development of mixed systems of welfare. Evers (1993) summarises the main features of the changes:

> More than a decade after the detection of the 'crisis of the welfare state', it seems there has been a clear resolution of one of the most important elements of the debate. The concept of dominant state-centred welfare has corroded and lost its hegemony. At no point along the political spectrum does it receive unqualified ideological support; even in the Nordic States scepticism has at least increased. Recently in most countries – especially the post-communist ones – economic liberalism has both in theory and practice filled the gap which arose.
>
> (p. 3)

Hill (1996) identifies the same process, although he is much more sceptical than Evers in his assessment of the impact of the shift. He argues that the main attraction for governments of the ideas stemming from mixed economies of welfare is their promise to restrict the costs of social policy: 'the globalisation of policy thinking is such that these ideas for curbing the costs of social policy travel rapidly around the world. They are seen as effective responses to the rising costs of social policy. There are grounds for scepticism about what they can achieve' (p. 315).

It should be clear from the introduction to this book and what has been said in subsequent chapters that mixed economies of welfare are not new. As was stated at the beginning, welfare states have always been mixed, and what has been happening since the late 1970s is a concerted attempt to shift the balance away from the state towards other sources of provision, finance and regulation. This has included attempts to shift the costs of provision to individuals, families and to some extent voluntary providers, by introducing and raising charges and co-payments and reducing subsidies and tax expenditures.

It is worth reiterating, however, the caution urged in the Preface about taking an entirely top-down approach in analysing mixed economies of welfare. While government policies and pressure from international financial institutions have played a central role in promoting mixed economies, there have been other influences from lower down the hierarchy. These include pressure groups, social movements (e.g. the consumers' movement and the women's movement) and, of course, the major changes in Central and Eastern Europe were brought about by popular discontent. More modestly, there have also been demands for greater citizen and user involvement and there has been a substantial growth of self-help. Furthermore, there have been demographic and social changes which were beyond the capacity of governments and international financial institutions to control.

The preceding chapters should have made it clear that the precise proportions of the welfare mix vary cross-nationally: a simple example is a comparison of the prominent role of the market and the voluntary sectors in the United States with their more limited role in Sweden. Another example stems from the principle of subsidiarity in Germany and the Netherlands which guarantees the voluntary sector a greater role in provision than is usual in other European countries. There may be further variations between the component units within federal states, especially when the sub-national units have the power to make decisions or modify the implementation of national policies. This is nowhere clearer than in the United States where Reagan's 'new federalism' and subsequent changes under Bush and Clinton have given the individual states more latitude in welfare spending and in determining their own approach to welfare reform

(O'Connor, 1998). Many other countries have implemented policies of decentralisation.

There are also variations in the mix as between one service area and another. It is difficult to be precise about the extent of this variation, but some very general comparisons may be made. The following examples are not intended to be even remotely comprehensive:

- Social assistance programmes are largely state-dominated.
- This is also mainly true of unemployment compensation but, since this is insurance based, employees and employers pay contributions and in Denmark, Germany and Sweden trade unions are heavily involved in administering the schemes.
- Pensions are a mixture of state, occupational and private market provision.
- Social care for elderly and disabled people typically involves all four sectors: state, commercial, voluntary and, most heavily of all, the informal sector (especially families).
- Education in most countries is predominantly a state responsibility, but frequently with private and voluntary sector participation.
- Health care, whether based on insurance or direct provision, may be either publicly financed as in Western Europe, or predominantly private, with a heavy reliance on private insurance, as in the United States, or it may be based on compulsory savings schemes as in Singapore; in some countries (notably, Japan and China) there is substantial occupational provision.

This book has demonstrated that the welfare mix is not fixed for all time. In stable democracies change tends to be gradual, but more rapid change may occur in periods of crisis or after major world events such as the Second World War. Revolutions, counter-revolutions and *coups d'états* will produce major change, but it may very well be that welfare reform is low on the new regime's priorities. It is instructive to compare the speed and scale of change in the welfare mix in the countries of Central and Eastern Europe or in Chile, under the repressive, military regime of Pinochet, with changes in Western Europe. The changes in Central and Eastern Europe have been particularly dramatic with the movement, in a matter of a very few years, away from a state-dominated system to a more mixed approach involving both commercial suppliers and voluntary agencies. However, merely looking at provision or delivery of services gives only a partial indication of change and is likely to produce a distorted picture of the balance between the four sectors: finance and regulation also have to be taken into account.

We have indicated that arguments for mixed economies of welfare are frequently arguments about reducing the role of the state. The position of nation states is being challenged from another direction – increasing globalisation. The growing power and influence of both multinational companies and international financial institutions may reduce the capacity of national governments to decide policies without reference to global economic pressures. Hill (1996, p. 53) says that 'multinational companies may tend to dictate policy choices in areas like social protection and the amelioration of the impact of unemployment'. Esping-Andersen (1996) takes a characteristically broad sweep:

> It may even be that governments' freedom to design discrete social policies has eroded, as contemporary pension reforms suggest. It is increasingly world finance which defines what is possible and desirable; not only in the ex-communist states or Latin America, but also recently in Italy and Sweden. There is the alarming prospect that globalization will eventually emasculate democratic choice.
>
> (p. 256–7)

Another recent example of international pressure on Western welfare states is the OECD's statement that Germany has not gone far enough in attempting to curb costs – especially in the field of health. In August 1997 The OECD's economic review of Germany recommended the replacement of its supplier-led health care system by a system based on the UK model of contracts and the purchaser-provider split. The International Monetary Fund (IMF) has been heavily criticised for protecting American interests rather than those of the countries which seek their assistance. More specifically, there have been criticisms of its response to the financial crisis in East Asia in 1997/98. Indonesia, South Korea and Thailand all received aid from the IMF, but the conditions attached to the emergency bailing out were severe: the IMF insisted on stringent recessionary monetary policies. However, to demonstrate that this is not an entirely new phenomenon, reference might be made to Britain in 1976. Britain, having experienced three years of mounting inflation and unemployment precipitating a sterling crisis, sought the assistance of the International Monetary Fund (IMF) which sent a team to Britain to examine the situation. The IMF eventually agreed to help on the strict condition that curbs would be imposed on both public expenditure and public sector borrowing.

Hutton (1997) is less pessimistic about the nation state's ability to decide policies, but his comment relates to multinational companies rather than to institutions such as the World Bank, the IMF and the OECD:

> The balance of power between the nation state and the world market is very complex. To the multinational, the new environment is as hazardous as it is to a national government.... While the nation state these days is clearly weaker in its capacity to run its national economy as it chooses, its ability to initiate partnerships, regulate activity, cut deals and even fix tax rates and spending levels is still significant. Indeed, there is no other player with the same power.
>
> (pp. 30–1)

Another aspect of globalisation is that open economies, an essential feature of global economics, increase competition. This was often related to the competition from the Far East, and its impact upon Western economies, and the downward pressure on wages and non-wage costs. At the time of writing (February 1998) it is still too early to say how the financial crisis will affect this equation, but the hardships being experienced by the populations of the countries in East Asia are all too apparent. Hill (1996) argues that policies should not be solely concerned with seeking competitive advantage by either adopting aggressive low-wage labour policies or trying to create a high quality labour force. He quotes Lipietz (1992) who argues that local solidarity must be based on national and international solidarity. Hill (1996) says that we need not always be in 'remorseless competition' and that 'the challenge for the modern world is to find ways which *either* distribute jobs *or* redistribute the benefits from production in ways which will enable all to share continuing global growth' (p. 200). Even supposing that the world needs growth, it is wrong to pursue it 'without attention to distributional and environmental consequences' (p. 317).

Esping-Andersen (1996) examines how different welfare states have responded to economic and social change over the past decade. Welfare states in the advanced industrial nations have taken one of three 'routes': the Scandinavian route, the neo-liberal route and the labour reduction route. Until the mid-1980s the Scandinavian route involved the creation of jobs, mainly for women and mostly part-time in the public sector. This eventually proved to be too costly, leading to high tax rates and the expansion of public sector employment came to an end. Sweden is now experiencing high unemployment rates. There are indications of a drift of the more prosperous members of the community away from public services towards private provision as public services languish. The Scandinavian countries, and Sweden in particular, have traditionally pursued a redistributive model aimed at broad equality of outcome. Redistribution of income is only one strand of this strategy, part of a policy of ensuring that 'all households have command over the bundle of resources deemed necessary in order to function in society the way everyone else does' (Esping-Andersen, 1996, p. 262). The problem with this approach is that it raises issues of equity or fairness. In the past Scandinavian countries have been able to contain equity problems because of their very high levels of labour market participation and their universal systems, providing high quality benefits for all, including, crucially, the middle classes. It is this consensus-building capacity, Esping-Andersen claims, which has been eroded and which needs to be re-established. Nevertheless, welfare states in Scandinavia, although they are experiencing difficulties, are not abandoning the principles of the welfare state as some of those countries following the neo-liberal route appear to be doing.

The main features of the neo-liberal approach, best exemplified by the United States the UK and New Zealand but also encompassing Australia and Canada, include: (i) a growing emphasis on markets in health and welfare; (ii) a move from welfare to workfare; (iii) greater emphasis on selectivity; (iv) a distinction between the deserving and undeserving poor; (v) cuts in social expenditure and reductions in social protection; (vi) deregulation of wages. When there was talk of the need for retrenchment in the neo-liberal states, a sub-text was the need to place more emphasis on private markets. This was undoubtedly the case in the UK and the United States which had conservative governments with strong New Right leanings through-out the 1980s and in Canada which had a similarly inclined government from 1985 to 1993. O'Connor (1998) says of the developments in America:

In trying to scale back the public sector, the administration ... looked toward marketising social welfare services. Believing that private, for-profit agencies could provide services in a more efficient manner, Reagan looked to marketisation as a way to lower expenditures, reduce government involvement and diversify service delivery.

(pp. 52–3)

It is ironic, however, that the most thoroughgoing neo-liberal policies occurred not in conservative America, Canada or Britain, but in New Zealand under a Labour Government. That New Zealand, one of the most stable and extensive welfare states, could so wholeheartedly embrace neo-liberal economics and begin to virtually dismantle its welfare system is an indication of the growing influence of the New Right during the 1980s.

Most of the countries of Western Europe, excluding the UK and Scandinavia, adopted a labour reduction strategy, principally by encouraging early retirement. However, as Esping-Andersen acknowledges, the labour reduction strategy has been considerably modified in the 1990s with most countries raising retirement ages and lengthening contribution requirements. Although New Right ideas have had some influence in Western Europe, their impact in terms of practical policy has been more limited as compared with the neo-liberal states. There has been no shortage of New Right rhetoric, however. For example, Mangen (1991) says:

The economic arguments of the radical right have been forcefully expressed in West Germany since the first oil crisis and, at least at the rhetorical level, have found an echo in the pronouncements of Chancellor Kohl and other leading politicians in the Christian Democratic Union (conservatives) and among the Free Democrats (liberals).

(p. 100)

Mangen argues that Kohl's much-trumpeted *wendepolitik* which promised neo-liberal economic policies combined with neo-conservative social policies which would curtail the welfare system and reduce the role of the state, was never really translated into action. There was a modest increase in self-help initiatives, some reductions in social protection, and a limited degree of privatisation, but there was no major restructuring of the welfare state. Since Mangen wrote this paper, there have been further cuts in benefits and the beginnings of a market-driven contracting system.

The recent tentative changes in Germany are mirrored in other European countries. For example, the European Commission (1995) says of health care reform in the European Union that, despite differences in detail, there is 'in nearly all countries . . . some tendency to adopt what might be termed a contractual approach' (p. 115). These developments suggest some caution about too rigid an application of Esping-Andersen's categorisation. The developments in most welfare states during the last decade were not along one of three clearly marked out routes. Governments, unaware of the routes, may follow several paths simultaneously or deviate from one to the another.

This brief analysis refers to welfare states in Western Europe, North America, Australia and New Zealand. There are three other areas where welfare states are less fully developed: Latin America, Central and Eastern Europe and South-East Asia. Any analysis of mixed economies of welfare in these areas has to be undertaken with caution because rapid economic, political and social change may be reflected in substantial shifts in the welfare mix over a relatively short time-span.

Enthusiasm for the neo-liberal approach was displayed by some of the governments in Latin America – most notably in Chile and to a lesser extent in Argentina (Borzutzky, 1991; Huber, 1996). However, a second trend, exemplified by Brazil and Costa Rica, is discernible in Latin America. As Huber (1996, p. 175) observes, Costa Rica merits attention 'because it is the only Latin American country that had built a pattern of social policy with social democratic aspirations, and because it is a rare case of a small country that could resist pressures for a move to a neoliberal model and instead could protect this pattern'. The progress of Brazil's welfare state has been rather more halting, but present policy objectives are to move towards a state-dominated universalist system. Benefit levels in Brazil, however, are very low and the system is characterised by considerable inequity.

After the fall of communism in Central and Eastern Europe, the New Right economists and business experts were quick to offer themselves as advisors and markets have begun to emerge in several sectors. Standing (1996, p. 245), for example, says that 'commercial private clinics and private access to better facilities have been spreading, while resources devoted to the public health care system have been curtailed and the private sector has been moving into the pharmaceutical industry'. It is difficult to predict the future development of welfare states in countries in which so much else is uncertain, but in the shorter term, the Czech Republic, Hungary, Poland, Slovenia and some of the republics of the former Soviet Union are likely to follow, to varying degrees, a neo-liberal approach. East Germany will follow patterns established in the Western part of Germany.

The countries of South-East Asia may be tentatively classified as neo-liberal, although Esping-Andersen's view (1997) is that we must await further developments before a reasoned judgement can be formed. He believes that there will be increasing pressure to provide social rights in these countries. Until the financial crises of 1997/98, some of the countries of South-East Asia were experiencing very rapid economic growth, and this may have silenced demands for increased state welfare, but now that growth has slowed down, demands may become irresistible. The case for at least a preliminary classification as neo-liberal rests on what appear to be relatively low levels of public expenditure on social and health care and the considerable resistance to any substantial extension of state-dominated social provision. However, this may be judging South-East Asian welfare states with western eyes, and in a study of Japan, South Korea, Hong Kong, Singapore and Taiwan, Goodman, White and Kwon (1997) argue that simply comparing proportions of GDP spent on welfare gives a misleading impression. They contend that 'state involvement in welfare provision is not as modest as some commentators suggest' (p. 373). The reason for the underestimate is 'the particular way in which the state participates in the financing of welfare' (p. 373). The state acts as a regulator, enforcing welfare programmes without providing direct finance. They conclude, however, that although the gap between South-East Asian states and those of Western Europe is not so wide as is sometimes supposed, the recalculation to take account of the state's regulative role does not eliminate the discrepancies:

> East Asian governments still play a welfare role which is less than their western counterparts. Instead, non-state agencies – community, firm and family – have been expected to play a major welfare role in an ideological context wherein self/mutual help is encouraged and dependence on the state discouraged, even stigmatised.
>
> (p. 374)

Since the mid-1970s, most countries have attempted to curb the growth of social expenditure, and the rate of growth has slowed down, not in absolute terms but as a percentage of GDP. In the European Community of twelve nations the increase in social expenditure as a percentage of GDP between 1970 and 1980 averaged 5.1 per cent, whereas between 1980 and 1990 the percentage increase was only 1.1 per cent. O'Connor (1998) shows a similar change in the United States. But although these figures represent a significant reduction in the rate of growth, it is not the scale of reduction that was sought by several governments.

The governments of the United States and the UK were among the keenest advocates of retrenchment, but Pierson (1994), in a detailed examination of the retrenchment policies of Reagan and Thatcher in the 1980s, concludes that the achievement of both administrations fell short of their ambitions. Pierson's analysis is very closely argued, and here we can give a taste of it only.

Governments' ability to achieve desired retrenchment depends upon the strategies employed and the obstacles encountered. Retrenchment strategies take several forms:

- Obfuscation which rests on the power of governments to control and manipulate information. If the size and nature of cuts can be obscured, or if the government's part in them can be minimised in people's minds, the strategies of retrenchment have less chance of meeting opposition. Gradual cuts have a better chance of escaping open and sustained opposition than larger cuts made over a shorter time-span. Myles (1996, p. 136) also talks about obfuscation, which he calls 'welfare by stealth', in Canada.
- Division of potential opposition by making the cuts affect some recipients of services/benefits, but not others. It may also be possible to create divisions between consumers and producers.
- Compensation offered to some of those losing from the cuts may help to dampen opposition.

In the United States and Britain there were some opportunities for employing politically low-risk strategies, but they were not by any means always available, and there could be no guarantees of success. Furthermore, there were several powerful limiting factors which may have outweighed the advantages of adopting the strategies even when opportunities arose.

Pierson (1994) comments on the resilience of the welfare state:

Despite the aggressive efforts of retrenchment advocates, the welfare state remains largely intact ... Any attempt to understand the politics of welfare state retrenchment must start from a recognition that social policy remains the most resilient component of postwar domestic policy.

(p. 179)

The most compelling reason for this is that the welfare state, as we saw in the Introduction, is for the most part popular and the political costs of damaging important parts of it may be high. Not only is the welfare state popular with the general public, but there are powerful interest groups who are opposed to cuts. Esping-Andersen develops this point:

Public choice economists ... point to the mutual complicity in favour of the status quo that welfare state bureaucrats and clients foster. Even residual or service-leaning welfare states employ a large proportion of the labour force: the Scandinavian public sector accounts for a third. These are also powerful, professionalized and highly organized lobbies. Ministers and governments come and go, the administrators remain. As a huge political science literature has shown, much of the really decisive policy-making occurs in bureaucracies, not in parliaments.

(pp. 265–6)

A second reason for the resilience of welfare states is, as Pierson (p. 181) says, 'the absence of attractive private alternatives'. Reagan was more successful than Thatcher in achieving cuts. According to O'Connor (1998) the Reagan administration achieved cuts in federal welfare spending as a proportion of total federal spending and cuts in federal spending as a proportion of GDP, but in specific programmes, the results were more equivocal. Combining the statistics from Pierson and O'Connor, it transpires that disability benefits, earned income tax credits and Medicare actually increased, but there were reductions in unemployment compensation, AFDC, food stamps, housing, education, training, employment and social services. As we saw in Chapter 2, AFDC recipients were among the biggest losers, although most of the losses occurred as a result of state rather than federal policies. In the UK there were cuts in pensions, housing (including housing benefits), unemployment benefits and child benefits, and there was a substantial increase in means-testing. European Commission figures (1995) indicate that the UK experienced the biggest rise in social expenditure as a percentage of GDP in the whole of the Union between 1980 and 1993: an increase of 6.8 percentage points as compared with an average for the EU of 3.6 percentage points. In three countries – Belgium, Germany and Luxembourg – social expenditure as a percentage of GDP actually fell between 1980 and 1993.

Prominence has been given to the ideologies of the New Right as an influence in welfare state change, but it should be noted that New Right philosophies are not always used as the main justification for cuts; the need to avoid increases in taxation and the alleged increased inability of the state to finance generous benefits and services are frequently cited, as is also the need for economic competitiveness in a global economy. For example, Lightman (1991) says that:

> Canada has never embraced neo-conservative or New Right ideology with the enthusiasm of Thatcher's Britain or Reagan's America. At the same time the Canadian welfare state, particularly since the onset of monetarism in the mid-1970s, has come under severe attack. The result has been a fundamental restructuring of the gains achieved through nearly half a century of struggle. This retreat has not primarily been based on ideology, at least on the surface, for radical right rhetoric has a singularly alien tone when applied in the Canadian context. Instead, the case to dismantle Canada's welfare state has been argued largely in terms of fiscal capacity and the need to reduce structural deficits within a federal budgetary process.
>
> (p. 141)

It is interesting to note that governments in Western Europe are currently justifying cuts in social expenditure on the grounds that they are needed in order to meet the requirements for entry into the European Monetary Union.

Furthermore, the success of retrenchment policies is not simply determined by the ideological commitment, enthusiasm and political astuteness of those implementing them. There are certain items of expenditure which are, in the short-term at least, outside of the government's control. Some of these are global matters – world recession and technological advance, for example – but there are also inescapable obligations based on past policies. Thus part of the UK's problem in seeking to cut expenditure was the higher than average unemployment during the early 1980s and again in the early 1990s. Thus, expenditure on social security rose sharply. This should serve as a warning not to read too much into total expenditure figures in specific areas of policy. It is quite possible to lower rates of individual benefit (as happened in the UK) and still be faced with a bigger total bill. Among the other factors contributing to higher spending totals in the long term, but beyond government control, is the increasing proportions of elderly people in the population.

The fact that only modest success was achieved in reaching retrenchment targets, should not lead to the comforting conclusion that large sections of the populations in the UK and the United States were no worse off in consequence of the policies pursued by Reagan and Thatcher. Pierson (1994) is adamant:

> To avoid any misunderstanding, I wish to distance myself at the outset from any claim that the Reagan and Thatcher administrations had little impact on the distribution of income. Indeed, the opposite is the case: income inequality increased sharply in both countries in the 1980s, and public policy played an important role in the process.
>
> (p. 5)

Some of the inequalities stem from taxation policies. Glennerster (1991) argues that the most decisive changes have been to taxation and the funding of social welfare. Some of the higher rates of income tax have been reduced and in some cases this has been balanced by increases in social security contributions. There is another point to be made about taxation. Political parties in every country seem locked into the view that electoral success is dependent upon promises not to increase taxation and in some cases to reduce it. Lower taxation is paid for by reduced services or by increased direct charges. I strongly endorse Hill's (1996) statement:

> ... people need to come to terms with the fact that social policy – broadly defined – offers in many cases the best way of socialising costs that will otherwise fall heavily, unpredictably and inequitably on individuals and families. ... The economic orthodoxy which terrifies politicians of the 'left' from championing public expenditure growth with its inevitable tax implications needs to be challenged.
>
> (p. 318)

Interestingly, a report in *The Observer* on 31 August 1997 (Vulliamy, 1997) indicated growing dissatisfaction in the United States with what has 'become the sacred cow of American politics': the pledge by political leaders to cut taxes and public spending. The complaints were from businessmen/women in conservative Virginia and Pittsburgh. The priority for extra spending in Pittsburgh is education, and the plan is to set up a pre-school education programme for poor children, but those funding the project are determined to put pressure on government to take over the funding as soon as feasible. In Virginia the spending priorities are again education, but also roads.

Inequality and poverty have increased, not only in the United States and the UK, as already indicated, but in a wide range of countries. High rates of unemployment create inequality between those in work and those not, although the degree of inequality thus created will depend on wage levels and the generosity of unemployment compensation. It is not insignificant that replacement rates have been reduced in several countries (see Chapter 2). Financial assistance is only part of the story, however; if attitudes and methods of service delivery stigmatise unemployed people, benefit recipients' sense of self-worth is diminished. Increasingly, citizens' status, rights and benefits are determined by their employment. An article on social exclusion by Levitas (1996) argues that:

> the concept of social exclusion, which was originally developed to describe the manifold consequences of poverty and inequality, has become embedded as a crucial element within a new hegemonic discourse. Within this discourse, terms such as social cohesion and solidarity abound, and social exclusion is contrasted not with inclusion but with integration, construed as integration into the *labour market*. . . . Within this discourse, the concept of social exclusion operates both to devalue unpaid work and to obscure the inequalities between paid workers, as well as to obscure the fundamental social division between the property-owning class and the rest of society.
>
> (p. 5) (emphasis added)

It also deepens the division between those in paid work and unemployed people. In the last twenty years there have been two periods of large-scale unemployment: the early 1980s and the early 1990s. After about 1995, unemployment in some countries began to decline, but the latest figures available in August 1997 showed Finland with a rate of 15 per cent and Belgium, France, Italy and Spain had rates in excess of 12 per cent. Germany's unemployment rate was 11.5 per cent, Sweden's was 9.1 per cent and Canada's was 9 per cent. By contrast, unemployment in Norway was 3.4 per cent, Japan had a rate of 3.5 per cent and the United States had a rate of 4.8 per cent. In

Central and Eastern Europe rates were high except in the Czech
Republic (3.8 per cent), Estonia (4.5 per cent), Lithuania (5.9 per
cent) and Ukraine (2.1 per cent). Economic reform and changing the
welfare mix in Central and Eastern Europe has so far widened
inequalities and increased poverty. Standing (1996, p. 231) says that
the result of what he classes as 'mass unemployment' in the absence
of a system of social security designed to deal with unemployment
and employment has been the development of 'widespread deprivation and impoverishment'.

Nobody, so far as I know, has suggested the use of the label 'underclass' to describe the very poor in Central and Eastern Europe; the
term has been used specifically in relation to the United States and
the UK. The idea has clear connections to ideas about problem
families in the 1950s, Oscar Lewis's (1964) work on the culture of
poverty and the notions of a cycle of deprivation popular in the
1970s. What these disparate approaches have in common is a belief
that poverty is in some way the result of the behaviour of the victims.
The concept of the 'underclass' has been popularised, but not
originated, by Murray (1984) who developed the idea in the United
States in the 1980s and then applied it to the UK in 1990 and 1994.
The important point about Murray's thesis is that there is a sizeable
group of people whose behaviour renders them poor. He asserts that
the underclass relates not to the degree of poverty but to a type of
poverty. The members of the underclass, described by Murray as the
'new rabble', are distinguished by a disinclination to work, a dependency on state benefits, illegitimate births (Murray's term), deviant
child-rearing practices, criminal behaviour (especially among young
males). Murray takes a high moral tone, but his work is rich in
vocabulary and assertions but poor in terms of hard evidence.
Dahrendorf (1987) and Field (1989) also use the term underclass,
but differ fundamentally with Murray in stressing structural causes
rather than behaviour. Critical commentary on Murray's two essays
relating to the UK is to be found in Lister (1996). Critics emphasise
the suspect nature of the evidence and the conclusions based on it.
There is also a criticism that by focusing on behaviour, the real
problems are being ignored. As Lister says:

> The danger is that in searching for the 'underclass', social scientists,
> politicians and the media will fail to see on the one hand the struc-
> tural forces which are pushing more and more people into poverty

and on the other the resourcefulness and resilience with which many of these 'victims' respond.

(1996, p. 12)

The connection between the debate about the underclass and mixed economies of welfare is to be found in the related debate on social exclusion. Whether there is an underclass or not, there are certainly people among the poor and very poor who are excluded from full citizenship rights. It is these people who will have been most adversely affected by 'rolling back the state', reducing benefits and introducing more restrictive, and sometimes punitive, eligibility criteria. They are also those most affected by the greater commodification that comes from increased reliance on markets. As was observed in Chapter 3, deprived people are excluded from any but the most marginal participation in market transactions. The voluntary sector (see Chapter 4) is often said to have the capacity to engender social solidarity and social integration, but it also has the capacity to foster exclusion and particularism. The poorer members of the community are on the periphery of community networks. Although it can be argued with less certainty and on scant evidence, it is possible that poorer people are less adequately served by the informal sector – if for no other reason than that the capacity to help relatives is constrained by lack of resources. The gender and financial inequalities in family care were outlined in Chapter 5.

Furthermore, the more fragmented systems resulting from mixed economies of welfare might be less rather than more accessible, and the state might find it more difficult to secure an equitable distribution and *guarantee* rights. Even so, the state is the *only* body which can guarantee rights, and if it is to do so, fairly detailed regulation may be required. There are some political obstacles to be overcome because most of the rhetoric is about deregulation. The whole subject of regulation in the provision and finance of health and welfare services requires much further study. Forms of regulation have to be sought which: (i) balance the need for probity in the spending of public money against the need for innovation and experimentation; (ii) preserve the independence of the voluntary sector and do not distort the activities of voluntary organisations; (iii) do not divert large amounts of financial resources or staff time from service provision to monitoring and evaluation; (iv) ensure quality; (v) involve service users; (vi) are backed up by effective sanctions and provisions for redress.

This suggests that the state's role in regulation may need to grow in volume and sophistication in the new welfare mixes, and that this may give rise to new forms of partnership between the state and the other sectors. The last twenty years has witnessed shifts in the welfare mix away from the state as a direct provider, and commercial and voluntary suppliers are more prominent than they were in the early 1970s. More too has been expected of the informal sector. But, despite these changes and increased globalisation, the state remains the major player in welfare states: not only does the state retain its role as regulator, but it also sets the rules, policies and priorities within which the other participants operate and it is the major source of finance. In fulfilling these roles, the state has the opportunity to pursue the broader aims of equity and egalitarianism (or achieving an appropriate balance between them). It might equally try to achieve greater inequality, as several governments did in the 1980s.

In summary, the changes associated with shifts in the welfare mix have included: (i) cuts in benefits and services and more circumscribed eligibility criteria; (ii) increases in charging and co-payments; (iii) increased privatisation in residential care, pensions, housing and health care; (iv) the spread of contracting from the United States and the UK to many other countries; (v) increasing inequality and poverty, particularly in those countries strongly influenced by neoliberal philosophies and the countries of Central and Eastern Europe experiencing rapid economic, political and social change; (vi) changes in the structure of government and in the nature of public service.

On the other hand, there is no question that the state-dominated welfare system had its faults and, while supported in general terms, was justly criticised for its over-bureaucratic inflexibility. If a shift in the welfare mix can bring about more sensitive and responsive services, empower users and give them more genuine autonomy and choice and ensure the robust defence of citizenship rights, then benefits will come from the reappraisal of the state and its role in welfare. All welfare states have to be judged by their results, but results do not have to be restricted to readily measurable phenomena such as income and wealth distribution, the quality of housing, education and health services or the adequacy of systems of social protection. These are all important, but there are other less tangible outcomes which are significant contributors to the quality of life. These include the protection of citizens' self-respect and autonomy, feelings of security and the sense of being valued.

The welfare state which is said to have been in crisis since the mid-1970s, seems to have survived. This suggests that crisis may not be an appropriate term: problems there undoubtedly are, but problems do not necessarily constitute a crisis. The resilience of the welfare state rests on its enormous general popularity, the support of powerful interest groups and the lack of a coherent and feasible alternative despite the efforts of the New Right to promote a market-driven system. These strengths have been sufficient to sustain the welfare state through a period of immense change; they should be sufficient to sustain it in the changes that lie ahead.

REFERENCES

Abrams, P. (1977) 'Community care: some research problems and priorities', *Policy and Politics*, no. 6, pp. 125–51.

Abrams, P. (1980) 'Social change, social networks and neighbourhood care', *Social Work Service*, no. 22.

Adams, R. (1990) *Self-help, Social Work and Empowerment*, Basingstoke: Macmilllan.

Alcock, P. (1996) *Social Policy in Britain: Themes and Issues*, Basingstoke: Macmillan.

Allan, G. (1985) *Family Life*, Oxford: Blackwell.

Althusser, L. (1972) *Lenin and Philosophy and Other Essays*, London: New Left Books.

Anheier, H.K. (1987) 'Indigenous voluntary associations, nonprofits and development in Africa', in Powell, W.W. (ed.) *The Nonprofit Sector: A Research Handbook*, New Haven: Yale University Press.

Anheier, H.K. and Knapp, M. (1990) 'An editorial statement', *Voluntas*, vol. 1, no. 1, pp. 1–12.

Anheier, H.K. and Seibel, W. (eds) (1990) *The Third Sector: Comparative Studies of Nonprofit Organizations*, Berlin: de Gruyter.

Anheier, H.K. and Seibel, W. (1993) *Defining the Nonprofit Sector: Germany*, Baltimore: The Johns Hopkins University.

Anheier, H.K. and Seibel, W. (1998) 'The nonprofit sector and the transformation of societies: a comparative analysis of East Germany, Hungary and Poland', in Powell, W. W. and Clemens, L. (eds) *Private Action and the Public Good*, New Haven: Yale University Press.

Archambault, E. (1993) *Defining The Nonprofit Sector: France,* Baltimore: The Johns Hopkins University.

Ashford, D.E. (1985) 'Governmental responses to budget scarcity: France', *Policy Studies Journal*, vol. 13, no. 3.

Atkinson, R. and Cope, S. (1997) 'Community participation and urban regeneration in Britain', in Hoggett, P. (ed.) *Contested Communities*, Bristol: Policy Press.

Atlas, J. and Dreier, P. (1983) 'Mobilize or compromise? The tenants' movement and American politics', in Hartman, C. (ed.) *America's Housing Crisis, What is to be Done?*, Boston: Routledge and Kegan Paul.

Bachrach, P. and Baratz, M. (1962) 'The two faces of power', *American Political Science Review*, vol. 56, no. 4, pp. 947–52.

Baldock, J. (1991) 'The frail elderly and the risks of a mixed economy of personal care services', paper prepared for international research project, *Shifts in the Welfare Mix; Social Innovations in Welfare Policies – A Case for the Elderly*, Vienna: European Centre for Social Welfare Policy and Research.

Baldwin, S. (1977) *Disabled Children – Counting the Costs*, London: Disability Alliance.

Baldwin, S. (1981) *The Financial Consequences of Disablement in Children: Final Report*, York: Social Policy Research Unit.

Baldwin, S. (1985) *The Costs of Caring*, London: Routledge and Kegan Paul.

Baldwin, S. and Twigg, J. (1991) 'Women and community care: reflections on a debate', in Maclean, M. and Groves, D. (eds) *Women's Issues in Social Policy*, London: Routledge, pp. 117–135.

Banting, K.G. (1995) 'The welfare state as statecraft: territorial politics and Canadian social policy' in Leibfried, S. and Pierson, P. (eds) *European Social Policy: Between Fragmentation and Integration*, Washington DC: The Brookings Institution, pp. 269–300.

Barrett M. (1981) *Women's Oppression Today*, London: Verso.

Barry, N. (1991) 'Understanding the market', in Loney, M., Bocock, R., Clarke, J., Cochrane, A., Graham, P. and Wilson, M. (eds) *The State or the Market: Politics and Welfare in Contemporary Britain* (2nd edn), London: Sage, pp. 231–41.

Bartlett, W. (1991) *Quasi-markets and Contracts: A Market and Hierarchies Perspective on NHS Reform*, Bristol: School for Advanced Urban Studies.

Bartlett, W., Propper, C., Wilson, D. and Le Grand (eds) (1994) *Quasi-Markets in the Welfare State*, Bristol: School for Advanced Urban Studies.

Basaglia, F. (1980) 'Problems of law and psychiatry: the Italian experience', *International Journal of Law and Psychiatry*, vol. 3, no. 3, pp. 17–37.

Bauer, R. (1996) 'Third sector and new social politics in Germany: A case study report', paper presented to international meeting, *Third Sector, the State and the Market in the Transformation of Social Politics in Europe*, Milan.

Baumol, W.J., Panzar, J.C. and Willig, R.D. (1982) *Contestable Markets and the Theory of Industry Structure*, New York: Harcourt Brace Jovanovich.

Bawden, D. and Palmer, J. (1984) 'Social policy: challenging the welfare state', in Palmer, J. and Sawhill, I. (eds) *The Reagan Record*, Cambridge: Ballinger Publishing Company.

Bayley, M. (1972) *Mental Handicap and Community Care*, London: Routledge and Kegan Paul.

Bell, D. (1993) *Communitarianism and its Critics*, Oxford: Clarendon Press.

Benington, J. (1974) 'Strategies for change at the local level: some reflections', in Jones, D. and Mayo, M. (eds) *Community Work One*, London: Routledge and Kegan Paul.

Ben-Ner, A. and Van Hoomison, J. (1993) 'Nonprofit organizations in the mixed economy: a demand and supply analysis', in A. Ben-Ner and B. Gui (eds) *The Nonprofit Sector in the Mixed Economy*, Michigan: Michigan University Press.

Bennett, F. (1987) 'What future for social security?', in Walker, A. and Walker, C. (eds) *The Growing Divide*, London: Child Poverty Action Group, pp. 120–8.

Bennett, R.J. (ed.) (1990) *Decentralisation, Local Governments and Markets: Towards a Post-Welfare Agenda?*, Oxford: Oxford University Press.

Bentley, A.F. (1908) *The Process of Government*, Chicago: University of Chicago Press.

Beresford, P. (1988) 'Consumer views: data collection or democracy?' in Allen, I. (ed.) *Hearing the Voice of the Consumer*, London: Policy Studies Institute.

Beresford, P. (1991) 'Against enormous odds', in Thompson, C. (ed.) *Changing the Balance: Power and People Who Use Services*, London: National Council for Voluntary Organisations.

Berger, B. (1993) 'The bourgeois family and modern society', in Davis, J., Berger, B. and Carlson, A. *The Family: Is it Just Another Lifestyle Choice?*, London: Institute of Economic Affairs, pp. 8–27.

Beveridge, W. (1948) Vol*untary Action: A Report on Methods of Social Advance*, London: Allen & Unwin.

Biggs, S.J. (1986) 'Bureaucratization and privatization of care for old people'. Paper presented at Conference on Bureaucratization and Debureaucratization of Social Welfare, Zurich.

Billis, D. and Glennerster, H. (1998) 'Human services and the voluntary sector: towards a theory of comparative advantage', *Journal of Social Policy*, vol. 27, pt. 1, pp. 79–98.

Billis, D. and Harris, M. (1992) 'Taking the strain of change: UK local voluntary agencies enter the post-Thatcher period', *Nonprofit and Voluntary Sector Quarterly*, vol. 21, no. 3, pp. 227–49.

Borzutsky, S. (1991) 'The Chicago Boys: social security and welfare in Chile', in Glennerster, H. and Midgley, J. (eds) *The Radical Right and the Welfare State: An International Assessment*, Hemel Hempstead: Harvester Wheatsheaf.

Bradshaw, J., Ditch, J., Holmes, H. and Whiteford, P. (1993) 'A comparative study of child support in fifteen countries', *Journal of European Social Policy*, vol. 3, no. 4, pp. 256–71.

Bradshaw, J., Kennedy, S., Kilkey, M., Hutton, S., Corden, A., Eardley, T., Holmes, H. and Neale, J. (1996) *Policy and the Employment of Lone Parents in 20 Countries*, York: Social Policy Research Unit, University of York.

Brandon, D. (1991) *Innovation Without Change?*, Basingstoke: Macmillan.

Brindle, D. 'NHS to sell private care plans', *The Guardian*, 25 March 1996.

Brittan, S. (1977) *The Economic Consequences of Democracy*, London: Temple Smith.

Brook, L., Hall, J. and Preston, I. (1996) 'Public spending and taxation', in Jowell, R., Curtice, J., Park, A., Brook, L. and Thomson, K. (eds) *British Social Attitudes, the 13th Report*, Aldershot: Dartmouth Publishing Company, pp. 185–202.

Browne, A.C. (1984) 'The mixed economy of day care: consumer versus professional assessments', *Journal of Social Policy,* vol. 13, pt. 3, pp. 321–39.

Buchanan, J.M. and Tullock, G. (1962) *The Calculus of Consent*, Ann Arbor: University of Michigan Press.

Bulmer, M. (1987) *The Social Basis of Community Care*, London: Allen & Unwin.

Burkitt, B. and Ashton, F. (1996) 'The birth of the stakeholder society', *Critical Social Policy*, vol. 16, no. 4, pp. 3–16.

Burns, D., Hambleton, R. and Hoggett, P. (1994) *The Politics of Decentralisation: Revitalising Local Democracy*, Basingstoke: Macmillan.

Cambridge, P. and Brown, H. (1997) 'Making the market work for people with learning disabilities: an argument for principled contracting', *Critical Social Policy*, vol. 17, no. 2, pp. 27–52.

Campling, J. (1985) 'Editor's introduction', in Gittins, D. *The Family in Question*, Basingstoke: Macmillan.

Carers National Association (1992) *Listen to Carers; Speak Up, Speak Out: Research Among Members of CNA*, London: Carers National Association.

Caring Costs Alliance (1996) *The True Cost of Caring: A Survey of Carers' Lost Income*, London: Carers National Association.

Carvel, J. (1993) 'EC urged to act as number of homeless reaches 2.5m', *The Guardian*, 25 September.

Castles, F.G. (1996) 'Needs-based strategies of social protection in Australia and New Zealand', in Esping-Andersen, G. (ed.) *Welfare States in Transition: National Adaptations in Global Economies*, London: Sage, pp. 88–115.

Cawson, A. (1982) *Corporatism and Welfare: Social Policy and State Intervention in Britain*, London: Heinemann.

Chamberlayne, P. (1990) 'Neighbourhood and tenant participation in the GDR', in Deacon, B. and Szalai, J. (eds) *Social Policy in the New Eastern Europe*, Aldershot: Avebury.

Chamberlin, J. (1977) *On Our Own: Patient-Controlled Alternatives to the Mental Health System*, New York: McGraw-Hill.

Charlesworth, A., Wilkin, D. and Durie, A. (1984) *Carers and Services: A Comparison of Men and Women Caring for Dependent Elderly People*, Manchester: Equal Opportunities Commission.

Chetwynd, J. (1985) 'Factors contributing to stress on mothers caring for an intellectually handicapped child', *British Journal of Social Work*, 15, pp. 295–304.

Clarke, J. and Newman, J. (1997) *The Managerial State*, London: Sage.

Clotfelter, C.T. (ed.) (1992) *Who Benefits from the Nonprofit Sector?*, Chicago: University of Chicago Press.

Cockburn, A. (1996) 'From new deal to great betrayal' *The Observer*, 4 August.

Commission of the European Communities (1982) *Report on Social Developments Year 1981*, Luxembourg: Office for Official Publications of the European Communities.

Commission of the European Communities (1983) *Report on Social Developments Year 1982*, Luxembourg: Office for Official Publications of the European Communities.

Commission on the Future of the Voluntary Sector (Chair: Deakin, N.) (1996) *Report of the Commission on the future of the Voluntary Sector*, London: NCVO Publications.

Craig, G. and Glendinning, C. (1993) 'Rationing versus choice: tensions and options. Cash and care for disabled and older people and their carers', in Page, R. and Deakin, N. (eds) *The Costs of Welfare*, Aldershot: Avebury, pp. 165–82.

Currie, E. (1990) 'Heavy with human tears: free market policy, inequality and social protection in the United States', in Taylor, I. (ed.) *The Social Effects of Free Market Policies*, Hemel Hempstead: Harvester Wheatsheaf, pp. 299–318.

Cutler, T. and Waine, B. (1997) 'The politics of quasi-markets: how quasi-markets have been analysed and how they might be analysed', *Critical Social Policy*, vol. 17, no. 2, pp. 3–26.

Dahl, R. (1956) *A Preface to Democratic Theory*, Chicago: University of Chicago Press.

Dahl, R. (1982) *Dilemmas of Pluralist Democracy: Autonomy Versus Control*, New Haven: Yale University Press.

Dahrendorf, R. (1987) 'The erosion of citizenship and its consequences for us all', *New Statesman*, June.

Dahrendorf, R. (1990) *Reflections on the Revolution in Europe*, London: Chatto and Windus.

Dale, J. and Foster, P. (1986) *Feminists and State Welfare*, London: Routledge and Kegan Paul.

Dalley, G. (1988) *Ideologies of Caring*, Basingstoke: Macmillan.

David, M. (1986) 'Moral and maternal: the family in the right', in Levitas, R. (ed.) *The Ideology of the New Right*, Cambridge: Polity Press.

Davidoff, P. and Gould, J. (1970) 'Suburban action: advocate planning for an open society', *Journal of the American Institute of Planners*, quoted in Higgins, J. (1978) *The Poverty Business: Britain and America*, Oxford: Blackwell.

Davis Smith, J. (1995) 'The voluntary tradition: philanthropy and self-help in Britain 1500–1945', in Davis Smith, J., Rochester, C. and Hedley, R. *An Introduction to the Voluntary Sector*, London: Routledge.

Deacon, B., Castle-Kanerova, M., Manning, M., Millard, F., Orosz, E., Szalai, J. and Vidinova, A. (1992) *The New Eastern Europe: Social Policy Past, Present and Future*, London: Sage.

Deakin, N. (1994) *The Politics of Welfare: Continuities and Change*, Hemel Hempstead: Harvester Wheatsheaf.

Deakin, N. and Walsh, K. (1996) 'The enabling state: the role of markets and contracts', *Public Administration*, vol. 74, no. 2, pp. 33–48.

Deakin, N. and Wright, A. (eds) (1990) *Consuming Public Services*, London: Routledge.

Dean, H. and Taylor-Gooby, P. (1992) *Dependency Culture: The Explosion of a Myth*, Hemel Hempstead: Harvester Wheatsheaf.

Delphy, C. and Leonard, D. (1992) *Familiar Exploitation: A New Analysis of Marriage in Contemporary Western Societies*, Cambridge: Polity Press.

Department of Health and Social Security (1981) *Growing Older*, London: HMSO.

DiMaggio, P. and Powell, W. (1983) 'The iron cage revisited: institutional isomorphism and collective rationality in organizational fields', *American Sociological Review*, 82, pp. 147–60.

Ditch, J., Barnes, H., Bradshaw, J., Commaille, J. and Eardley, T. (1996a) *A Synthesis of National Family Policies 1994*, York: Social Policy Research Unit.

Ditch, J., Bradshaw, J. and Eardley, T. (1996b) *Developments in National Family Policies in 1994*, York: Social Policy Research Unit.

Domberger, S. and Hall, C. (1996) 'Contracting for public services: a review of Antipodean experience', *Public Administration*, vol. 74, no. 2, pp. 129–47.

Dowler, E. and Calvert, C. (1995) *Nutrition and Diet in Lone-parent Families in London*, London: Family Policy Studies Centre.

Downs, A. (1957) *An Economic Theory of Democracy*, New York: Harper and Row.

Downs, A. (1967) *Inside Bureaucracy*, Boston: Little, Brown.

Dunleavy, P. (1991) *Democracy, Bureaucracy and Public Choice*, Hemel Hempstead: Harvester Wheatsheaf.

Dunleavy, P. and O'Leary, B. (1987) *Theories of the State: The Politics of Liberal Democracy*, Basingstoke: Macmillan.

Durkheim, E. (1893) *The Division of Labour in Society*, translated by Simpson, G. (1933) New York: Free Press.

Easton, D. (1953) *The Political System: An Inquiry into the State of Political Science*, New York: Knopf.

Edwards, S. (1996) 'Opening Doors to the Community', *The Guardian*, 22 May.

Ehrenreich, B. and English, D. (1979) *For Her Own Good: 150 Years of the Experts' Advice to Women*, London: Pluto Press.

Emms, P. (1990) *Social Housing: A European Dilemma?*, Bristol: School for Advanced Urban Studies.

Enthoven, A.C. (1985) *Reflections on the Management of the NHS*, London: Nuffield Provincial Hospitals Trust.

Enthoven, A.C. (1993) 'The history and principles of managed competition', *Health Affairs*, Summer Supplement.

Esping-Andersen, G. (1990) *The Three Worlds of Welfare Capitalism*, Cambridge: Polity Press.

Esping-Andersen, G. (1996) 'After the golden age? Welfare state dilemmas in a global economy', in Esping-Andersen, G. (ed.) *Welfare States in Transition: National Adaptations in Global Economies*, London: Sage, pp. 1–31.

Esping-Andersen, G. (ed.) (1996) *Welfare States in Transition: National Adaptations in Global Economies*, London: Sage.

Esping-Andersen, G. (1997) 'Hybrid or unique? The Japanese welfare state between Europe and America', *Journal of European Social Policy*, vol. 7, no. 3, pp. 179–89.

Estrin, S. and Le Grand, J. (1989) 'Market socialism', in Le Grand, J. and Estrin, S.(eds) *Market Socialism*, Oxford: Clarendon Press, pp.1–24.

Estrin, S. and Winter, D. (1989) 'Planning in a socialist market economy', in Le Grand, J. and Estrin S.(eds) *Market Socialism*, Oxford: Clarendon Press.

Etzioni, A. (1988) *The Moral Dimension: Towards a New Economics*, New York: Free Press.

Etzioni A. (1995) *The Spirit of Community*, London: Fontana Press.

European Commission (1994) *Social Protection in Europe*, Luxembourg: Office for Official Publications of the European Communities.

European Commission (1995) *Social Protection in Europe*, Luxembourg: Office for Official Publications of the European Communities.

European Commission (1996) *Social Protection in the Member States of the European Union*, Luxembourg: Office for Official Publications of the European Community.

Evans, R. and Harding, A. (1997) 'Regionalisation, regional institutions and economic development', *Policy and Politics*, vol. 25, no. 1, pp. 19–38.

Evers, A. (1990) 'Shifts in the welfare mix. The case of care for the elderly – mapping the field of a cross-national research project', paper prepared for international research project, *Shifts in The Welfare Mix; Social Innovations in Welfare Policies – The Case of Care for the Elderly*, Vienna: European Centre for Social Welfare Policy and Research.

Evers, A. (1993) 'The welfare mix approach: understanding the pluralism of welfare systems', in Evers, A. and Svetlik, I. (eds) *Balancing Pluralism: New Welfare Mixes in Care for the Elderly*, Aldershot: Avebury.

Evers, A., Pijl, M. and Ungerson, C. (eds) (1994) *Payments for Care: A Comparative Overview*, Aldershot: Avebury.

Evers, A. and Svetlik, I. (eds) (1993) *Balancing Pluralism: New Welfare Mixes in Care for the Elderly*, Aldershot: Avebury.

Ferriman, A. (1992) 'Private patients swamp hospitals and insurers', *The Observer*, 21 June.

Field, C. (1996) 'New Zealand Labour repents love affair with market', *The Observer*, 21 April.

Field, F. (1989) *Losing Out: The Emergence of Britain's Underclass*, Oxford: Blackwell.

Filer, J. H. (1975) *Giving in America: Toward a Stronger Voluntary Sector*, Washington DC: Report of the Commission on Private Philanthropy and Public Needs.

Finch, J. (1984) 'The deceit of self-help: preschool playgroups and working class mothers', *Journal of Social Policy*, vol. 13, pt. 1, pp. 1–20.

Finch, J. (1989) *Family Obligations and Social Change*, Cambridge: Polity Press.

Finch, J. (1993) 'The concept of caring: feminist and other perspectives', in Twigg, J. (ed.) *Informal Care in Europe*, York: University of York.

Finch, J. and Groves, D. (1980) 'Community care and the family: a case for equal opportunities?', *Journal of Social Policy*, vol. 13, pt. 4.

Finch, J. and Mason, J. (1993) *Negotiating Family Responsibilities*, London: Routledge.

Finn, D. (1994) *A New Parnership? Training and Enterprise Councils and the Voluntary Sector*, London: London Boroughs Grants Committee.

Fitzgerald, T. (1983) 'The new right and the family', in Loney, M., Boswell, D. and Clarke, J. *Social Policy and Social Welfare*, Milton Keynes: Open University Press.

Flora, P. (1985) 'On the history and current problems of the welfare state', in Eisenstadt, S.N. and Ahimeir, O. (eds) *The Welfare State and its Aftermath*, London: Croom Helm.

Forder, J., Knapp, M. and Wistow, G. (1996) 'Competition in the Mixed Economy of Care', *Journal of Social Policy*, vol. 1, pt. 2, pp. 201–21.

Fox Harding, L. (1996) *Family, State and Social Policy*, Basingstoke: Macmillan.

Freeman, R. and Clasen, J. (1994) 'The German social state: an introduction', in Clasen, J. and Freeman, R. (eds) *Social Policy in Germany*, Hemel Hempstead: Harvester Wheatsheaf.

Friedman, M. and Friedman, R. (1980) *Free to Choose*, Harmondsworth: Penguin.

Froland, C., Pancoast, D.L., Chapman, N.J. and Kimboko, P.J. (1981) *Helping Networks and Human Services*, Beverly Hills: Sage.

Gamble, A. (1988) *The Free Economy and the Strong State: The Politics of Thatcherism*, Basingstoke: Macmillan.

George, V. and Wilding, P. (1994) *Welfare and Ideology*, Hemel Hempstead: Harvester Wheatsheaf.

Gidron, B., Kramer, R.M. and Salamon, L.M. (eds) (1992) *Government and the Third Sector: Emerging Relationships in Welfare States*, San Francisco: Jossey-Bass.

Gilbert, N. and Gilbert, B. (1989) *The Enabling State*, New York: Oxford University Press.

Ginsburg, N. (1992) *Divisions of Welfare*, London: Sage.

Glendinning, C. (1989) *The Financial Needs and Circumstances of Informal Carers: Final Report*, York: Social Policy Research Unit.

Glendinning, C. (1992) *The Costs of Informal Care: Looking Inside the Houshold*, London: HMSO.

Glendinning, C. and McLaughlin, E. (1993) 'Paying for informal care: lessons from Finland', *Journal of European Social Policy*, vol. 3, no. 4, pp. 239–53.

Glendinning, C. and Millar, J. *Women and Poverty in Britain: The 1990s*, Hemel Hempstead: Harvester Wheatsheaf.

Glennerster, H. (1991) 'The radical right and the future of the welfare state', in Glennerster, H. and Midgley, J. *The Radical Right and the Welfare State: An International Assessment*, Hemel Hempstead: Harvester Whearsheaf, pp. 163–74.

Glennerster, H. (1992) *Paying for Welfare: The 1990s*, Hemel Hempstead: Harvester Wheatsheaf.

Glennerster, H. (1995) *British Social Policy Since 1945*, Oxford: Blackwell.

Glennerster, H. and Midgley, M. (eds) (1991) *The Radical Right and the Welfare State: An International Assessment*, Hemel Hempstead: Harvester Wheatsheaf.

Glenny, M. (1990) *The Re-birth of History*, Harmondsworth: Penguin.

Goffman, E. (1961) *Asylums: Essays on the Social Situation of Mental Patients and Other Inmates*, New York: Doubleday.

Goffman, E. (1968) *Stigma: Notes on the Management of Spoiled Identity*, Harmondsworth: Penguin Books.

Goodin, R.E. (1988) *Reasons for Welfare: The Political Theory of the Welfare State*, Princeton: Princeton University Press.

Goodman, R. and Peng, I. (1996) 'The East Asian welfare states: peripatetic learning, adaptive change and nation-building', in Esping-Andersen, G. (ed.) *Welfare States in Transition: National Adaptations in Global Economies*, London: Sage, pp. 192–224.

Goodman, R., White, G. and Kwon, H-J (1997) 'East Asian social policy: a model to emulate?', in May, M., Brunsdon, E. and Craig, G. (eds) *Social Policy Review 9*, London: Social Policy Association.

Gornick, J.C., Meyers, M.K. and Ross, K.E. (1997) 'Supporting the employment of mothers: policy variation across fourteen wefare states', *Journal of European Social Policy*, vol. 7, no. 1, pp. 45–70.

Gough, I., Bradshaw, J., Ditch, J., Eardley, T. and Whiteford, P. (1997) 'Social assistance in OECD countries', *Journal of European Social Policy*, vol. 7, no. 7, pp. 17–43.

Gould, A. (1993) *Capitalist Welfare Systems: A Comparison of Japan, Britain and Sweden*, London: Longman.

Graham, H. (1983) 'Caring: a labour of love', in Finch, J. and Groves, D. (eds) *A Labour of Love: Women, Work and Caring*, London: Routledge and Kegan Paul.

Gramsci, A. (1971) *Selections from the Prison Notebooks*, edited by Hoare, Q. and Nowell-Smith, G., London: Lawrence and Wishart.

Gray, J. (1992) *The Moral Foundations of Market Institutions*, London: Institute of Economic Affairs Health and Welfare Unit.

Gray, J. (1994) *The Guardian*, 9 June. Quoted in Lister, R. (1996) *op. cit.*

Gray, J. (1996) *After Social Democracy*, London: Demos.

Green, D.G. (1996) *Community Without Politics: A Market Approach to Welfare Reform*, London: Institute of Economic Affairs.

Green, D.G. (1997) 'From National Health monopoly to National Health guarantee', in Gladstone, D. (ed.) *How to Pay for Health Care: Public and Private Alternatives*, London: Institute of Economic Affairs Health and Welfare Unit, pp. 30–56.

Habermas, J. (1976) *Legitimation Crisis*, trans. McCarthy, T., London: Heinemann.

Habermas, J. (1984) 'Legitimation problems in late capitalism', in Connolly, W. (ed.) *Legitimacy and the State*, Oxford: Blackwell.

Ham, C. (1996) *Public, Private or Community: What Next for the NHS?*, London: Demos.

Hambleton, R. (1994) 'The contract state and the future of public management', paper presented to Unemployment Research Unit conference, *The Contract State and the Future of Public Management*, Cardiff.

Hansmann, H. (1980) 'The role of the nonprofit enterprise', *Yale Law Journal*, 89, pp. 839–901.

Hansmann, H. (1987) 'Economic theories of nonprofit organizations', in W.W. Powell (ed.) *The Nonprofit Sector: A Research Handbook*, New Haven: Yale University Press.

Hantrais, L. (1994) 'Comparing family policy in Britain, France and Germany', *Journal of Social Policy*, vol. 23, pt. 2, pp. 135–160.

Harris, M. (1996) 'Do we need governing bodies?', in Billis, D. and Harris, M. (eds) *Voluntary Agencies: Challenges of Organisation and Management*, Basingstoke: Macmillan, pp. 149–65.

Hartman, C. (1983) (ed.) *America's Housing Crisis: What is to be Done?*, Boston: Routledge and Kegan Paul.

Havas, E. (1995) 'The family as ideology', *Social Policy and Administration*, vol. 29, no. 1.

Hayek, F.A. (1944) *The Road to Serfdom*, London: Routledge and Kegan Paul.

Hayek, F.A. (1976) *Individualism and Economic Order*, London: Routledge and Kegan Paul.

Health Care Information Services (1994) *The Fitzhugh Directory of Independent Healthcare*, London: Health Care Information Services, cited in Laing and Buisson (1994).

Hedley R. and Rochester, C. (1992) *Understanding Management Committees*, Berkhamsted: Volunteer Centre.

Heidenheimer, A.J., Heclo, H. and Adams, C.T. (1983) *Comparative Public Policy*, New York: St Martin's Press.

Henry J. Kaiser Family Foundation (1994) *Uninsured in America*, Washington DC: Kaiser Health Reform Project.

Hernes, H. (1987) *Welfare State and Woman Power: Essays in State Feminism*, Oslo: Norwegian University Press.

Higgins, J. (1989) 'Defining Community Care', *Social Policy and Administration*, vol. 23, no. 1, pp. 3–16.

Hill, M. (1993) *The Welfare State in Britain: A Political History Since 1945*, Aldershot: Edward Elgar.

Hill, M. (1996) *Social Policy: A Comparative Analysis*, Hemel Hempstead: Prentice Hall/Harvester Wheatsheaf.

Hirst, P. (1994) *Associative Democracy: New Forms of Economic and Social Governance*, Cambridge, Polity Press.

Hodgkinson, V.A. and McCarthy, K.D. (1992) 'The voluntary sector in International perspective: An overview', in McCarthy, K.D., Hodgkinson, V.A. and Sumariwalla, R.D. (eds) *The Nonprofit Sector in the Global Community: Voices from Many Nations*, San Francisco: Jossey-Bass.

Hood, C. (1991) 'A public management for all seasons?, *Public Administration*, vol. 69, no. 1, pp. 3–20.

Horton, C. and Berthoud, R. (1990) *The Attendance Allowances and the Costs of Caring*, London: Policy Studies Institute.

Horton, S. and Jones, J. (1996) 'Who are the new public managers? An initial analysis of "next steps" chief executives and their managerial role', *Public Policy and Administration*, vol. 11, no. 4, pp. 18–44.

Huard, P., Mossé, P. and Roustang, G. (1995) 'France', in Johnson, N. (ed.) *Private Markets in Health and Welfare: An International Perspective*, Oxford: Berg, pp. 65–90.

Huber, E. (1996) 'Options for social policy in Latin America: neoliberal versus social democratic models', in Esping-Andersen (ed.) *Welfare States in Transition: National Adaptations in Global Economies*, London: Sage, pp. 141–91.

Hughes, N.S. and Lovell, A.M. (1986) 'Breaking the circuit of social control: Lessons in Public Psychiatry from Italy and Franco Basaglia', *Social Science and Medicine*, vol. 23, no. 2, pp. 159–78.

Hughes, O.E. (1994) *Public Management and Administration: An Introduction*, Basingstoke: Macmillan.

Hutton, W. (1997) *The State to Come* (Extracts), London: Vintage.

Institute for Policy Studies (1994) *Towards a Vital Voluntary Sector I: A Statement of Principles*, Baltimore: The Johns Hopkins University.

James, E. (1987) 'The nonprofit sector in comparative perspective', in W. W. Powell (ed.) *The Nonprofit Sector: A Research Handbook*, New Haven: Yale University Press.

Johansson, L. (1993) 'The state and the family: policy, services and practice in Sweden', in Twigg, J. (ed.) *Informal Care in Europe*, York: Social Policy Research Unit, pp. 103–08.

Johansson, L. and Sundström, G. (1994) 'Sweden', in Evers, A., Pijl, M. and Ungerson, C. (eds) *op. cit.*, pp. 87–100.

Johnson, L. (1991) *Contracts for Care: Issues for Black and Other Ethnic Minority Voluntary Groups*, London: National Council for Voluntary Organisations.

Johnson, N. (1987) *The Welfare State in Transition: The Theory and Practice of Welfare Pluralism*, Brighton: Wheatsheaf.

Johnson, N. (ed.) (1995) *Private Markets in Health and Welfare: An International Perspective*, Oxford: Berg.

Jones, H. and Millar, J. (eds) (1996) *The Politics of the Family*, Aldershot: Avebury.

Joshi, H. (1987) 'The cost of caring', in Millar, J. and Glendinning, C. (eds) *Women and Poverty in Britain*, Brighton: Wheatsheaf.

Joshi, H. (1991) 'Sex and motherhood as handicaps in the labour market', in Maclean, M. and Groves, D. (eds) *Women's Issues in Social Policy*, London: Routledge, pp. 179–93.

Jowell, R., Brook, L. and Dowds, L. (1993) *International Social Attitudes: The 10th BSA Report*, Aldershot: Dartmouth.

Judge, K. and Knapp, M. (1985) 'Efficiency in the production of welfare: the public and private sectors compared', in Klein, R. and O'Higgins, M. (eds) *The Future of Welfare*, Oxford: Blackwell, pp. 131–49.

Kamerman, S.B. and Kahn, A.J. (eds) (1978) *Family Policy: Government and Families in Fourteen Countries*, New York: Columbia University Press.

Kempson, E. (1996) *Life on a Low Income*, York: Joseph Rowntree Foundation.

Kendall, J. and Knapp, M. (1996) *The Voluntary Sector in the UK*, Manchester: Manchester University Press.

King, A. (1975) 'Overload: problems of governing in the 1970s', *Political Studies*, vol. 23, nos. 2 and 3.

King, D.S. (1987) *The New Right: Politics, Markets and Citizenship*, Basingstoke: Macmillan.

Kirkpatrick, I. and Lucio, M.M. (1996) 'Introduction: the contract state and the future of public management', *Public Administration*, vol. 74, no. 2, pp. 1–8.

Knapp, M., Wistow, G., Forder, J. and Hardy, B. (1994) 'Markets for social care: Opportunities, Barriers and Implications', in Bartlett, W., Propper, C., Wilson, D. and Le Grand (eds) *Quasi-Markets in the Welfare State*, Bristol: School for Advanced Urban Studies, University of Bristol.

Knight, B. (1993) *Voluntary Action*, London: Centris.

Kohl, J. (1981) 'Trends and problems in postwar public expenditure development in Western Europe and North America', in Flora, P. and Heidenheimer, A.J. (eds) *The Development of Welfare States in Europe and America*, New Brunswick: Transaction Books.

Kolberg, J.E. (1991) 'The gender dimension of the welfare state', *International Journal of Sociology*, vol. 21, no. 2, pp. 119–148.

Kramer, R.M. (1981) *Voluntary Agencies in the Welfare State*, Berkeley: University of California Press.

Kramer, R.M. (1987) 'Voluntary agencies and the personal social services', in Powell, W.W. (ed.) *The Nonprofit Sector: A Research Handbook*, New Haven: Yale University Press.

Kramer, R.M., Lorentzen, H., Melief, W.B. and Pasquinelli, S. (1993) *Privatization in Four European Countries: Comparative studies in government–third sector relationships*, Armonk, New York: M.E. Sharpe.

Kuhnle, S. (1981) 'The growth of social insurance programs in Scandinavia', in Flora, P. and Heidenheimer, A.J. (eds) *The Development of Welfare States in Europe and America*, New Brunswick: Transaction Books.

Kuhnle, S. and Selle, P. (eds) (1992) *Government and Voluntary Organizations: A Relational Perspective,* Aldershot: Avebury.

Kuti, E. (1993) *Defining the Nonprofit Sector: Hungary*, Baltimore: The Johns Hopkins University.

Kuti, E. (1996) *The Nonprofit Sector in Hungary*, Manchester: Manchester University Press.

Kvist, J. and Sinfield, A. (1997) 'Comparing tax welfare states', in May, M., Brunsdon, E. and Craig, G. (eds) *Social Policy Review 9*, London, Social Policy Association, pp. 249–75.

Laing, R.D. (1959) *The Divided Self*, London: Tavistock.

Laing, R.D. (1961) *The Self and Others*, London: Tavistock.

Laing and Buisson (1994) *Laing's Review of Private Healthcare, 1994*, London: Laing and Buisson Publications.

Laming, H. (1985) *Lessons from America: The Balance of Services in Social Care*, London: Policy Studies Institute.

Laslett, P. (1980) 'Characteristics of the Western European family', *London Review of Books*, 16 October–5 November.

Lawrence, R. (1983) 'Voluntary action: a stalking horse for the right?', *Critical Social Policy*, vol. 2, no. 3, pp. 14–30.

Leadbetter, C. (1997) *The Rise of the Social Entrepreneur*, London: Demos.

Leat, D. (1988) *Voluntary Organisations and Accountability*, London: National Council for Voluntary Organisations.

Leat, D. (1990a) 'Voluntary organisations and accountability: theory and practice', in Anheier, H.K. and Seibel, W. (eds) *The Third Sector: Comparative Studies of Nonprofit Organizations*, Berlin: De Gruyter.

Leat, D. (1990b) 'Overcoming voluntary failure: strategies for change', in Sinclair, I., Parker, R., Leat, D. and Williams, J. *The Kaleidoscope of Care: A Review of Research on Welfare Provision for Elderly People*, London: HMSO.

Leat, D. (1996) 'Are Voluntary Organisations Accountable?', in Billis, D. and Harris, M. (eds) *Voluntary Agencies: Challenges of Organisation and Management*, Basingstoke: Macmillan.

Le Grand, J. (1991) *The Theory of Government Failure*, Studies in Decentralisation and Quasi-Markets, Bristol: School for Advanced Urban Studies.

Le Grand, J. and Bartlett, W. (eds) (1993) *Quasi-Markets and Social Policy*, Basingstoke: Macmillan.

Le Galès, P. and John, P. (1997) 'Is the grass greener on the other side? What went wrong with French regions, and the implications for England', *Policy and Politics*, vol. 25, no. 1, pp. 51–60.

Leira, A. (1993) 'Concepts of care: loving, thinking and doing', in Twigg, J. (ed.) *Informal Care in Europe*, York: Social Policy Research Unit, pp. 23–40.

Leung, J.C.B. (1994) 'Dismantling the iron rice bowl: welfare reform in the People's Republic of China', *Journal of Social Policy*, vol. 23, pt. 3, pp. 341–62.

Levacic, R. (1991) 'Markets and government: an overview', in Thompson, G., Frances, J., Levacic, R. and Mitchell, J. (eds) *Markets, Hierarchies and Networks*, London: Sage, pp. 35–47.

Levin, E., Sinclair, I. and Gorbach, P. (1989) *Families, Services and Confusion in Old Age*, Aldershot: Gower.

Levitas, R. (1996) 'The concept of social exclusion and the new Durkheimian hegemony', *Critical Social Policy*, vol. 16, no. 1, pp. 5–20.

Lewis, J. (1989) 'Introduction to Part III: Social Policy and the Family', in Bulmer, M., Lewis, J. and Piachaud, D. (eds) *The Goals of Social Policy*, London: Unwin Hyman, pp. 131–40.

Lewis, J. (1992) 'Gender and the development of welfare regimes', *Journal of European Social Policy*, vol. 2, no. 3, pp. 159–73.

Lewis, J. and Meredith, B. (1988) *Daughters Who Care*, London: Routledge.

Lewis, O. (1964) *The Children of Sanchez*, Harmondsworth: Penguin.

Lightman, E. (1991) 'Caught in the middle: the radical right and the Canadian welfare state', in Glennerster, H. and Midgley, J. (eds) *The Radical Right and the Welfare State: An International Assessment*, Hemel Hempstead: Harvester Wheatsheaf, pp. 141–60.

Lindblom, C. (1977) *Politics and Markets*, New York: Basic Books.

Lingsom, S. (1994) 'Norway', in Evers, A., Pijl, M. and Ungerson C. (eds) *op. cit.*, pp. 67–86.

Lipietz, A. (1992) *Towards a New Economic Order*, Cambridge: Polity Press.

Lister, R. (ed.) (1996) *Charles Murray and the Underclass: The developing debate*, London: The Institute of Economic Affairs and *The Sunday Times*.

Lister, R. (1996) 'Back to the family: family policies and politics under the Major government', in Jones, H. and Millar, J. (eds) *op. cit.* pp. 11–32.

Lorenz, W. (1994a) *Social Work in a Changing Europe*, London: Routledge.

Lorenz, W. (1994b) 'Personal social services', in Clasen, J. and Freeman, R. (eds) *Social Policy in Germany*, Hemel Hempstead: Harvester Wheatsheaf.

Lowe, R. (1993) *The Welfare State in Britain Since 1945*, Basingstoke: Macmillan.

Lukes, S. (1974) *Power: A Radical View*, Basingstoke: Macmillan.

Lundström, T. and Wijkström, F. (1995) *Defining the Nonprofit Sector: Sweden*, Baltimore: The Johns Hopkins University.

Lyons, M. (1995) 'The development of quasi-vouchers in Australia's community sevices', *Policy and Politics*, vol. 23, no. 2, pp. 127–40.

Mangen, S. (1991) 'Social policy, the radical right and the German welfare state', in Glennerster, H. and Midgley, J. (eds) *The Radical Right and the Welfare State: An International Assessment*, Hemel Hempstead: Harvester Wheatsheaf, pp. 124–40.

Marmor, T.R., Schlesinger, M. and Smithey, R.W. (1987) 'Nonprofit organizations and health care', in Powell, W.W. (ed.) *The Nonprofit Sector: A Research Handbook*, New Haven: Yale University Press, pp. 221–39.

Marsland, D. (1996) 'Community care as an alternative to state welfare', *Social Policy & Administration*, vol. 30, no. 3, pp. 183–88.

Marx, K. and Engels, F. (1977) *The Communist Manifesto*, Moscow: Progress Publishers.

Mayo, M. (1994) *Communities and Caring: The Mixed Economy of Welfare*, Basingstoke: Macmillan.

MacAdam, E. (1934) *The New Philanthropy*, London: Allen and Unwin.

McGlone, F. and Cronin, N. (1994) *A Crisis in Care? The Future of Family Life and State Care for Older People in the European Union*, London: Family Policy Studies Centre.

McGlone, F., Park, A. and Roberts, C. (1996) 'Relative values: kinship and friendship', in Jowell, R., Curtice, J., Park, A., Brook, L. and Thomson, K. (eds) *British Social Attitudes, the 13th Report*, Aldershot: Dartmouth, pp. 53–72.

McLean, I. (1987) *Public Choice: An Introduction*, Oxford: Blackwell.

Meekosha, H. and Mowbray, M. (1995) 'Activism, service provision and the state's intellectuals: community work in Australia', in Craig, G. and Mayo, M. (eds) *Community Empowerment: A Reader in Participation and Development*, London: Zed Books.

Melief, W.B. (1993) 'The Netherlands: institutionalized privatization', in Kramer, R.M., Lorentzen, H., Melief, W.B. and Pasquinelli, S. *Privatization in Four European Countries: Comparative Studies in Government–Third Sector Relationships*, New York: M.E. Sharpe, pp. 67–86.

Michels, R. (1911) *Political Parties: A Sociological Study of the Oligarchical Consequences of Modern Democracy*, trans. Paul, C. and Paul, E. (1959), New York: Dover.

Miliband, R. (1969) *The State in Capitalist Society*, London: Weidenfeld and Nicholson.

Millar, J. (1996) 'Women, poverty and social security', in Hallett, C. (ed.) *Women and Social Policy*, Hemel Hempstead: Prentice Hall/Harvester Wheatsheaf.

Millar, J. and Warman, A. (1996) *Family Obligations in Europe*, London: Family Policy Studies Centre.

Miller, D. (1989) 'Why markets?', in Le Grand, J. and Estrin, S. (eds) *Market Socialism*, Oxford: Clarendon Press, pp. 25–49.

Miller, D. (1990) *Market, State and Community: Theoretical Foundations of Market Socialism*, Oxford: Clarendon Press.

Miller, S.M., Rein, M. and Levitt, P. (1995) 'Community action in the United States', in Craig, G. and Mayo, M. (eds) *Community Empowerment: A Reader in Participation and Development*, London: Zed Books.

Mills, C. W. (1956) *The Power Elite*, Oxford: Oxford University Press.

Milne, R.G. (1987) 'Competitive tendering in the NHS: an economic analysis of the early implementation of HC(83)H8', *Public Administration*, vol. 15, no. 2, pp. 145–60.

Mishra, R. (1984) *The Welfare State In Crisis*, Brighton: Wheatsheaf.

Mishra, R. (1989) 'Riding the new wave: social work and the neo-conservative challenge', *International Social Work*, no. 32.

Moore, B. (1966) *Social Origins of Dictatorship and Democracy: Lord and Peasant in the Making of the Modern World*, Boston: Beacon Press.

Morgan, P. (1995) *Farewell to the Family? Public Policy and Family Breakdown in Britain and the USA*, London: Institute of Economic Affairs.

Mosca, G. (1896) *The Ruling Class*, trans. Kahn, H.D. (1939), New York: McGraw-Hill.

Murray, C. (1984) *Losing Ground: American Social Policy, 1950–1980*, New York: Basic Books.

Murray, C. (1990) *The Emerging British Underclass*, London: Institute of Economic Affairs.

Murray, C. (1994) *Underclass: The Crisis Deepens*, London: Institute of Economic Affairs.

Myles, J. (1996) 'When markets fail: social welfare in Canada and the United States', in Esping-Andersen, G. (ed.) *Welfare States in Transition: National Adaptations in Global Economies*, London: Sage.

National Consumer Council (1995), *Budgeting for Food on Benefits*, London: National Consumer Council.

National Council for Voluntary Organisations (1984) *Voluntary Organisations*, London: Bedford Square Press.

Navarro, V. (1994) *The Politics of Health Policy: The US Reforms, 1980–1994*, Oxford: Blackwell.

Niskanen, W.A. (1971) *Bureaucracy and Representative Government*, Chicago: Aldine-Atherton.

Niskanen, W.A. (1978) 'Competition among government bureaus', in Buchanan, J.M. (ed.) *The Economics of Politics*, London: Institute of Economic Affairs.

Nissel, M. and Bonnerjea, L. (1982) *Family Care of the Handicapped Elderly: Who Pays?*, London: Policy Studies Institute.

Noden, S. and Laczco, F. (1993) 'Combining paid work with eldercare', *Health and Social Care*, 1, pp. 81–9.

Novak, M. (1991) *The Spirit of Democratic Capitalism*, Lanham, Maryland: Madison Books and London, The Institute of Economic Affairs Health and Welfare Unit.

Nowak, J. (1988) *Soziale Probleme und Soziale Bewegungen*, Basle: Beltz. Cited in Lorenz, W. (1994b).

Nozick, R. (1984) *Anarchy, State and Utopia*, Oxford: Blackwell.

Nuffield Provincial Hospitals Trust (1993) *Looking Forward to Looking After*, London: Nuffield Provincial Hospitals Trust.

O'Connor, J. (1973) *The Fiscal Crisis of the State*, New York: St Martin's Press.

O'Connor, J. (1984) *Accumulation Crisis*, New York: Blackwell.

O'Connor, J. (1998) 'US social welfare policy: the Reagan record and legacy', *Journal of Social Policy*, vol. 27, pt. 1, pp. 37–61.

O'Connor, P. (1992) *Friendships Between Women*, Hemel Hempstead: Harvester Wheatsheaf.

OECD (1984) *The Employment and Unemployment of Women in OECD Countries*, Paris: OECD.

OECD (1985) *Social Expenditure 1960–1990*, Paris: OECD.

OECD (1993) *Managing with Market-Type Mechanisms*, Paris: OECD.

OECD (1994) *New Orientations for Social Policy*, OECD Social Policy Studies, no. 12, Paris: OECD.

OECD (1996) *Tax Expenditures: Recent Experiences*, Paris: OECD.

Offe, C. (1984) *Contradictions of the Welfare State*, ed. Keane, J., London: Hutchinson.

Okazaki, Y., Tsuji, T., Otomo, E., Hayakawa, K., Ibe, H. and Furuse, T. (1990) *Responding to the Needs of an Aging Society*, Tokyo: Foreign Press Center.

Olsson Hort, S.E. and Cohn, D. (1995) 'Sweden', in Johnson, N. (ed.) *Private Markets in Health and Welfare: An International Perspective*, Oxford: Berg, pp. 169–202.

OPCS (1992) *General Household Survey 1990*, London: HMSO.

Orosz, E. (1995) 'Hungary', in Johnson, N. (ed.) *Private Markets in Health and Welfare: An International Perspective*, Oxford: Berg.

Osborne, D. and Gaebler, T. (1992) *Reinventing Government: How the Entrepreneurial Spirit is Transforming the Public Sector From Schoolhouse to Statehouse, City Hall to the Pentagon*, Reading, MA: Addison-Wesley.

Owen, D. (1965) *English Philanthropy, 1660–1960*, Cambridge, MA: Harvard University Press.

Pahl, J. (1989) *Money and Marriage*, Basingstoke: Macmillan.

Palmer, J.L. and Sawhill, I.V. (eds) *The Reagan Record*, Cambridge, MA: Ballinger.

Pareto, V. (1916) *The Mind and Society*, London: Cape.

Parker, G. (1990) *With Due Care and Attention: A Review of the Literature on Informal Care*, 2nd edition, London: Family Policy Studies Centre.

Parker, G. (1993) *With This Body: Caring and Disabilty in Marriage*, Buckingham: Open University Press.

Parker, G. and Lawton, D. (1994) *Different Types of Care, Different Types of Carer: Evidence from the General Household Survey*, London: HMSO.

Parker, R.A. (1980) *The State of Care*, Jerusalem: Brookdale Institute of Gerontology and Adult Human Development in Israel.

Parker, R.A. (1981) 'Tending and social policy', in Goldberg, E.M. and Hatch, S. (eds) *A New Look at the Personal Social Services*, London: Policy Studies Institute.

Peele, G. (1984) *Revival and Reaction: The Right in Contemporary America*, Oxford: Oxford University Press.

Petracca, M.P. (1992) *The Politics of Interests: Interest Groups Transformed*, Boulder, CO: Westview Press.

Phillips, A. (1996) 'Faltering Reform', *Maclean's*, 2 December, 1996.

Phillipson, C. (1988) *Planning for Community Care: Facts and Fallacies in the Griffiths Report*, Centre for Social Gerontology, University of Keele.

Pierson, P. (1994) *Dismantling the Welfare State? Reagan, Thatcher and the Politics of Retrenchment*, Cambridge: Cambridge University Press.

Piven, F. and Cloward, R. (1993) *Regulating the Poor*, New York: Vintage Books.

Polanyi, M. (1951) *The Logic of Liberty*, Chicago: University of Chicago Press.

Pollitt, C. (1993) 'The struggle for quality: the case of the National Health Service', *Policy and Politics*, vol. 21, no. 3. pp. 161–70.

Poulantzas, N. (1973) *Political Power and Social Classes*, London: New Left Books.

Poulantzas, N. (1978) *State, Power, Socialism*, London: New Left Books.

Qureshi, H. (1990) 'Boundaries between formal and informal care-giving work', in Ungerson, C. (ed.) *Gender and Caring: Work and Welfare in Britain and Scandinavia*, Hemel Hempstead: Harvester Wheatsheaf, pp. 59–79.

Qureshi, H. and Simons, K. (1987) 'Resources within families: caring for elderly people', in Brannen, J. and Wilson, G. (eds) *Give and Take in Families: Studies in Resource Distribution*, London: Allen and Unwin.

Ramon, S. (1985) 'The Italian psychiatric reform', in Mangen, S. P. (ed.) *Mental Health Care in the European Community*, Lodon: Croom Helm.

Randon, A. and 6, P. (1994) 'Constraining campaigning: the legal treatment of non-profit policy advocacy across 24 countries', *Voluntas*, vol. 5, no. 1, pp. 27–58.

Ranson, S. and Stewart, J. (1994) *Management for the Public Domain: Enabling the Learning Society*, Basingstoke: Macmillan.

Rawls, J. (1972) *A Theory of Justice*, Oxford: Clarendon Press.

Richardson, A. (1984) *Working with Self-help Groups*, London: Bedford Square Press.

Richardson, J. (1993) *Reinventing Contracts: Transatlantic Perspectives on the Future of Contracting*, London: NCVO publications.

Riches, G. (1990) 'Market ideology and welfare reform: the breakdown of the public safety net in the new Canada', in Taylor, I. (ed.) *The Social Effects of Free Market Policies*, Hemel Hempstead: Harvester Wheatsheaf.

Ross, G. (1987) 'From one left to another: *Le social* Mitterrand's France', in Ross, G., Hoffman, S. and Malzacher, S. (eds) *The Mitterrand Experiment*, Cambridge: Polity Press.

Salamon, L.M. (1987) 'Partners in public service: the scope and theory of government–nonprofit relations', in Powell, W.W. (ed.) *The Nonprofit Sector: A Research Handbook*, New Haven: Yale University Press.

Salamon, L.M. (1992) *America's Nonprofit Sector: A Primer*, New York: The Foundation Center.

Salamon, L.M. (1993) 'The nonprofit sector and democracy: prerequisite, impediment, or irrelevance? paper prepared for the Aspen Institute Nonprofit Sector Research Fund symposium, Wye MD.

Salamon, L.M. and Anheier, H.K. (1992) *In Search of the Nonprofit Sector 1: The Question of Definitions*, Baltimore: The Johns Hopkins University.

Salamon, L.M. and Anheier, H.K. (1994) *The Emerging Sector: An Overview*, Baltimore: The Johns Hopkins University.

Salamon, L.M. and Anheier, H.K. (1996) 'Explaining the nonprofit sector: a cross-national analysis', Paper presented to the Second Annual Conference of the International Society for Third Sector Research, Mexico City.

Sandford, C. (1993) *Successful Tax Reform*, Bath: Fiscal Publications. Quoted in Kvist, J. and Sinfield, A. (1997) 'Comparing tax welfare states', in May, M., Brunsdon, E. and Craig, G. (eds) *Social Policy Review 9*, London, Social Policy Association.

Savas, E.S. (1987) *Privatization: The Key to Better Government*, Chatham, N.J.: Chatham House.

Schumpeter, J. (1944) *Capitalism, Socialism and Democracy*, London: Allen and Unwin.

Schwarzmantel, J. (1994) *The State in Contemporary Society: An Introduction*, Hemel Hempstead: Harvester Wheatsheaf.

Seibel, W. (1992) 'Government-nonprofit relationships in comparative perspective: The cases of France and Germany', in McCarthy, K.D., Hodgkinson, V.A. and Sumariwalla, R.D. (eds) *The Nonprofit Sector in the Global Community: Voices from Many Nations,* San Francisco: Jossey-Bass.

Selbourne, D. (1994) *The Principle of Duty*, London: Sinclair-Stevenson.

Seyd, R., Simons, K., Tennant, A. and Bayley, M. (1984) *Community Care in Dinnington: Informal Support Prior to the Project*, Sheffield: University of Sheffield.

Shackle, G.L.S. (1972) *Epistemics and Economics: A Critique of Economic Doctrines,* Cambridge: Cambridge University Press.

Shaw, I. (1995) 'The quality of mercy: the management of quality in the personal social services', in Kirkpatrick, I. and Lucio, M. (eds) *The Politics of Quality in the Public Sector*, London: Routledge.

Shirley, I. (1990) 'New Zealand: the advance of the New Right', in Taylor, I. (ed.) *The Social Effects of Free Market Policies*, Hemel Hempstead: Harvester Wheatsheaf.

Shorter, E. (1975) *The Making of the Modern Family*, New York: Basic Books.

Siegal, D. and Yancey, J. (1992) *The Rebirth of Civil Society: The Development of the Nonprofit Sector in East Central Europe and the Role of Western Assistance*, New York: Rockefeller Brothers Fund.

Sipilä, J. and Anttonen, A. (1994) 'Finland', in Evers, A., Pijl, M. and Ungerson, C. (eds) *op. cit.*, pp. 51–66.

Smart, V. (1996) 'Mighty regions unnerve Brussels', *The European*, 15 August.

Smith, B.H. (1993) 'Non-governmental organizations in international development: trends and future research priorities', *Voluntas*, vol. 4, no. 3, pp. 326–44.

Smyth, M. and Robus, N. (1989) *The Financial Circumstances of Families with Disabled Children Living in Private Households*, London: HMSO.

Social Security Advisory Committee (1988) *Sixth Report*, London: HMSO.

Sosin, M. (1986) *Private Benefits: Material Assistance in the Private Sector*, London: Academic Press.

Spicker, P. (1991) 'The principle of subsidiarity and the social policy of the European Community', *Journal of European Social Policy*, vol. 1, no. 1.

Standing, G. (1996) 'Social protection in Central and Eastern Europe: a tale of slipping anchors and torn safety nets', in Esping-Andersen, G. (ed.) *Welfare States in Transition: National Adaptations in Global Economies*, London: Sage, pp. 225–55.

Stephens, J.D. (1996) 'The Scandinavian welfare states: achievements, crisis and prospects', in Esping-Andersen, G. (ed.) *Welfare States in Transition: National Adaptations in Global Economies*, London: Sage, pp. 32–65.

Stoesz, D. and Midgley, J. (1991) 'The radical right and the welfare state', in Glennerster, H. and Midgley, J. (eds) *The Radical Right and the Welfare State: An International Assessment*, Hemel Hempstead: Harvester Wheatsheaf.

Sullivan, M. (1996) *The Development of the British Welfare State*, Hemel Hempstead: Prentice Hall/Harvester Wheatsheaf.

Summer, L. and Shapiro, I. (1994) *Trends in Health Insurance Coverage, 1987 to 1993*, Washington, DC: Center on Budget and Policy Priorities.

Svetlik, I. (1991) 'Welfare pluralism, welfare mix, social innovation and the fall of "real socialism"', in Huston, L. (ed.) *Shifts in the Welfare Mix: The Case of Care for the Elderly*, Eurosocial Report 38, Vienna: European Centre for Social Welfare Policy and Research.

Swane, C.E. (1994), 'Denmark', in Evers, A., Pijl, M. and Ungerson, C. (eds) *op. cit.*, pp. 101–24.

Szalai, J, and Orosz, E. (1992) 'Social Policy in Hungary', in Deacon, B. *et al.*, *The New Eastern Europe: Social Policy Past Present and Future*, London: Sage.

Szasz, T. (1961) *The Myth of Mental Illness*, New York: Harper.

Taylor, I. (ed.) (1990) *The Social Effects of Free Market Policies*, Hemel Hempstead: Harvester Wheatsheaf.

Taylor, M. (1995) 'Community work and the state: the changing context of UK practice', in Craig, G. and Mayo, M. (eds) *Community Empowerment: A Reader in Participation and Development*, London: Zed Books.

Taylor, M. (1996) 'Between public and private: accountability in voluntary organisations', *Policy and Politics*, vol. 24, no. 1, pp. 51–72.

Taylor, M. and Hoggett, P. (1994) 'Trusting in networks? The third sector and welfare change', in 6, P. and Vidal, I. (eds) *Delivering Welfare: Repositioning non-profit and co-operative action in Western Europe*, Barcelona: Centre d'Iniciatives de l'Economia Social.

Taylor-Gooby, P. (1985) *Public Opinion, Ideology and State Welfare*, London: Routledge and Kegan Paul.

Taylor-Gooby, P. (1991) *Social change, Social Welfare and Social Science*, Hemel Hempstead: Harvester Wheatsheaf.

Taylor-Gooby, P. (1993) 'What citizens want from the state', in Jowell, R., Brook, L. and Dowds, L. (eds) *International Social Attitudes*, Aldershot: Dartmouth Publishing Company, pp. 81–102.

Timmins, N. (1995) *The Five Giants: A Biography of the Welfare State*, London: HarperCollins.

Titmuss, R.M. (1967) *Choice and the Welfare State*, London: Fabian Society.

Titmuss, R.M. (1970) *The Gift Relationship: From Human Blood to Social Policy*, London: Allen and Unwin.

Toft, C. (1996) 'Constitutional choice, multi-level government and social security systems in Great Britain, Germany and Denmark', *Policy and Politics*, vol. 24, no. 3, pp. 247–61.

Tönnies, F. (1887) *Community and Association*, translated by Loomis, C.P. (1955), London: Routledge and Kegan Paul.

Townsend, P. (1957) *The Family Life of Old People*, London: Routledge and Kegan Paul.

Traynor, I. (1997) 'Democracy proves dire for children', *The Guardian*, 22 April.

Truman, D. (1951) *The Governmental Process*, New York: Knopf.

Ungerson, C. (1983) 'Why do women care?', in Finch, J. and Groves, D. (eds) *A Labour of Love: Women, Work and Caring*, London: Routledge and Kegan Paul.

Ungerson, C. (1987) *Policy is Personal: Sex, Gender and Informal Care*, London: Tavistock.

Ungerson, C. (ed.) (1990) *Gender and Caring: Work and Welfare in Britain and Scandinavia*, Hemel Hempstead: Harvester Whearsheaf.

Ungerson, C. (1995) 'Gender, cash and informal care: European perspectives and dilemmas', *Journal of Social Policy*, vol. 24, pt. 1, pp. 31–52.

Vulliamy, E. (1997) 'Read our lips – don't cut taxes', *The Observer*, 31 August.

Wærness, K. (1990) Informal and formal care in old age: what is wrong with the new ideology in Scandinavia today?', in Ungerson, C. (ed.) *Gender and Caring: Work and Welfare in Britain and Scandinavia*, Hemel Hempstead: Harvester Wheatsheaf, pp. 110–32.

Walby, S. (1990) *Theorising Patriarchy*, Oxford: Blackwell.

Walker, A. (1984) *Social Planning: A Strategy for Socialist Welfare*, Oxford: Blackwell.

Walker, A. (1990) 'The strategy for inequality: poverty and income distribution in Britain 1979–89', in Taylor, I. (ed.) *The Social Effects of Free Market Policies*, Hemel Hempstead: Harvester Wheatsheaf.

Walker, A. (1993) 'A cultural revolution? Shifting the UK's welfare mix in the care of older people', in Evers, A. and Svetlik, I. (eds) *Balancing Pluralism: New Welfare Mixes in Care for the Elderly*, Aldershot: Avebury.

Walker, M. (1996) 'Electrifying Issue for US', *The Guardian*, 27 January.

Walsh, K., Deakin, N., Smith, P., Spurgeon, P. and Thomas, N. (1997) *Contracting for Change*, Oxford: Oxford University Press.

Watts, R. (1990) 'Jam every other day: living standards and the Hawke governmnent 1983–9', in Taylor, I. (ed.) *The Social Effects of Free Market Policies*, Hemel Hempstead: Harvester Wheatsheaf.

Weale, A. (1983) *Political Theory and Social Policy*, Basingstoke: Macmillan.

Weisbrod, B. (1977) *The Voluntary Nonprofit Sector*, Lexington, MA: Lexington Books.

Whelan, R. (ed.) (1995) *Just a Piece of Paper? Divorce Reform and the Undermining of Marriage*, London: Institute of Economic Affairs.

Wiewel, W. and Gills, D. (1995) 'Community Development Organizational Capacity and US Policy: Lessons from the Chicago Experience 1983–1993', in Craig, G. and Mayo, M. (eds) *Community Empowerment: A Reader in Participation and Development*, London: Zed Books.

Wilding, P. (1992) 'Social policy in the 1980s', *Social Policy and Administration*, vol. 26, no. 2, pp. 107–16.

Wilensky, H.L. and Lebeaux, C.N. (1965) *Industrial Society and Social Welfare*, New York: The Free Press.

Williams, F. (1989) *Social Policy: A Critical Introduction*, Cambridge: Polity Press.

Willmott, P. (1986) *Social Networks: Informal Care and Public Policy*, London: Policy Studies Institute.

Willmott, P. (1989) *Community Initiatives*, London: Policy Studies Institute.

Willmott, P. and Young, M. (1960) *Family and Class in a London Suburb*, London: Routledge and Kegan Paul.

Wistow, G., Knapp, M., Hardy, B. and Allen, C. (1994) *Social Care in a Mixed Economy*, Buckingham: Open University Press.

Wolch, J. (1990) *The Shadow State: Government and Voluntary Sector in Transition*, New York: The Foundation Center.

Wolf, C. (1988) *Markets or Governments*, Cambridge, MA: MIT Press.

Wolfenden, J. (1978) *The Future of Voluntary Organisations*, London: Croom Helm.

Wollert, R. and Barron, N. (1983) 'Avenues of collaboration', in Pancoast, D.L., Parker, P. and Froland, C. (eds) *Rediscovering Self-help: Its Role in Care*, Beverly Hills: Sage.

World Bank (1994) *Averting the Old Age Crisis: Policies to Protect the Old and Promote Growth*, New York: Oxford University Press.

Young, H. (1994) 'Only Blair dares to admit that the good old days are gone', *The Guardian*, 16 June.

Young, M. and Willmott, P. (1957) *Family and Kinship in East London*, London: Routledge and Kegan Paul.

Zimmerman, S. (1988) *Understanding Family Policy: Theoretical Approaches*, Newbury Park: Sage.

Zimmerman, S. (1992) *Family Policies and Family Well-being*, Newbury Park: Sage.

6, P. (1994) 'Conclusion: will anyone talk about 'the third sector' in ten years time?', in 6, P. and Vidal, I. (eds) *Delivering Welfare: Repositioning non-profit and co-operative action in Western Europe*, Barcelona: Centre d'Iniciatives de l'Economia Social.

6, P. (1995) 'The voluntary and non-profit sectors in continental Europe', in Davis Smith, J., Rochester, C. and Hedley, R. (eds) *An Introduction to the Voluntary Sector*, London: Routledge.

6, P. and Vidal, I. (eds) (1994) *Delivering Welfare: Re-positioning Non-profit and Co-operative Action in Western European Welfare States*, Barcelona: Centre d'Iniciatives de l'Economia Social.

INDEX

304   *Index*

308   *Index*

Index compiled by Annette Musker